THE
Mindbody
DICTIONARY

By Ronald B. Wayman
with Denise Wayman Scholes

Copyright © 2024
West Jordan, UT 84088
& West Plains MO 65692

Disclaimer:

This book is intended for informational purposes only and should not be considered as medical advice, diagnosis, or treatment.

The material in this book is intended to provide information that may provide insights into your life. Any suggestions for techniques, treatments, or lifestyle changes referred to or implied in this book should be undertaken only with the guidance of a licensed medical professional, therapist, healthcare or wellness practitioner. The ideas, suggestions, and techniques in this book should not be used in place of professional advice.

The author and publisher are not responsible for any adverse effects or consequences resulting from the use of information in this book. Any lifestyle or health-related changes should be discussed with a healthcare provider.

Copyright © 2024 Mind Body Dictionary, LLC

All rights reserved. No part of this book may be reproduced, stored in a retrieval system, or transmitted in any form or by any means, electronic, mechanical, photocopying, recording, or otherwise, without the prior written permission of the copyright owner, Ronald B. Wayman & Denise Wayman Scholes.

Mindbodydictionary.com

ISBN: 978-1-947176-07-2
Imprint: Independently Published

Author: Ronald B. Wayman
Contributing Author: Denise Wayman Scholes
Illustrator: Elizabeth R. Whitmore

An Introduction...	xii
How to Use this Book...	xiv
Look It Up..	xiv
Read it Cover to Cover...	xiv
Consider Contributing Conditions........................	xiv
Use the Drama Triangle..	xv
Step-by-Step Procedure...	xvii
Ask and Listen...	xviii
Connect and Calm...	xx
Process with Gratitude..	xxii
Abdominal Pain...	1
Abscess...	3
Accidents...	5
Acne..	8
Addictions...	10
Addison's Disease...	13
Adenoids...	15
ADHD...	17
Adrenal Problems...	20
Aging Problems..	23
AIDS..	25
Alcoholism..	27
Allergies..	29
Alzheimer's Disease..	32
Amnesia..	35
Anemia...	37
Ankle Problems..	39
Anorectal Bleeding...	41
Anorexia...	43
Anus..	45
Anxiety...	47
Appendicitis..	51

Appetite: Excessive	53
Appetite: Loss of	55
Arm Problems	57
Arm: Left	59
Arm: Right	61
Arteries	63
Arthritis	65
Asthma	67
Back Problems	71
Back: Lower	73
Back: Lower Area Pain	75
Back: Middle	78
Back: Upper	81
Bad Breath / Halitosis	84
Bed-Wetting (Nocturnal Enuresis)	87
Biting Fingernails	90
Bladder Problems	93
Bleeding Gums	96
Blisters	99
Bloated (Body Wide Water Retention)	101
Blood	104
Blood Clots	107
Blood Pressure: High	109
Blood Pressure: Low	112
Body Odor	115
Boils, Cuts, Fevers, Sores, Inflammations	117
Bones	119
Bowel	122
Brain Problems	125
Breast Problems	128
Bronchitis	131
Bruises	134

Bulimia	136
Burn	139
Burning Tears	142
Burnout	144
Buttocks Problems	147
Cancer	149
Candida	153
Canker Sores	156
Carpal Tunnel Syndrome	158
Cervix	161
Chest Pain	163
Cholesterol	166
Chronic Fatigue Syndrome	170
Chronic Illnesses	173
Claustrophobia	176
Cold	179
Cold Extremities	182
Cold Sores	184
Colon Problems: Large Intestine	187
Colon Problems: Small Intestine	191
Constipation	194
COPD (Chronic Obstructive Pulmonary Disease)	197
Corns	200
Cough	202
Cramps	205
Craving: Breads	208
Craving: Chocolate	211
Craving: Cold Dairy	214
Craving: Gluten	217
Craving: Ice Cream	220
Craving: Salty Foods	223
Craving: Sex	226

Craving: Spicy Foods	229
Cravings: Sugar	232
Cysts	236
Dandruff	238
Dehydration	240
Depression	243
Diabetes	247
Diarrhea	250
Dizziness (Vertigo)	252
Drug Addiction	254
Dry Lips	256
Duodenum Problems	259
Dyslexia	262
Ear	266
Elbows	269
Emotion: Anger	272
Emotion: Bitter	275
Emotion: Fear	278
Emotion: Greed	282
Emotion: Guilt	285
Emotion: Hatred	288
Emotion: Irritation	291
Emotion: Shame	294
Emotion: Worry	297
Emphysema	300
Endometriosis	302
Epilepsy	305
Eyes	308
Eyes: Red / Blood Shot	311
Eyes: Stye / Suffering	314
Face	317
Fainting	320
Fatigue	322

Feet	325
Fever	328
Fibromyalgia	330
Flu (Influenza)	334
Fungus	336
Gallbladder	338
Gallstones	341
Gangrene	344
Gas/Flatulence	346
Hair Loss	348
Hands	350
Hands Chapped	353
Hay Fever	356
Head	359
Headache	364
Heart Problems	367
Heartburn	368
Hemorrhoids	370
Hepatitis	374
Hernia	377
Hiccups	380
Hip Problems	382
Hives	385
Hodgkin's Disease	388
Hyper-Activity	391
Hypoglycemia	393
Immune Issues	395
Impotence	399
Incontinence	402
Indigestion	405
Infection	408
Inflammation	412

Insomnia	415
Itching	417
Jaundice	419
Jaw Problems	422
Joint Pain	425
Kidney Stones	428
Kidneys	431
Kleptomania / Stealing	434
Knee Problems	437
Laryngitis	439
Leg Problems	441
Liver	444
Lung Problems	448
Lyme Disease	450
Manic	453
Mast Cell Disease	456
Memory	459
Meningitis	463
Menstrual Problems	467
Migraine	471
Miscarriage	474
Morning Sickness	476
Motion Sickness	479
Mouth	480
Multiple Sclerosis	484
Nausea	487
Neck Problems	490
Nerve Problems	493
Nose	496
Nosebleeds	498
Numbness	501
Osteoporosis	504

Overweight	507
Pancreas	511
Parasites	514
Parkinson's Disease	516
Phobias	519
Pneumonia	522
Post-Nasal Drip	525
Premenstrual Syndrome (PMS)	528
Prostate	532
Receding Gums	535
Restless Leg Syndrome	538
Rheumatism	541
Ribs	544
Sciatica	547
Scoliosis (Curvature of the Spine)	550
Shin	554
Shingles	557
Shortness of Breath	560
Shoulder Pain / Tension	563
Sinuses	566
Skin: Cancer	569
Skin: Dry / Irritations	572
Skin: Eczema	576
Skin: Issues	579
Skin: Rashes	583
Sleep Apnea	586
Sleepwalking	589
Sneezing	592
Snoring	595
Spleen	598
Sprains	602
Stiffness	606

Stomach Problems (Digestive)	609
Stroke	613
Stuttering	616
Suicidal	619
Swelling/ Edema	622
Tailbone	625
Teeth Grinding	628
Tendon	631
Throat Problems	635
Throat Problems: Specific	638
Thymus Gland	641
Thyroid	644
Tinnitus (Ringing in the Ear)	649
Toes	651
Tongue	654
Tonsillitis	657
Toothache	660
Tumors	663
Ulcers	667
Ulcerative Colitis or Colitis	672
Underweight	675
Urinary Tract Infections	678
Varicose Veins	681
Venereal Disease	684
Viruses	687
Virus, Corona	690
Vitiligo	694
Vomiting	697
Warts	700
Wrist Problems	702
About the Author - Ronald B. Wayman	706
About the Contributing Author - Denise W. Scholes	709
Additional Resources	710

An Introduction

If I were to distill the essence of the Mind Body Dictionary, I'd describe it as much more than a discourse on maintaining a healthy mindset—it's deeply rooted in the wisdom of heart-based connections and nourishing relationships. Focusing primarily on the relationship we have with ourselves and extends to the connections we maintain with others as well as the divine, vital source we all depend on.

For many, self-love remains uncharted territory. Indeed, the life journey, from birth to death, might be a quest to 'find' ourselves, a discovery of our divine value in love. Along the way we may experience moderate to challenging health situations. As we relate positively to these challenges, we will see that they provide an opportunity to deepen and expand our awareness and self-love.

A truly integrated mind, heart, and body create a simple and beautiful harmony, with each part working in concert with the others. When living in harmony with oneself, your awareness can soften into a state of awe towards the majesty of creation, encompassing all living things, radiating through every cell, including reaching into each part of you. This state and space of alignment is peaceful and filled with wonder; it's an incredible way to live.

A basic Google search reveals that over 80% of doctor visits are attributed to illnesses induced by stress. Our bodies are designed for wellness; we are made to heal and be whole. Often, it's the dramas and traumas of life—or more accurately, our response and interpretation of these drama/traumas—that hinder our wholeness and well-being.

By allowing the maturation process to heal the parts of ourselves that got stuck, through a higher, deeper, and more charactered perspective, we can address old wounds and let the body's natural healing process take its course.

Incorporate this information as you go about the necessary treatments for your wellbeing. Allow yourself time, patience, and nourishment as you seek to understand the internal stresses giving rise to maladaptive patterns, resulting in heightened stress within your body. View these alarms with gratitude; your body loves you enough to communicate what's happening. Show love in return by tenderly caring for your body.

You are a child of light and goodness. Embrace that truth as you explore these pages, witness your transformation from a caterpillar into a butterfly—the natural process of evolving into who we are meant to be as we walk the path into greater light.

-Denise Wayman Scholes

How to Use This Book

The Mind Body Dictionary offers several ways to integrate its information into your mind, heart, and life. Consider the following suggestions:

Look It Up:
When facing a physical symptom, condition, or issue, refer to the dictionary.
1. Read both the troubled and healing mindsets.
2. Connect with meanings or parts that are relevant to your specific circumstances and mindset.
3. Bookmark or make note of the definition for easy reference to the healing mindset and/or affirmations.

Read Cover to Cover:
Explore the Mind Body Dictionary from beginning to end.

You may be surprised to stumble upon insights you relate to, but you are not manifesting those conditions in your life. This does not necessarily indicate issues that are underlying, energetic or yet-to-be-manifested in the physical realm, but it could. Whether seeking mental, emotional and/or physical balance, you'll find themes and details that will contribute to your alignment with your true self and overall well-being.

Consider Contributing Conditions:
Recognize that many conditions result from a build up of underlying issues.

Sinus issues may be related to issues found in the liver, colon, and experiences of anger. Explore interconnected aspects to address each piece of the overall puzzle.

The Mind Body Dictionary App *includes related conditions in the search function.*

Use the Drama Triangle:
Sometimes illness is a result of an interconnected constellation of waring parts. We call these types of conflicts the Drama Triangle within the body.

Recognize that internal conflicts often contribute to illness, each with its own "story." Identify internal roles of 'hero,' 'victim,' and 'villain' to clarify the dynamic playing out in your body. For example, heart issues may involve a heart - hero, liver - villain, and kidney/pancreas - victim.

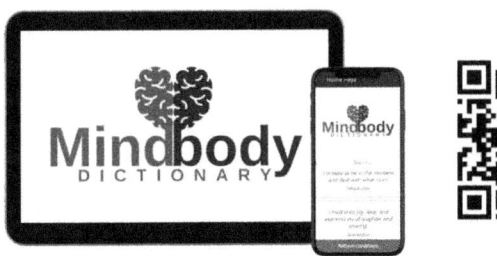

The **Mind Body Dictionary App** search function helps bring related conditions and organs. We also offer an online class about the Drama Triangle that provides additional insights. You can find more information on these resources at mindbodydictionary.com.

A note to the reader: Foods are general recommendations. Foods of the highest quality is advised. Not all recommended foods apply in all situations. Consider needs on a case by case basis.

Step-by-Step Procedures

We will briefly cover three main possible procedures to process conditions:

1. Ask and Listen
2. Connect and Calm
3. Process with Gratitude

We have created a workbook that goes into greater depth for each of these healing process pathways.

Go to mindbodydictionary.com to learn more.

Ask and Listen

If only your body spoke in a language you were used to hearing. The truth is, it does. It's like learning a new language—one that's not entirely unfamiliar. Your body communicates using what it has: pain, discomfort, tears, blushing, changes in breathing, itches, gut movements, tightness—need I go on? Pay attention. Ask questions and listen to what your body is saying. What's the message? What does it mean? Look it up in the Mind Body Dictionary and find out.

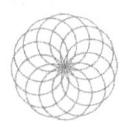

Simple Procedure

1. Close your eyes.
2. Take a deep cleansing breath.
3. Calm the mind and allow messages from the body to flow up to the conscious mind.
4. Ask, "What does my body want me to know about _____ condition?"
5. Write down what comes up.
    - Even if it seems random, consciously asking often yields answers. Listen.
    - The messages may include memories, beliefs, words, emotions, images, or physical sensations.
    - Continue to ask questions to uncover the meaning of the messages. Write down your insights.
6. Once you understand the message, seek to release the energy, feeling, thought, etc. using the Connect and Calm or Gratitude Processes. Repeat as often as necessary.

TIP
Reprogram Your Response

Whenever you experience the discomfort of the condition —be it pain, emotion, or certain thoughts—avoid responding negatively. Instead, greet the sensation with calm awareness or gratitude. For instance, you might say, *"Ouch! Thank you for the reminder that I am doing it differently now."* Appreciate your body for communicating, teaching, and emphasizing the significance of the changes, expansion, and growth you are undergoing.

Offer gentle care. Take the discomfort as a signal to repeat one of the affirmations from the definition. Extend your appreciation to your body for these valuable reminders. Connect your awareness, ease the response with your breath, and release with gratitude.

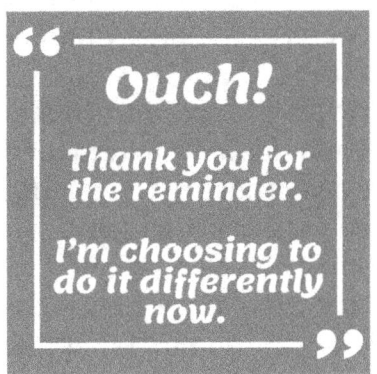

Connect and Calm

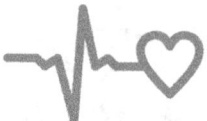

Sometimes the information found in the conditions of The Mind Body Dictionary can be painful, scary, or angering to observe. If we want to heal, transform, and release, it is vital that we choose to see the truth, and come to acceptance, calming the reaction/response to the troubles in our life.

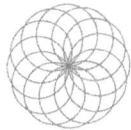

Connect and Calm Procedure

1. Look up the condition and read through the **Troubled Mindset.**
2. Choose one or two bullet point items that resonate, trigger, hurt, or create curiosity for you the most.
3. Calm yourself as you observe.
    - Sit up, perhaps you stretch, put your feet flat on the ground, take a deep breath, root into the ground, imagine a waterfall helping your energy flow deep into the earth.
    - Observe the conflict, ground your energy, and breathe in and out for a minute or two as you settle into a new awareness of the mindset or conflict you've been entertaining that is connected to the issue.
4. Now focus on the area of your body or the condition that you are trying to tend to. What does it feel like? What do you notice?

- What are the physical sensations? Write them down.
- What are the emotions you experience as you pay attention to this condition? Write them down.
- What thoughts come to your mind? Even if they seem random, write them down, then search for the connection.

5. Once you can see the personal resistance and the inner conflict more clearly, read the **Healing Mindset** page.
    - Connect to what that coaching means to you.
        - What does it look like in your life with this specific conflict?
        - What will you change in order to align with a higher vision?

6. Look at the **Affirmation** page.
    - Choose your top two favorite affirmations today. Write them on the affirmation page; perhaps reference them each day, once or twice a day, for a day, a week, or a month, as long as needed.
    - Breathe in and out as you focus on the affirmation.
    - Journal, align, release the old, replace with the new.
    - Consciously choose your beliefs. Observe any beliefs as they come to the surface, write them down. Clean out negative/harmful beliefs or belief patters. Clarify, or deepen positive reinforcing beliefs. Consider the healing mindset and affirmation pages to replace those beliefs.

7. Repeat the process.
    - Sift through the troubled mindset as well as the other affirmations and concepts; does anything new stand out to you more than before?
    - Repeat steps 1 through 6 as many times as needed to feel aligned and connected. When you integrate these new beliefs into your heart and mind, they will naturally emerge anytime time you are faced again with a question, challenge or related issue.

Process with Gratitude

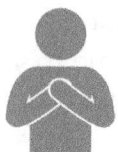

Gratitude – the 'Great Attitude' isn't contingent on having all the answers or being free from challenges. It's not a whimsical wish fulfilled by fantasies or magical entities. Gratitude emerges when the mind surrenders to the potential for personal growth amid struggles and conflicts. It recognizes that the process of developing one's character, building your "character muscle" so to speak, is more significant and important than the conflicts themselves.

What if you've experienced job loss, business setbacks, the end of a friendship, or betrayal? Each of these challenges can offer incredible opportunities for growth and understanding if you're open to the idea that life has its seasons. Just as the earth goes through winters, embracing these difficult times without overwhelming complaints can serve as a stepping stone into a new spring and summer, bringing forth experiences that might not have unfolded without the preceding winter.

Within the Mind Body Dictionary, physical problems reveal gems of insights, understandings, and opportunities for growth. Each condition highlighted in this dictionary signifies the potential for both personal development and healing.

You can read more and get a more thorough process by getting the Mind Body Dictionary workbook. Go to mindbodydictionary.com to learn more.

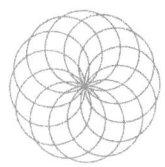

Gratitude Procedure

1. Notice an issue you are having with your body, mind, or heart.
2. Read the description of the problem and the suggestions.
3. Write the thoughts and feelings you have about the negative and positive aspects of the condition.
    - If needed, write or express your emotions to ensure that the part of you that feels wounded is honored. (If you are unsure about the emotional aspects or contributions to the condition, proceed anyway).
    - The goal is not to wallow in pain and stubbornness of feeling horrible or wronged. The goal is to put those thoughts or scripts you tell yourself, including the attached emotions, fears, resentments, etc. in a space where you can observe them.
4. Reflect what you have done to deal with the problem and your reactions.
    - Ask yourself:
        - Have you created space and time to learn and grow from the problem?
        - Have you found new character-building aspects in the process?
    - If yes, close your eyes and allow your heart and mind a moment to appreciate the value of the process of living this experience.
    - If no, go to step 6.
5. Be grateful.

6. If you need more time because you don't feel that you are learning at all or that your condition is hurting others, producing feelings of guilt – then you are holding onto the problem as if it is more important than growing from it.
- Ask yourself the following and start to accept the possibility of finding value from your life experiences of negative and positive nature:
    - What is it that is more precious to you than finding peace inside?
    - What is more valuable to you than finding amazing character-building attributes?
    - What is more important than your ego and pride?
- Return to step 5 and be grateful.

> Gratitude doesn't indicate you have solved your life's problems. It indicates you are learning and experiencing value by living your life path with insight and purpose.
>
> Your healing and change are so much easier with a sincere heart and clear mind of gratitude.

THE
Mindbody
DICTIONARY

Abdominal Pain

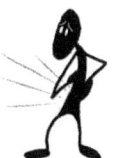

Troubled Mindset

- In a world that often feels competitive, you might sense a struggle to maintain your true self.
- Trust issues may constrict your energy, leading to a defensive or territorial demeanor.
- The yearning for love drives you to seek validation through your accomplishments.
- Recognizing these challenges is a key step towards fostering more balanced connections and acknowledging your inherent worth beyond achievements.

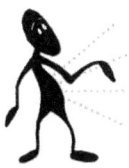

Healing Mindset

Embrace every moment in each day as a precious gift and a chance to encounter love and joy. Release any physical or emotional pain with each exhale, and inhale the tranquility that resonates with your true essence. Reflect on your actions, learning and growing from every experience. Trust that life will support you as you honor yourself and your unique gifts. Prioritize self-support, savoring the moments when others can also be a source of support in your journey.

Abdominal Pain

Affirmations:
- I am grateful for every moment of life and my experience.
- I respect myself and my gifts.
- I stand up for myself.
- I trust that life will support me.
- I am motivated to find peace that is based on oneness with God, my values, and my identity.
- I am flexible.
- Wisdom is natural and ever-present.
- I am touched by the transformation of awesome insights.

Supporting Foods:
- Fermented foods
- Kombucha
- Bananas
- Fibrous foods
- Fish
- Meats (moderate amounts & not fried)
- Green peppers
- Kale
- Barley
- Beans
- Beets
- Cabbage
- Carrots
- Apples
- Asparagus
- Citrus fruits
- Millet
- Okra
- Rice
- Romaine lettuce
- Watermelon

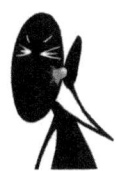

Abscess

Troubled Mindset

- Your emotional pains are erupting.
- You are rejecting your situation.
- When you fail to learn and grow from experiences, your mental progress comes to a standstill. Consequently, you find yourself emotionally festering, searching for an escape.
- You may feel lonely and long for something more in your life.
- You tend to hide secrets and suppress your expression.

Healing Mindset

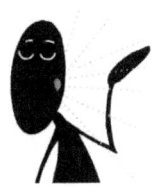

During moments of conflict, seize the opportunity to grow and change. Foster self-awareness without judgement, catching yourself when you slip into real negative thinking.

Consciously observe these thoughts and recognise that you don't need them. Detach from them, then return to the present moment with an honest acknowledgement of reality. Establish this as a daily routine. Through consistent practice of this three-step process, you'll naturally develop a pattern of confronting and releasing negative emotions.

Abscess

Affirmations:
- I hope, I pray, and I stay focused on what is real and helpful.
- I release the pain and hurt.
- I recognise the value in transforming resentment and fear into positive actions and making simple daily changes.
- I am prepared to achieve wellness and remain true to myself.

Supporting Foods:

- Garlic
- Lemons
- Orange
- Fermented foods
- Green leafy vegetables
- Spinach
- Seeds
- Squash
- Broccoli
- Ginger
- Avocado
- Citrus fruits

Accidents

Troubled Mindset

- You're feeling really stressed out, and it's making it hard for you to stay grounded.
- Perhaps your mind is scattered, making it difficult to pay full attention or to stay calm and focused.
- The stress is making it tough for your body and mind to communicate clearly.
- It's possible that your energy field is not as strong, and that's making you more vulnerable.
- Blaming others and being hard on yourself because of the stress is making things worse. You need to open your heart and mind to a perspective so you can behave differently when handling life's trials.
- You may feel out of place and sometimes have a difficult time taking a firm stand on particular topics.

Accidents

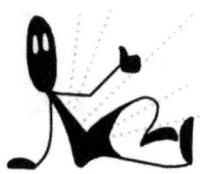

Healing Mindset

Be present in THIS moment. Without judgment, calm yourself by self-soothing and re-centre as you breathe through any thoughts, emotional tugs, or concerns unrelated to this moment.

Release them. If they persist, focus in or get assistance to heal the emotional wound that keeps triggering these persistent thoughts. Consider how that experience is trying to help you grow. What is it that you have not yet understood? Be aware of the areas where you are lost, hurt, blaming, or injuring yourself; this can be an indicator of where to focus your attention to heal. See the body area for more information.

Accidents

Affirmations:

- I am here, right now.
- I breathe and ground into the earth easily.
- There is nowhere else for me to be.
- I love being present, alive, and well.
- I focus on what is real and enjoyable, in the clear, and present.
- When I am off, I easily come back to myself and my life.

Supporting Foods:

- Papaya
- Pineapple
- Apples
- Eggs
- Watermelon
- Buckwheat
- Green leafy vegetables
- Bone broth for strengthening
- Go to the relevant body area for specific foods
- AVOID: Sugary foods, processed foods, chemicals, or food additives.

Acne

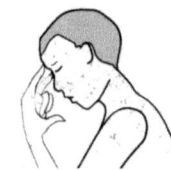

Troubled Mindset

- You haven't been kind or accepting of yourself. Perhaps you're avoiding a certain situation, or perhaps it's a combination of both.
- Your feelings of upset and embarrassment are creating an inner conflict between pleasing others and honoring yourself. You can't do both.
- You might be experiencing loneliness, yearning for something more, or keeping secrets instead of expressing yourself honestly and freely.
- Distaste towards yourself, your expressions, and your physical self can result in unnecessary stress and a rejection of love.

Healing Mindset

Choose today to love and cherish yourself. Be true to who you are. Choose each moment to be the best version of yourself.

Release any anger and resentment tied to past mistakes or upsets. Beating yourself up isn't helping you grow. Accept yourself where you are now, with hope for growth and positive change. Choose to express yourself lovingly to others while maintaining your honesty and connection. Be reflective as you gradually and continually grow into your strength and compassion.

Acne

Affirmations:

- I can balance the need to expand and the need to reflect.
- I have strong self-esteem.
- I move toxins out and heal from within.
- I resolve conflicting communications.
- I have mercy for myself and others.
- I open my expressions.
- I speak the truth, and I respect myself.

Supporting Foods:

- Water/Get hydrated
- Apples
- Asparagus
- Bananas
- Barley
- Beans
- Beets
- Cabbage
- Carrots
- Citrus fruits
- Fish
- Green peppers
- Kale
- Millet
- Okra
- Rice
- Romaine lettuce
- Watermelon
- Cayenne pepper
- Ginger
- Meats (moderate amounts and not fried)
- Fibrous foods if safe; otherwise, steam the fibrous vegetables.

Addictions

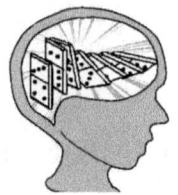

Troubled Mindset

- You are masking feelings of emotional pain that you do not want to feel.
- You seriously question whether you are a good person or not.
- This deep fear drives you away from confronting any negative feeling that might reinforce that horrifying conclusion.
- You seek love everywhere else, but instead of healing, you end up nourishing the insecurity.
- You are compensating, attempting to fill the void of love, but it's not working. You do it again and again, hoping that the short relief will last, but it doesn't.
- Rational thought takes a back seat as you run from issues and emotions. Not believing in your inherent worth and not accepting yourself sustains the persistent pains. You're putting a square peg into a round hole.

Addictions

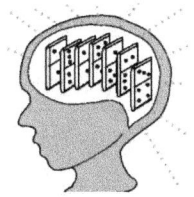

Healing Mindset

The key to discovering relief resides within you, by offering genuine care for every aspect of yourself: mental, emotional, physical, and spiritual. Consider forming a deep and personal connection with a divine source.

Beating yourself up during low moments isn't helpful. Love yourself through your mistakes to nurture your way back to strength, hope, and health. Confront the hidden negative belief patterns and emotions. As you face yourself and honor the divine part within you, you can truly grow into your authentic self. Reach out for help and acknowledge the need for genuine self-responsibility.

Addictions

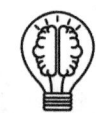

Affirmations:

- I am ready to uncover what I am hiding.
- I can see clearly the precious emotions and habits that actually hurt me.
- I create new steps, new paths, and new patterns that nourish my soul, mind, and body.
- I let my heart rest and then vibrate to the beat and pattern of habits that support every part of my soul and body.
- I no longer submit to immature fears and cravings.
- I surrender to true personal responsibility.
- My response to life includes respect for my body, mind, and heart.
- I am empowered every moment to bring sweetness into my life that no substance ever can.
- Real joy is real connection and true action that supports all parts of myself.

Supporting Foods:

- Eat a well-balanced, nutrient-dense diet that emphasizes fresh, raw foods, fresh fruits, and vegetables.
- Legumes
- Bananas
- Cereal grasses
- Seaweeds
- Sprouts
- Wild blue-green algae
- Leafy green vegetables
- Flax seeds/oil
- Salmon
- Cod
- Trout
- Goat's milk

Addison's Disease

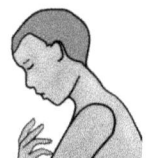

Troubled Mindset

- Being perfectionistic is contributing to a feeling of anxiety about life. It hasn't turned out the way that you had imagined.
- You may find it difficult to understand your own experiences or emotions.
- You worry about what you don't understand.
- You struggle to trust emotional nourishment from others, so you resist opening your heart to healthy connections.

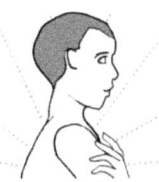

Healing Mindset

Forgive, be kind, and be flexible with yourself through mistakes or life's challenges. Support others appropriately, without insisting on carrying their burdens for them. Cultivate positive connections by maintaining healthy boundaries. Bring laughter back into your life and go with the flow of life's current instead of resisting what comes into your path. Take time for yourself to unwind and do what you love.

Addison's Disease

Affirmations:
- I create a life of order without spinning out of control.
- I cultivate patterns of peace throughout my day.
- I feel safe being myself, living life.
- I sleep with the trust that the next day will be a wonderful experience.

Supporting Foods:

- Millet
- Mulberry
- Parsley
- Quinoa
- Radish
- Sesame seeds (black)
- Sunflower seeds
- Spinach
- String beans

Adenoids

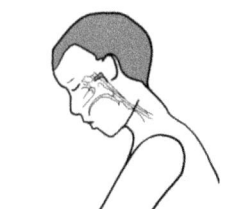

Troubled Mindset

- Home life feels distressing.
- A child may perceive themselves as the source of the conflict.
- They might feel like a burden or unwelcome.
- Subtle blame emerges as ripples of regret and self-shame.
- They may wish it could be different, quietly resenting what could have been.

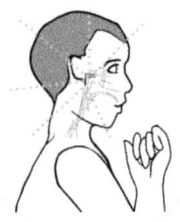

Healing Mindset

Nourish an attitude of self-love amid heavy feelings. With gratitude, direct your attention to the positive aspects of your life. Express these sentiments regularly, particularly to children grappling with this issue. Consider life as an opportunity for discovery, as it teaches and helps us grow each day.

Adenoids

Affirmations:
- I turn the pity to self-care.
- I enjoy what is positive in my life.
- Life struggles are my teachers, and I discover new ways of growing every day.
- I turn the fear into the assertive action of taking care of myself and going for the best part of the day and life.

Supporting Foods:
- Garlic
- Lemon
- Orange
- Ginger
- Fermented foods
- Seeds
- Green leafy vegetables
- Spinach
- Broccoli
- Avocado
- Squash

ADHD

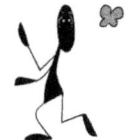

Troubled Mindset

- You are uncomfortable or discontented with your current situation.
- You have too many things to do and don't know what to do first or last.
- You feel pressure from others all the time, so it is easier to be scattered or hyper-focused on something that intrigues you.
- Your mind is in constant need of entertainment or something to focus on.
- You'd rather be busy with something fun or something that can be accomplished than be bothered by others telling you what to do.
- You ask, "Why does everyone want something and why do they tell me what to do and think?"
- You tell yourself, "I just want to be left alone" and "I can be the one to decide what I want and when I want it."

ADHD

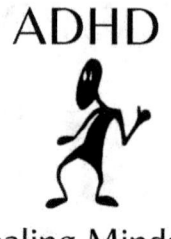

Healing Mindset

It may be beneficial to explore what's happening beneath the surface. Different parts of your brain may be out of sync with each other, leading to different speeds within yourself. When these parts aren't aligned and working together as one, you may feel like you're spinning out of control while desperately seeking control.

Take moments throughout the day to "pause" your life. You may consider setting an alarm or timer for these breaks. During these pauses, practice breathing in intervals of 7 long breaths followed by 2 short breaths for 2 minutes.

Look or imagine looking into nature during these pauses—observe trees, hills, and clouds. Appreciate the beauty and wonder. Then, focus on your hand or a nearby flower with a sense of wonder. Return to the moment and engage your heart with exercises, followed by calming down with some push-ups.

Apply a similar approach for your mind. Quickly jot down what you're excited or hyper about, then write slowly about the purpose behind it all. Choose one item from the list and enjoy the action. Remember, life isn't about doing everything; it's an experience of discovering your true nature in each moment and living as one, not many.

ADHD

Affirmations:
- I am awesome and cool.
- I embrace all aspects of myself as one person in one moment, engaging in one activity, thinking clearly about one thought.
- I am connected to all through one focused filter.
- I appreciate the opportunity to be challenged.
- I find joy in discovering clarity and integrity in every thought and action.
- I channel my creativity in a balanced, clear, and focused manner each and every day.

 ## Supporting Foods:

- Fresh vegetables
- Almonds raw or raw sprouted
- Apples
- Avocado
- Bananas
- Banana squash
- Black beans
- Blackberries
- Blueberries
- Boysenberries
- Brown rice
- Celery & carrot
- Crenshaw melon
- Oranges
- Cucumber
- Custard
- Delicata squash
- Green beans
- Green peas
- Hummus
- Jicama
- Kiwi
- Kumquat
- Lentils
- Mango
- Marion berries
- Millet
- Mung beans
- Papaya
- Perch
- Pineapple
- Plums
- Pumpkin seeds
- Quinoa
- Quinoa & lentils
- Raspberries
- Salmon
- Strawberries, organic
- Sunflower seeds sprouted
- Trout
- Tuna
- Yellow squash
- Watermelon
- Wild rice
- Zucchini

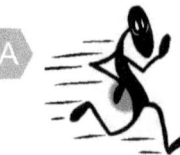

Adrenal Problems

Troubled Mindset

- Feeling stressed, tense or anxious, and possibly having a panic attack; your lack of loyalty to yourself is having a detrimental impact on you.
- You doubt yourself.
- Perhaps you are prioritising perfection over self-acceptance.
- At some level, you have believed that you must suffer to succeed in life.
- You ultimately feel tired, run-down, and emotionally unbalanced.
- You need to keep going, keep pushing, keep trying, keep finding ways to get things done, keep hoping that if you keep doing and wishing, things will work out.
- Whether you know it or not, your internal engine is constantly idling too fast.
- Your mind is consumed with worry and concern about potential and possible outcomes; stressing your thoughts, mind, and heart.
- Your body is trying to keep up with your need to be on constant alert.
- You wish things were perfect in some area of your life.
- Maybe you want everyone else or yourself to be okay and safe.
- Anticipating the possible worst, or working so hard to prevent your feared outcomes of the future, is taking its toll.
- The adrenals, your body's best defence, are being strained with too much, too big, too long, too crazy.

Adrenal Problems

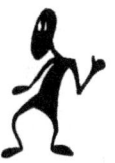

Healing Mindset

Consider more sleep, more quiet, more trust. The body's fatigue and tiredness are trying to get a message through to you: "pause, trust, and enjoy the moment." Appreciate each moment and stop rushing through life.

There's nothing to prove except to see if you can pause, appreciate, and discover the adventure of moving through your obstacles without stress or worry or pushing all the time. The most significant obstacle is your overwhelm, and learning to deal with your internal struggle is key to turning obstacles into opportunities. When push comes to shove, take a walk and reconnect with your authentic self. Create 3 to 5 minutes each hour to quietly pause your life. Joyfully move with the flow of life as you reach toward your goals.

Adrenal Problems

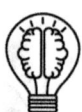

Affirmations:

- I follow my goals with ease.
- I am motivated to turn obstacles into opportunities.
- I am motivated by choice, by joy, and by intrigue.
- I pause, listen, and experience the moment.
- Life is an adventure full of new discoveries.
- I create a new view every time I sense any worry or concern.
- I let the anxiety flow back to the earth.
- I breathe in refreshing new life and new thought.
- I realize that my fears make me aware and faith makes me act.
- I take one step at a time with each new breath.
- I anticipate that the future is positively intriguing.

Supporting Foods:

- Beets
- Black beans
- Carrots
- Garlic
- Grapes with carrots
- Green beans
- Hummus
- Kidney beans
- Lentils
- Millet
- Mulberry
- Onion
- Parsley
- Peas
- Quinoa
- Radish
- Salmon
- Sesame seeds (black)
- Sunflower seeds
- Spinach
- String beans
- Tilapia

Aging Problems

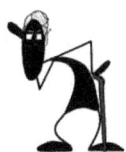

Troubled Mindset

- You fear the changing of the times and losing your value.
- Your resistance towards change contributes to your anxiety about the future.
- You're struggling to share who you are because of past hurts.
- You may carry a belief that age equals illness.

Healing Mindset

The most constant thing in the world is change. Flow with it with trust and joy. Open your heart and mind to the adventure of the unfolding changes through time.

Learn to love life and yourself, nurturing the teacher and leader within you. Enjoy each moment as a gift, and time will be yours.

Aging Problems

Affirmations:
- I live in this moment, and now this one. Embracing and flowing with each moment as a gift.
- I gracefully mature my cells to maintain vitality and joy.
- I experience the amazing discoveries of life every day, keeping my youthful bliss in all that I do and say.
- I thoroughly enjoy life.
- My heart is full.

Supporting Foods:

- Salmon
- Soybeans
- Garlic
- Onions
- Pearl barley
- Broccoli
- Cauliflower
- Cabbage
- Chia seeds
- Flax seeds
- Quinoa
- Parsley
- Amaranth
- Sunflower seeds
- Sprouts
- String beans
- Zucchini squash

- Water/Get hydrated
- Eat a well-balanced diet that includes raw vegetables, fruits, whole grains, nuts and seeds, and quality protein.

AIDS

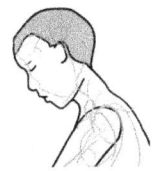

Troubled Mindset

- You've been really hard on yourself.
- Feelings of not being good enough provoke you.
- Your personal attacks are weakening your immune system.
- Your immune system is being kept down by feelings related to self-disgust and an overall unwillingness to see yourself as acceptable.
- You are experiencing feelings of guilt about sexuality and your past.
- Denying the issues and concerns hasn't helped.

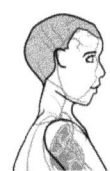

Healing Mindset

Make reconciliation with the past. Forgive yourself and anyone else you harbor animosity towards. Recognize that those negative emotions are not serving you. Seek to identify with and cherish your authentic self. Get to know your core values and needs. Then, find the path that honors and respects the needs of every aspect of your mental, emotional, physical, and spiritual self. Discover and release the inner conflict, bringing a sense of peace through love and self-acceptance.

AIDS

Affirmations:

- Whatever happens is immaterial to what really matters—the matter of my heart.
- I choose to let go of my inner critic to make room for my purpose in living.
- I choose to live each day where I matter to someone.
- I make a difference in my own life and the lives of others.
- I am loved, and the divine loves me.

Supporting Foods:

- Red beets
- Garlic
- Onion
- Leeks
- Shallots
- Zucchini squash
- Quinoa
- Amaranth
- Kimchi
- Sauerkraut
- Radishes
- Watermelon
- Sprouted sunflower seeds
- Sprouted almonds
- Soaked chia seeds

Alcoholism

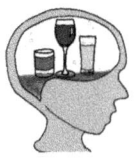

Troubled Mindset

- You are struggling with feelings of uselessness.
- You sense that people don't want you around, and you carry unresolved negative emotions.
- Discussing these issues becomes challenging for you because any criticisms feel overwhelming. You're already engaging in self-degradation and can't endure more of it.
- You may seek relaxation through substances like alcohol, yet this choice often results in a loss of control, transferring that control to someone else. Consequently, this intensifies the tension you feel, establishing a vicious cycle as you return to alcohol for relaxation once again.

Healing Mindset

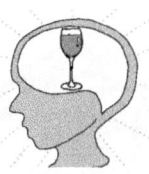

Start by firmly facing the self-degradation and offering yourself compassion. Search your own heart and mind for kindness and offer it to yourself, especially in those normally harsh, critical moments. Acknowledge your mistakes with honesty and tenderness; this will strengthen you to grow and choose your actions with more responsibility. Trust that life will support you as you seek the highest good for all.

Alcoholism

Affirmations:
- I enjoy managing the comings and goings of life in its vast matrix.
- I choose my actions responsibly.
- I show compassion for myself as I grow.
- I empower myself with positive thinking.
- I trust life will support me.
- I am my own true best friend.
- I come out of hiding and gladly associate with those who are true to themselves and not to old habits.
- I love creating new habits every day that support me and my family.

Supporting Foods:

- Jackfruit
- Kudzu
- Garlic
- Onions
- Grapefruit
- Red beets
- Celery juice
- Citron fruit
- Salted prunes (Umeboshi)
- Leafy greens with sprouts
- Quinoa
- Salmon
- Sprouts
- Zucchini squash
- Broccoli
- Jicama
- Rutabaga
- Red pepper
- Green pepper
- Yellow pepper
- Orange pepper
- Watermelon

Allergies

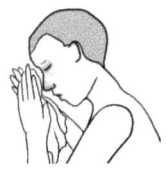

Troubled Mindset

- You've bottled up so many of your emotions.
- You find it hard to believe that sharing your feelings could bring positive change, mainly because the fear of sharing outweighs your faith in the possibility of change.
- Your negative reaction to unpleasant feelings, whether directed towards yourself or others, is ultimately making the problem worse.
- The reluctance to face conflict partly arises from the raw sensitivity of emotional pains.
- You are relinquishing your personal power each time you allow unresolved emotions to remain unchecked within your heart or mind.
- You are allowing someone or something to keep you feeling trapped, controlled, and unable to experience true freedom or peace.
- Your fear of honestly facing and addressing these issues within yourself or with another person prevents you from being your authentic self.

Allergies

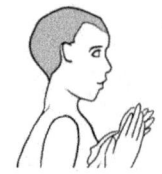

Healing Mindset

Confront the emotional annoyances, irritations, or upsets in your life. Recognize when you've judged yourself or others, then soothe the sensitivities by being kind and gentle. Learn how, then focus on developing healthy mental, emotional, and/or physical boundaries. Differentiate between what is you and what is not you.

Take responsibility for your own emotions and avoid carrying an excess burden of someone else's emotions. Be conscientious and considerate of how your words and actions influence and impact others, but do not take responsibility for the thoughts and behaviors of others. Open up and release negative feelings as you seek resolution for past upsets. This will help you understand and identify with your true self, fostering authentic and balanced feelings.

Allergies

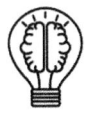

Affirmations:

- I seek to understand the pains and sorrows in my life.
- I am real with what is.
- I have a clear sense of my identity.
- My authenticity shines when I share my heart.
- I release my burdens to God.
- I feel secure as I embrace this wonderful life.
- I enjoy gradually adapting to my amazing environment.

Supporting Foods:

- Water/Get hydrated
- Soaked chia seeds
- Sprouted lentils
- Sprouted spelt
- Wheat/barley grass
- Foods that support your heart
- Citrus fruits
- Turmeric
- Endive
- Sprouts
- Celery
- Microalgae
- Microgreens
- Papaya
- Mango
- Kamut
- Oats
- Parsley
- Tomatoes
- Onions
- Ginger

Alzheimer's Disease

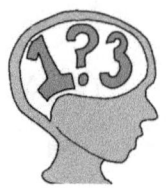

Troubled Mindset

- Life has felt overwhelming, and it has now reached a point where it is officially over the top.
- You might have been frustrated for not being or feeling in control, now hope is fading away.
- At times, you've seen yourself as 'less than' others.
- Your abilities and contributions haven't felt appreciated, leading to deep hurt and simmering anger.
- The idea of creating your own alternative reality has been tempting, and in the process, you've overlooked the good moments, fixating on the bad.
- It seems like you're caught between not truly living and fearing the unknown of death. So now, you are stuck in between.

Alzheimer's Disease

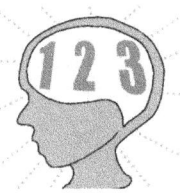

Healing Mindset

The universe is rooting for you, not against you. You can trust that there is a loving purpose behind all your experiences, including the emotions that you have experienced or are experiencing. Stop suppressing them. Face your emotions so you can release them.

Allow yourself to see things as they really are and trust the process of life. If you believe you are loved and can trust a divine purpose, then you will not need to control it. Remember the good in your life. Remember your positive contributions without neglecting the positive lessons learned from the hard times. Do activities that bring you joy.

Alzheimer's Disease

Affirmations:
- What has happened has happened.
- What will happen will happen.
- I find comfort in the fact that history is, and stories have character, but I let go of the regret and anger that tries to change the colourful stories of my past.
- I am ready to live each day without the pain of the past.
- I am grateful for my life.
- It is amazing that I have made it this far. So, I forgive myself and others and hope to God that everyone will feel His enduring love.

Supporting Foods:
- Water/Get hydrated
- Chia seed
- Flax seed
- Salmon
- Leafy greens
- Avocados
- Jicama
- Sprouted sunflower seeds

Amnesia

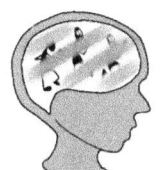

Troubled Mindset

- You may be harboring feelings of guilt and have a hard time standing up for yourself.
- Guilt and fear may lead you to not want to deal with your past, so you're trying to erase certain memories.
- You don't know your true value.

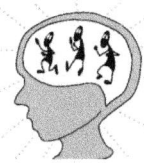

Healing Mindset

Cherish and honor your value. Separate that from what has happened. Work to find fulfillment and embrace the now and your emotional experiences. Empower your intuition and purpose and focus on what is real. Let go of what is in the past and experience each moment with love, courage, and passion.

Amnesia

Affirmations:
- I live with enriched emotional experiences.
- I have stability of health, immunity, and inner self-knowing.
- I empower my intuition and purpose.
- I am focused on what is real.
- I let go of the past and tap into positive inner resources to complete each moment with love, courage, and passion.
- I have fun with what I do have.

Supporting Foods:

- Chia seeds
- Flax seeds
- Red beets
- Carrots
- Celery
- Radishes

- Apples
- Oranges
- Watermelon
- Figs
- Leafy greens
- Romaine lettuce

- Red leaf lettuce
- Broccoli
- Cauliflower
- Jicama
- Dragonfruit
- Pomegranate

Anemia

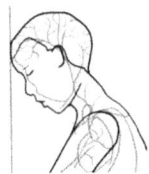

Troubled Mindset

- You may be having a hard time loving yourself and find that you're focusing on someone else's well-being over your own.
- You struggle with not being able to control things in your life and worry that you aren't enough.
- You feel a lack of strength to deal with the big challenges.
- Your will feels challenged by the massive responsibilities in life.
- You feel a need to compartmentalize life so it is not overwhelming.

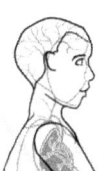

Healing Mindset

Learn to love yourself completely, free from judgment. You are human and you always will be. You weren't meant to have all the answers for everyone. Find your strength and change what you can. Seek to learn from the pains of the past and forgive yourself and others for perceived wrongs. You are a divine soul, and so are they. Restore order to return to joy in your life.

Anemia

Affirmations:
- I love myself completely.
- I now release all judgment.
- I easily feel loved.
- I forgive and trust in the process of life.
- I choose to find my strength from within and my truth.
- I accept my weaknesses as my learning and clearly change what I can.

Supporting Foods:

- Leafy greens
- Red beets
- Jicama
- Chia seeds
- Flax seeds
- Sprouted almonds
- Sprouted sesame seeds
- Sprouted sunflower seeds
- Brazil nuts
- Hazel nuts
- Broccoli
- Peas
- String beans
- Pole beans
- Black beans
- Turnips
- Celery
- Eggs
- Protein from meat
- Fish
- Poultry

Ankle Problems

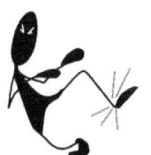

Troubled Mindset

- You are a little nervous about which path to take, so you have tried to take both, which twists you up and makes you unsure.
- You have a habit of trying to please others, making it difficult to honor your own needs, goals, and desires.
- Pleasing and accommodating habits are creating too much flexibility and weakness.
- The challenges and burdens above, in your heart and mind, are making you ungrounded and unstable below.

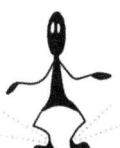

Healing Mindset

Identify then honor your true needs, desires, values, and aspirations. You may want to write them down and reference them. Caring about others is a virtue, but in a balanced way and not at your own expense. Find the courage to be your true divine self each day. Left ankle: You feel as if you are overwhelmed with life and your responsibilities. Wisely choose what you bring into your life and honor your choice. Right ankle: You are doing something that conflicts with your morals. Focus on standing up for what you believe in. It is OK to say, "no."

Ankle Problems

Affirmations:
- I listen to my inner core self, and I begin each day honoring the person inside.
- I walk my path, honoring and respecting my values and passions.
- I take the chance to be me and have the courage to live the "me" every day.
- I feel an inner direction and follow that path.
- I seek universal friendship, while maintaining a quality friendship with myself.

Supporting Foods:

- Carrots
- Jicama
- Peas
- Sesame seeds
- Sprouted sunflower seeds
- Sprouted almonds
- Slow-cooked cereal grains
- Butter
- Salmon
- Grass-fed beef
- Papaya
- Fermented foods
- Slow-cooked eggs
- High-quality cheese

Anorectal Bleeding

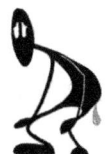

Troubled Mindset

- You are frustrated by the way life is going.
- Due to a lack of trust in life's experiences, you keep attempting to control and force fate instead of going with the flow of life.
- You push through the troubles, hoping they'll just go away, or go your way, rather than dealing with them honestly.

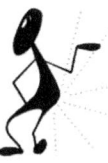

Healing Mindset

Release the need for control. When challenging memories come to the surface, breathe and release tension in your mind and body to resolve past difficulties that are still affecting you today. As you relax into accepting what is, you will begin to flow with life. Choose to trust in a higher purpose to life's experiences.

Anorectal Bleeding

Affirmations:

- I face my fears, which are too near, giving me a chance to turn them into courage and strength.
- That pesky negative self-talk and worry is now my buddy because I turn any shadow into humor, fun, and something to learn from.
- I pause when I eat, and I eat with clarity and calm.
- I pause often and feel gratitude for life.
- I bring authentic courage back into my life.

Supporting Foods:

- Chia seeds, sprouted
- Flax seeds, sprouted
- Pineapple
- Papaya
- Peppers
- Cucumbers
- Leafy greens
- Onions
- Peas
- Radishes
- Alfalfa
- Dark green leafy vegetables
- Molasses

Anorexia

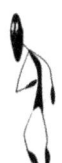

Troubled Mindset

- Fear may stem from struggling to live up to the standards of others - either real or imagined.
- You might feel like you can't please your parent(s) enough.
- You are angry with yourself for not being 'enough,' and you deal with it by self-punishing.
- You grasp at a sense of control through not eating. However, you are losing your strength to have healthy control by not nourishing yourself emotionally or physically.

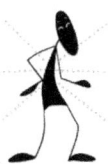

Healing Mindset

Turn the fear into strength and courage. Learn to trust what you can change, and truly give up on being overly responsible for the saving of others. Choose to love yourself and nourish your body, so your soul won't want to leave. Trust, love, and care for yourself. Nourish yourself spiritually. Seek divine love for you personally.

Anorexia

Affirmations:

- I let the wishes go like fishes, and let my negative self-thoughts calmly float away.
- I replace wishes and stories with encouraging self-talk.
- I find one small piece of life that is simple and I embrace that.
- I take each moment and find safety in it.
- I don't have to solve everything, just notice and do what I can.
- I create boundaries that keep me safe while creating feelings and thoughts that are beneficial and full of light.

Supporting Foods:

- Watermelon
- Lemon
- Orange
- Lime
- Rutabaga
- Carrot
- Leafy greens
- Chia seeds, soaked
- Sprouts
- Wheatgrass juice
- Red beets
- Cucumbers
- Bananas
- Pineapple
- Alfalfa sprouts
- Pumpkin seeds
- Raw fruits
- Steamed vegetables
- Tomatoes

Anus

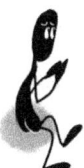

Troubled Mindset

- Powerlessness or embarrassment may lead to living in survival mode.
- It's been hard to let go of the 'unspoken' family creeds that are no longer cultivating the best for you.
- As you reflect on actions or decisions, you carry a heaviness or regret for whatever has happened.
- You are very critical of yourself and others.
- Instead of learning from life and letting things go, you hold on for fear of what will happen if you no longer have that familiar crap in your life.
- You feel people cross your boundaries often.
- You are not holding a boundary for yourself.
- All of this leaves you feeling vulnerable and angry.

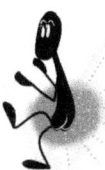

Healing Mindset

It starts with you. Seek to understand the part you have played in all of your unpleasant experiences. Stop beating yourself up. Have compassion for yourself as you seek learning and change. Learn about maintaining healthy boundaries and identify what you believe will bring the highest and best for all.

Anus

Affirmations:

- I enjoy moving forward.
- The pressures of the past are dissipating into ease of movement.
- My inner voice is one of strength, comfort, and encouragement.
- All other voices are not mine, only those that build my inner strength and truth.

Supporting Foods:

- Chia seeds, sprouted
- Flax seeds, sprouted
- Pineapple
- Papaya
- Peppers
- Cucumbers
- Leafy greens
- Onions
- Peas
- Radishes

Anxiety

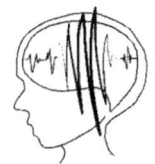

Troubled Mindset

- Coping with stress makes you feel that life is dangerous and not safe to communicate freely and openly.
- You want to relax but your body takes over with tightness of breath, shakiness, tight muscles, and head pressure.
- Rather than trusting life, you try to control it with your thoughts, feelings and actions.
- You are struggling to connect to your capacity to create positive change in your life, and this makes the future seem particularly frightening.
- You fear your own anger, as well as any conflict it may bring, so you suppress it.
- You are frustrated and angry with the way things are, but fear overrides the confidence to address it.
- Your worries tighten muscles in your body as if you are afraid to run, but you wish you could just go and be somewhere else without all the concerns that haunt you.
- You want to say what is on your mind, but your heart believes it will only get worse if you do.
- You use your anxiety to stay alert and busy so that you can avoid looking at something that might be overwhelming.

Anxiety

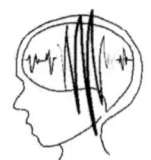

Troubled Mindset
(Continued)

- If you keep being too perfectionistic, you become overly "procrastinistic" to deal with what is most important.
- It is so difficult to see the forest from the trees because your thoughts branch off into scattered thoughts and feelings just trying to avoid what is scaring you. Thus, you are hiding within your tangled-up forest of life experience.

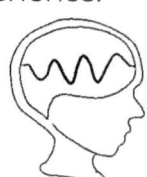

Healing Mindset

The goal is to embrace each moment in life as an opportunity to experience and learn. Even though it is difficult to see the bigger picture, it is helpful to take moments to stop and pause your life. Permit yourself to feel each emotion that flows through your life's experience. Learn from these experiences. As you do this, face your anger; don't fear it, suppress it, or give in to it in a way that will cause harm to yourself or others. Rather, allow it to motivate you with the courage that it takes to make the positive changes that you seek. This may be a challenge, and it takes practice, but you will get

Anxiety

Healing Mindset
(Continued)

better as you remain aware of what is going on within you.

When someone tells you to "go with the flow," you might resist it and become more stressed. Because you need to be in so much control that your body and mind thinks "being in control" is more important than feeling calm and relaxed. It is time to decide what is safe for you.

Start simple. Start with feeling safe with the earth and nature. Start with feeling safe with breath and awareness. Do some interval paced breathing where you breathe 5 slow breaths, 1 regular breath, and then 1 quick breath. Do this interval for 3 to 4 times to reset your breathing pattern. Touch your body on the arms, legs, belly to let yourself feel you. Take moments to honor your simple thoughts.

Anytime you are in a tight spot inside, find a safe place in your life. Most of what you fear is your mind and body trying to find a way to make you safe. But it doesn't work because it is not based on reality or truth. It is based on perceptions and possibilities that spin you into fear. Take the crazy spiral of excessive thinking and gradually slow the spin to a calm wave. Visualize the ocean calmly moving a wave back and forth washing over you and through you, bringing you into a nice simple movement of peaceful energy.

Anxiety

Affirmations:
- I enjoy each moment fully.
- I am safe.
- It is okay to be afraid.
- I give myself permission to feel.
- I give myself permission to let go and enjoy.
- Life offers exciting adventures.
- I am united with myself.
- I feel that I have a place, and I belong.
- I allow worry for a few moments a day and allow rest and peace many moments a day.
- I send the scattered thoughts to the wind and ground with peace to mother earth.
- Peace comes when I take a calming breath and smile at myself.
- I pause my worried self and take a nice calm breath for my real self.

 ### Supporting Foods:

- Water
- Alfalfa sprouts
- Algae
- Beetroot
- Black beans
- Celery
- Chlorophyll
- Egg
- Fennel
- Fish
- Globe artichoke
- Greens
- Kidney beans
- Lamb
- Lettuce
- Mushrooms
- Rhubarb
- Romaine lettuce
- Sesame seeds
- Sprouts
- Walnuts
- Watermelon
- Wheat grass

Appendicitis

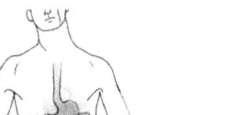

Troubled Mindset

- You are aiming for something that you do not sincerely believe you can achieve.
- Your fears related to your own feelings, an authority figure, or of rejection are stuck inside of you.
- Your fear of facing a certain individual or group causes a great deal of inner conflict.
- You hold onto inner conflict as a way of leveraging control over yourself and what you might do.

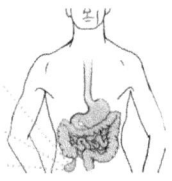

Healing Mindset

Trust in the process of life. Tap into your intuition and trust in the life path that is meant for you. Breathe in positive thoughts and emotions and breathe out the negative ones as you ground yourself. Trust that you can deal with conflict in a way that will bring about positive change and resolution. Ground your energy in who you are, not what others might think of you or what they might do to you.

Appendicitis

Affirmations:

- I let go of the need for junk food and junk emotional thoughts.
- I can face my fears and not let them rule my mind and lifestyle.
- I gain strength each time I face my conflict with faith in the process.
- I am a functional, communicative, fun-loving person.
- I enjoy my life and relationships and let go of inner conflicts that block my inner joy.

Supporting Foods:

- Fresh lime juice
- Manuka honey
- Milk
- Steamed non-gasing forming vegetables
- Fresh carrot juice
- Fresh celery juice
- Fresh beet juice
- Fresh cucumber juice
- Tea of fenugreek seeds

Appetite: Excessive

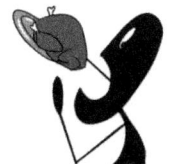

Troubled Mindset

- You are replacing an emotional void with food, using it to feel "safe" or protected.
- You judge your own emotions, and you fear the judgement of others.
- You struggle to calm down because there is too much going on inside.
- You are using food to stuff the chaos down.
- You are not being real with the true inner conflict, those emotions seem too frightening.

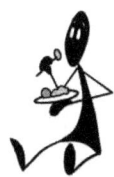

Healing Mindset

Breathe. Pause.
There is another path that is far more fulfilling. Be ready to stop and pause your "crazy" self. Then feel it. It is time to be real with it all. It is time to find true safety inside yourself so you can relax and not strain through life. You truly can deal with your emotions and fears. Love and accept yourself; your strength could be in living with awareness.

Appetite: Excessive

Affirmations:

- I am ready to stop and look around.
- I see beauty everywhere.
- I am safe.
- I am grateful for what I have, who I am, my gifts, and my family.
- I have everything I need.
- I am enjoying slowing down and receiving the nourishment that is right in front of me.
- I am nourished by life, air, water, and a smile.

Supporting Foods:

- Water/Get hydrated
- Watermelon
- Chia seeds, soaked
- Flax seeds, soaked
- Steamed carrots
- Slowly chewed carrots
- Celery juice
- Celery
- Red beets
- Cucumber
- Lime
- Sprouted almonds

Appetite: Loss of

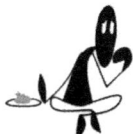

Troubled Mindset

- You are depressed, have lost interest mentally, or your body is protecting you physically and needs a rest.
- You may be lacking trust in yourself and others.
- You feel as if you need to keep a constant guard up.

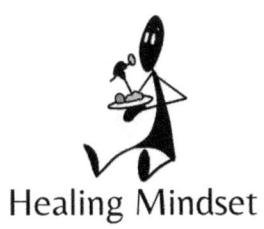

Healing Mindset

Take a moment to pause, reflect, rest, and rejuvenate before moving ahead. Believe that everything that has happened in your life is meant to empower you.

Life can throw curveballs at us when we least expect it, and it can seem like things are falling apart. Every experience is an opportunity for growth and learning. Taking a moment to pause, reflect, rest, and rejuvenate can help us gain perspective and renew our energy for the road ahead. Believe in yourself and your ability to overcome obstacles. You are stronger than you realise, and every challenge you face is a chance to become a better, more resilient version of yourself. So take a deep breath, trust the journey, and keep moving forward with confidence and grace.

Appetite: Loss of

Affirmations:

- I'm taking the time to rethink, refresh, and renew my body with rest and self-care before eating.
- I am ready to step back into life, eating that which is truly beneficial to my body and soul.
- I easily overcome obstacles.
- I am stronger than I realise.
- Every challenge is an opportunity to become better and more resilient.
- I breathe in confidence and trust.

Supporting Foods:

- Warm chicken broth soup
- Corn
- Strawberries
- Whitefish
- Applesauce
- Berries
- Grapefruit
- Orange
- Tomato
- Apple
- Alfalfa sprouts

Arm Problems

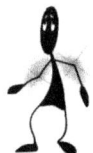

Troubled Mindset

- You are trying to carry the burden and do the work.
- You are strong, but sometimes that is deceptive because you are relying on yourself and have a fear of letting others be a part of the daily tasks of life.
- You find it challenging to connect to your heart/feelings, let alone articulate them.
- It's difficult to determine and express what is important to you.
- Fear of change is causing you to hold back or resist.

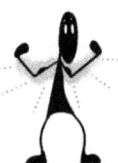

Healing Mindset

Follow your dream, but include others. Learn to be strong together. You can be open and let your fear of being overwhelmed serve as the catalyst for changing your life and doing your daily tasks with wisdom, insight, and mutual cooperation with others and your inner self.

Learning to be strong together means acknowledging that we all have unique skills and perspectives that can help us achieve our goals. As you do, you will enjoy new and exciting opportunities.

Arm Problems

Affirmations:
- I embrace life and others with a sharing attitude.
- I open my heart feelings instead of fearing them.
- I am capable.
- I am strong.
- I can do this.
- I trust others to be involved.
- I have the courage to be honest with my real capacity.
- I see the future, it is bright, and I enjoy doing the tasks to get me to where I want to go and be.

Supporting Foods:
- Dark green leafy vegetables
- Okra
- Broccoli
- Cauliflower
- Wheat/barley juice
- Soaked chia seeds
- Soaked almonds
- Celery stalks
- Grass-fed beef
- Romaine lettuce
- Endive
- Parsley
- Cilantro
- Kelp
- Fresh pineapple

Arm: Left

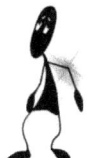

Troubled Mindset

- You have a sense of powerlessness in your life.
- You do not feel like you are in control of your own life and are not content with it.
- You may feel like your efforts to express what's really in your heart are insufficient because nothing's working or changing.
- The struggle may have more to do with spiritual matters or females in your life.
- You resist vulnerability as you fear it will be used against you.
- See arm problems.

Healing Mindset

Observe what you are doing in your life that is affecting you spiritually. Consider changing your actions to match the core truths you feel inside. Perhaps you need to resolve inner discord towards a mother, sister, or female teacher, friend, or coworker. Consider combining your strengths with theirs, rather than battling. Seek cooperation. You may need to have a higher spiritual understanding to accomplish this well. Be creative and open to the possibilities.

Arm: Left

Affirmations:
- I use my inner personal strength to become stronger every day.
- I let the need to force life be replaced with becoming balanced and grounded, and then using my strength to carry on.
- My heart has what it takes to be a positive force for good and action.
- I trust in positive change as I practice expressing my heart as clearly as I can.
- I feel more and more confident as I courageously express my needs and desires.

Supporting Foods:
- Green leafy vegetables
- Okra
- Broccoli
- Cauliflower
- Wheat/barley juice
- Soaked chia seeds
- Soaked almonds
- Celery stalks
- Grass-fed beef
- Romaine lettuce
- Endive
- Parsley
- Cilantro
- Kelp
- Fresh pineapple

Arm: Right

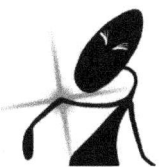

Troubled Mindset

- You may be experiencing difficulties with being assertive and confident; this may come across as controlling, or you may feel controlled.
- Your fear of underperforming or being wrong is holding you down.
- You may fear that you are not enough.
- You are unsure of how to get your needs met.
- The struggle may have more to do with physical matters and males in your life.
- See arm problems.

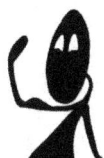

Healing Mindset

Your right arm is related to having compassion for others and true personal success. Release the aggression and open your heart to help balance your actions. Observe what you are doing in your life that is affecting you physically. Consider changing your actions to match the core truths inside of you. Perhaps you need to resolve inner discord towards a father, brother, or male teacher, friend, or coworker. Consider combining your strengths with theirs, rather than battling. Be cooperative. Be creative and open to the possibilities.

Arm: Right

Affirmations:
- I am aware of connecting to my whole body and using core strength to accomplish the tasks of life.
- My core is deeper than proving myself to others.
- I am capable and strong because of who I am, not whom I am proving.
- I am grateful for the use of my arms.
- I can do so much good and accomplish so many tasks.
- I coordinate my efforts with my mind/heart/body so that my intentions are not forced but completed with fun, discovery, and positive drive.
- I easily release discord and replace it with cooperation.
- I trust the answer is just around the corner.
- I act in alignment with my values.

Supporting Foods:

- Green leafy vegetables
- Okra
- Broccoli
- Cauliflower
- Wheat/barley juice
- Soaked chia seeds
- Soaked almonds
- Celery stalks
- Grass-fed beef
- Romaine lettuce
- Endive
- Parsley
- Cilantro
- Kelp
- Fresh pineapple

Arteries

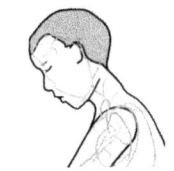

Troubled Mindset

- You have been driven to perfectionism rather than flowing with and honoring your true feelings.
- You are trying to squeeze things out of life.
- You want to feed all your interests, but there is not enough energy or capacity.
- You eat too much junk or think too much junk.
- Your distrust toward others collides with your notion of love and creates a disconnect with your heart.
- You push yourself too hard to compensate.
- You may have a tendency towards seriousness rather than being light-hearted and enjoying life.
- You may be trying to feel everything and have stopped honoring yourself, your limits and boundaries.

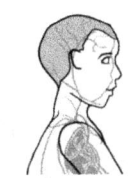

Healing Mindset

It's time to focus on your creativity, lighten up, and be open with others to free these avenues to your heart. You don't need to have all the answers to life's troubles to relax and smile. Try on the experience of trusting your interactions with others so you can be receptive to love and focus on the positive aspects of your life. It is great to feel alive; thus, sense that zest in every cell of your body.

Arteries

Affirmations:
- I am open to love and focus on the positive in life.
- I express my joy in living every day.
- I love being fed by life, and I offer my passion for living back to myself and others.
- I love being creative.
- I enjoy focusing on the positive nature of life.
- I am open to sharing.
- I smile and feel the sunlight and love of the universe.
- I easily release junk thoughts and replace them with wonder and awe.
- I wonder what my next thought will be.

Supporting Foods:
- Apples
- Black beans
- Broccoli
- Brown rice
- Butter (organic)
- Cabbage
- Cauliflower
- Corn
- Garbanzo beans
- Fenugreek
- Fenugreek sprouts
- Kale
- Lentils
- Oats
- Red legumes
- Romaine lettuce
- Shiitake mushroom
- Wheat (if not gluten sensitive)

Arthritis

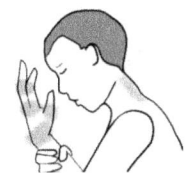

Troubled Mindset

- You wish things and/or people were different.
- You may often come across as nice on the surface, but inwardly you are being critical.
- You may feel like a victim to people and events, which has led you to tighten up with tension, resentment, anger, and/or bitterness deep inside.
- You have been holding on to these unhealthy emotions for an extended period.
- Your negativity is calcifying in your mind and body.
- Sadness has now set in because you can't manipulate change in others.
- Your immune system is struggling to do what you want due to your conflicting emotions.

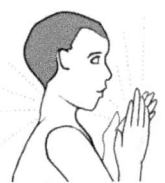

Healing Mindset

It is necessary to take time for yourself. Give yourself permission to breathe, release, and find emotional peace in the storms of your life. Learn from life and embrace an attitude of change, rather than insisting that life learns from you. Let go of the judgments and resentments and allow your true, joyful self to emerge. You may consider a meditative approach with breathwork.

Arthritis

Affirmations:

- I am free to feel.
- I am free to move and express myself.
- I let go of all emotional judgments and resentments.
- I learn from life.
- All things work for my good.
- I am reflective without judgment.
- I am clear, hopeful, not wishful.
- I enjoy a path of simple giving and let go of complicated emotional thinking.
- I receive the healing of nature and open the channels within to receive support from the unseen, such as those who unconditionally care about me; thus, I offer love to my body and soul.
- I appreciate all that my body and soul are and do for me.

Supporting Foods:

- Alfalfa
- Cabbage
- Celery
- Flaxseed soaked
- Oats & oat brain
- Rice Bran
- Green leafy vegetables
- Fresh pineapple
- Brown rice
- Wheat
- Rye
- Asparagus
- Farm fresh eggs
- Garlic
- Onions
- Oatmeal
- Fish
- Amaranth
- Salmon
- Ginger
- Parsley

Asthma

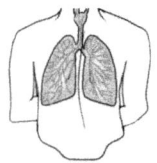

Troubled Mindset

- It feels as if you are being held hostage from within.
- Your automatic reflex of holding your breath is based on a deep fear of losing someone, being abandoned, or being smothered.
- In addition, eventually there is an obvious fear that there won't be enough air, love, space, time, and connection.
- In your fear of abandonment or smothering, you think that you have only one option, that is to hold on tight.
- You are in a closed loop of panic and concern.
- The thoughts of "what if" come storming in, but you already are having a storm inside, so there is no room left for more turmoil.
- The anxiety is overtaking your mind and is becoming your single focus.

Asthma

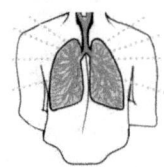

Healing Mindset

Try embracing the moment of fear and high stress with some simple mindfulness techniques. First, use some reverse psychology on yourself by embracing the fear, holding your breath for 3 seconds, and then letting go. Do it again and then let go. Watch the tightness and fear reduce as you flow with the fear and then release it. Your brain thinks that you are getting enough oxygen, when in reality you are not letting go of the excess carbon dioxide.

Holding on to the fear of being abandoned is keeping you isolated inside from others and from life. Embrace your fear by increasing it intentionally in order to show the brain that the fear is worse than reality. Letting go is scary if you are a small child that is subconsciously needing to be attached to something because some people are unpredictable, but the mind thinks that holding on to the breath is going to keep you aware and safe.

Asthma

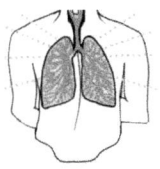

Healing Mindset
(continued)

Take this one step and one breath at a time. Breathe in a little and walk a little. Breathe in and out a little longer and walk a little farther. Doing an interval breath that allows you to breathe a few long breaths and two short breaths while walking a few long slow steps and then a couple of fast steps, helps reset the mind and the body.

Trust in your body is difficult if your body doesn't trust you and your mind. Taking the time to listen to your body and learning intuition helps establish good rapport.

Establishing a positive connection and respecting the body will help build the bridge between your emotions, feelings, body reactions, and your mind. Your best friend can be your very own body, if you decide to listen and respond with understanding to you and your body.

Asthma

Affirmations:
- I easily face and release my fears.
- I am open to flow with life.
- I open to the next part of my life.
- I embrace this moment, then release it, and embrace the next.
- God is always there for me.
- I am safe and secure. I am loved.
- I trust in my body and mind that we can get through this together.
- I embrace my fear as a traffic cop but not as my permanent boss.
- I listen to my body and calmly let the scattered thoughts fly away with the wind.
- I am learning to respect my real self and lessen my reaction to the fear self.
- I take one breath and one step at a time.

 ### Supporting Foods:

- Water/Get hydrated
- Apple
- Carrots
- Cauliflower
- Celery
- Chard
- Chickweed: for some
- Citrus
- Fenugreek seeds
- Fennel
- Fish
- Garlic
- Greens
- Kelp
- Onions
- Papaya
- Peach
- Pear
- Persimmon
- Pumpkin
- Radish
- Seaweed
- Tomato
- Turkey: for some
- Yam
- Possibly brown rice
- Cantaloupe: for some - if candida or fungus, do not use
- Use garlic & onion to sniff when there is lung congestion

Back Problems

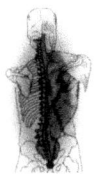

Troubled Mindset

- The back has to do with feeling supported or supporting yourself.
- You are torn because your thoughts and actions do not line up.
- You may be feeling guilt, resentment, or distaste towards your own actions.
- The spine is responsible for supporting you, but it compromised by the tug-a-war between honoring your true feelings and your ego. For example, you may be either dominating or over-dependent with others. This indecisiveness has led to undue stress and is taking its toll on your body.

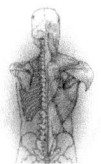

Healing Mindset

It's time to recenter. Drop 'the rope' or the fight with yourself. Find your footing with who you are from a higher perspective, the perspective of the true self. Realign your beliefs and actions to relieve your discomfort. Be fully present rather than divided in your support of this moment's actions.

Back Problems

Affirmations:
- I feel a deep inner support.
- I am clear of twisted worries and excess concerns.
- I turn worries into clarity, strength, courage, and love.
- I am ready to face the world but not take it on.
- I live within my capacity and encourage myself to go forward with vision and discovery.
- I am grateful for the challenge and step forward with self-support first.

Supporting Foods:
- Water/Get hydrated
- Papaya
- Pineapple
- Watermelon
- Red beets
- Radishes
- Apples
- Oranges
- Red bell pepper
- Yellow bell pepper
- Black beans
- Applesauce w/o sugar
- Poached farm fresh eggs
- Flax seed, soaked

Back: Lower

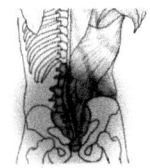

Troubled Mindset

- You feel your burden is too heavy, and your support is too little.
- You fear the past events, the audacious people, and your own capacity to move forward.
- You may feel unable to support yourself and hold insecurity about your financial stability.
- You worry about your burdens, yet you are reluctant to seek help from others.
- You live in survival mode, along with struggles to feel that you are of worth.
- There is a continual inner control to keep from running away or attacking others for the resentments you feel.

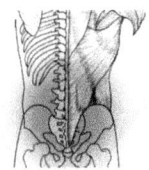

Healing Mindset

Dig deep within and find the possibility that your own courage develops because of your fears. Take a chance to embrace your learning, and to release your fears and blames. There is no better time than now to relax, move, stretch your mind and your body, and step forward with new intentions to experience each moment with simple faith, and discovery.

Back: Lower

Affirmations:

- I approve of myself and open my heart to the values of others.
- I take the fears of the past and let go of the need to hold onto everything and every feeling.
- I am free to move my thoughts, my feelings, and the energy of my body like a river through a forest of life.
- Each experience has value.
- Each experience released opens me to discover new adventures and learning every day.
- I fear no evil.
- I need no blame or shame.
- I believe in myself with courage, trust, understanding, and strength.

Supporting Foods:

- Purple or orange colored natural foods
- Eggplant
- Carrots
- Orange pepper
- Black beans
- Black sesame seeds
- Grass-fed beef
- Red beets
- Carrot juice
- Celery juice
- Watermelon

Back: Lower Area Pain

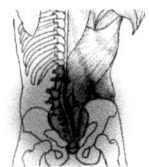

Troubled Mindset

- "Why can't I make it?" or "Why won't you help me?" kind of thinking. It's like you are playing tug-of-war between your true feelings that will support you and your negative thoughts and emotions that are not serving you.
- This includes the struggle with feeling safe and supported financially or within relationships.
- You've been living in "survival mode."
- You have focused on how you can't get things right instead of allowing your creativity to show you how you can.
- The limitation on success is in part due to not trusting in your self-worth and therefore feeling low personal value.
- You hang on to your negative emotions of guilt, frustration, sorrow, and being over-burdened/under-supported to reinforce this false negative belief about yourself.
- You may feel unable to support yourself and insecure about your financial stability.
- You are afraid that you won't make it, so you push harder.
- Your fear of finances or people is not real. They may push, but you don't have to pull them to you.
- You are living too much in survival and self-blame.

Back: Lower Area Pain

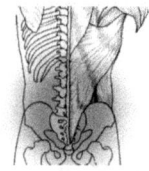

Healing Mindset

Support can be found in unexpected ways, including true support that arises from within you through healing. As you honor the need to support yourself with value and honesty, you can open creatively to resources or opportunities that you have not yet considered or embraced, including divine support.

Embrace a sense of adventure as you take on everyday life challenges. You need to move past your fears that increase when you revert to being afraid of taking the risk of being real with the inner monster. The monster inside wants to push you to stand up for yourself, to be more responsible with money, work, and relationships. But you are afraid of your own messenger. So take a deep breath and calmly work through your inner fear of yourself. Then, you will find it easier to deal with the external enemies.

Back: Lower Area Pain

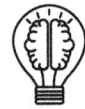

Affirmations:

- I see and feel my personal value.
- I observe the amazing value in others.
- I choose to create mutually honoring relationships.
- I have courage when confronted by those with agendas.
- I let any guilt be a reminder that I am not responsible for the judgments they put on others.
- I am responsible for my own feelings and thoughts.
- I enjoy realizing that I am in control of my own life and thoughts.
- "I release the past and make room for beneficial change."
- I am unwinding my old feelings and renewing my abundant life.

Supporting Foods:

- Drink lots of water
- Millet
- Barley
- Black beans
- Black soybean
- Water chestnut
- Mung beans and sprouts
- String beans
- Legumes
- Melons
- Blackberry
- Mulberry
- Wheat germ
- Potato
- Tofu
- Seaweeds
- Sardines
- Crab
- Clam
- Eggs
- Cheese

Back: Middle

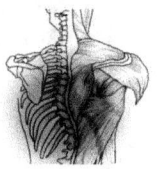

Troubled Mindset

- You keep your heart guarded because of the pain of the past and the fear of the future.
- Feelings of betrayal and now higher sensitivity keeps you on guard.
- You have added resentment, guilt, worry, and fear as conflicting emotions that tie up the muscles of your middle back.
- You fear that if you let go and open up your tender heart, you will be stabbed in the back.
- There is a high sensitivity to the judgments and criticisms of others.
- Part of the sensitivity is because of a lack of self-confidence. You fear taking life in fully, living wholly, and embracing all experiences. Your shallow breathing is another manifestation of this fear.

Back: Middle

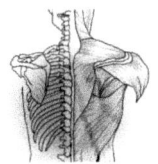

Healing Mindset

Become aware of your highly sensitive nature. You are burning sugar just by worrying too much about life and the possible outcomes.

Enjoy moments of peace and quiet. You need it. Let your mind practice coming back to the "now" moments. That doesn't include the "would have," "could have," and "should have." Those don't exist. They are figments of scattered thoughts that are causing you to run from what actually matters; connection, love, warmth, trust, courage, and experiencing life fully.

Back: Middle

Affirmations:
- I love myself when I feel scared, lonely, betrayed, or worried.
- I am doing the best that I can with what I have.
- I am not going to solve the world's problems by waiting for others to change, or by trying to please them into changing.
- I let worry fly away like a butterfly and deeply breathe in the sunshine of the day.
- I can breathe freely, without any price or cost.
- I can think freely, without worry or concern about another's response.
- I can feel freely, without regretting what could or should happen.
- I let go of sorrow and open to simple joy, simple thought, and simple connection between me, myself, and I.
- I gradually open to those who love and care for me.
- I am good, and I am love.

Supporting Foods:
- Purple or orange colored natural foods
- Eggplant
- Carrots
- Orange pepper
- Black beans
- Black sesame seeds
- Grass-fed beef
- Red beets
- Carrot juice
- Celery juice
- Watermelon

Back: Upper

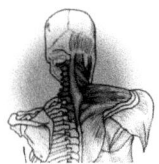

Troubled Mindset

- The overbearing stresses of life are weighing down on you.
- The frustrations that lead you to tighten your shoulders and upper back are running your life.
- You are doing your best, but your body is responding to the belief that it's not enough and the belief that you should carry some burden.
- You're blocking the pathway to give or receive love; it feels too vulnerable.
- You feel there is a lot to do, but you believe you deserve nothing in return.
- Letting go is difficult because you don't believe that it will help.
- Of course, letting go of the burden won't change the outcome of another person or any emotional weather outside of your control.

Back: Upper

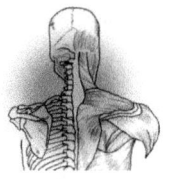

Healing Mindset

Letting go of the burden will allow you to be present and aware. Then your body can relax and get the fuel and nutrition necessary to think and sense your surroundings clearly. Worry and burden inhibit your awareness and your ability to deal with life situations. Faith, courage, hope, and calm thinking allow you to open your body and your mind to be clear and ready to deal with situations. Your heart will work less and more efficiently to provide the blood and nutrients to the body, and the emotions of courage and love to yourself and then to others.

Be open to life as an experience and then take action. Your response to life determines your experience, not the other way around. Breathe and trust through the weight of responsibility and share appropriately, your value isn't based on the load you carry. In truth, the burden is your belief, not reality. Your positive experience is the adventure you can take.

Back: Upper

Affirmations:

- I feel alive and ready to experience life in all its wonders.
- Every day of ups and downs makes the adventure that more amazing.
- I let the "shoulds" turn into interesting designs like the grain of wood.
- The negative worries are showing patterns that I can learn from and then release.
- I am free of the need to worry and carry burdens. I am responsible or able to respond with clarity, focus, excitement, and joy.
- I enjoy the challenge and let go of anything that takes me into the shadows of life's forest paths.
- My path is to be, do, and observe life.

Supporting Foods:

- Purple or orange colored natural foods
- Eggplant
- Carrots
- Orange pepper
- Black beans
- Black sesame seeds
- Grass-fed beef
- Red beets
- Carrot juice
- Celery juice
- Watermelon

Bad Breath / Halitosis

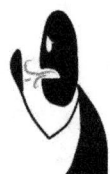

Troubled Mindset

- You tend to worry about things too much, especially the relationships in your life.
- You let these worries build up and turn your mood sour.
- You feel like you don't belong in some areas and therefore repel others.
- It is like your body is partially asleep, and when challenged, it suppresses the emotions and the toxins and performs 'in part.'
- You may be clueless about the bad taste in your mouth and how life is turning out, so there is a warning to others that you are not to be trusted. But the trust is not about honesty; it is about the two sides of life that you are living.
- You are pleasing others and storing frustrations about life, but not realizing that your mind has two agendas, and your heart has another two agendas. The liver is just trying to keep up with all the suppressed conflicts and intentions.

Bad Breath / Halitosis

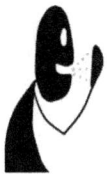

Healing Mindset

If something doesn't feel right in your life, take a look inside yourself. Acknowledge that you can't control others or magically alter your situation with a wish or an outburst.

Pause and give your mind and body a stretch several times a day. Guide your thoughts and actions towards what you can change and let go of what you can't. Be kind to yourself, recognizing your value, especially when life gets tough. Embrace the lessons from your experiences instead of resisting them.

Bad Breath / Halitosis

Affirmations:

- I challenge myself to admit to what is real and what I can do and be each and every day.
- I engage my whole self throughout each day.
- I let my fears of what could happen change into courage to face each day with the thought that life is an opportunity to grow, learn, and become renewed and fresh in body, mind, and soul.
- I engage my inner resources to learn how to assimilate my experiences for my good.
- I learn from the reflections of others.
- I now take time for myself to recharge my inner self and body.

Supporting Foods:

- Ginger
- Green foods
- Micro-greens
- Alfalfa sprouts
- Parsley
- Lemon and lime
- Millet
- Watercress
- Cilantro
- Beets

Bed-Wetting
(Nocturnal Enuresis)

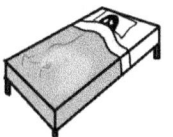

Troubled Mindset

- You've held fear towards authority and desire compassionate attention.
- You've accepted a belief of low self-worth.
- You are anxious about the unpredictable future; "Will I be punished?" or "Will something bad happen?"
- You can't seem to sort out what you want and how to get it.
- You can't control the outcomes or your insecurity about them.
- Check with how you relate to your father or father figure.

Bed-Wetting
(Nocturnal Enuresis)

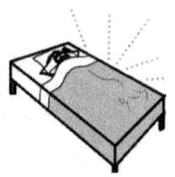

Healing Mindset

Take the moments before bed to be real with the day. Breathe, write, draw, scribble and let go of fears, frustrations, and burdens.

If it is a child, then connect to the earth and be real with life as it showed up that day. Be honest with your own inabilities, fears, and embarrassments. Embarrassments are feelings that are trying to protect your innocence and tenderness. Checking out at night, and running from your body while you sleep, creates a problem that not even your bladder can keep up with.

Visualize the brain waves of your mind and bring them into sync. Take time to practice deep meditation where you barely move or tighten individual muscles, one at a time, throughout your body. Your fears are signs to learn to practice courage in the day and experience peace at night.

Bed-Wetting
(Nocturnal Enuresis)

Affirmations:

- I flow with the adventures in life.
- I look deep inside to find direction.
- I choose compassion and strength.
- I honor myself and my infinite worth.
- I connect to all the brain wave patterns of my mind. Each one is important.
- I'm safe to be intelligent and innocent.
- The night is my renewal, and my body is aware of changes.
- I let my muscles move in the night, and I allow the messages to be conveyed so that I recycle my body fluids with little effort.
- I am mentally integrated with my surroundings, and the fears around me are sent to the earth to be calmed.
- Life is happening softly and gently.
- The sweet things of life are found in my experience.
- I turn the need for excitement into balanced adventures.

 ### Supporting Foods:

- Oats
- Watercress
- Soaked chia seeds
- Soaked almonds
- Soaked flax seeds
- Walnuts
- Micro-greens
- Dark green vegetables
- Sprouts

Biting Fingernails

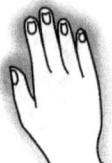

Troubled Mindset

- You are uncomfortable with life from the beginning of the day to the end.
- Your discomfort is being laid at the tips of your fingernails because each finger has energy that relates to different parts of oneself.
- That includes emotional, biochemical, physical, and more.
- Thus, your mind is trying to bite off more than it can chew and you are worried about all the upset and overwhelm.
- You feel that you don't have much choice but to go forward with excess concern and worry.

Biting Fingernails

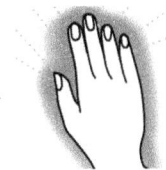

Healing Mindset

Be open to the possibility that life is never really settled completely. There will always be something out of place, not resolved, and in conflict. The goal of living is not to have complete peace and no conflict. The goal of life is to firmly and boldly deal with daily issues with hope, trust, courage, and a sense of confidence that life will work itself out.

You are often worried about outcomes. Change to enjoying the moment that you are living right now. Breathe new air that has little worry and more adventure.

Inhale as if it were spring today.
Exhale as if it were autumn.

Take the details of your worry, write them down, and walk away from them for one hour with calm and relaxing thoughts. After an hour, ask yourself - "Did I survive?" If you did, do it again, and again, until the details don't spin you into an internal worry cycle.

Live long and prosper your happy thoughts.

Biting Fingernails

Affirmations:

- I am calm, cool, collected.
- I enjoy this awesome moment of life.
- I pray with gratitude for life and all of its experiences.
- I pause and notice what a wonderful life.
- I feel amazing.
- I am clearly curious and curiously clear.
- I thank the good Lord for all the blessings of what has happened, what is happening, and what will happen.
- I learn from my experiments in living life.

Supporting Foods:

- Broccoli
- Carrots
- Celery
- Cabbage
- Kimchi
- Sauerkraut
- Red beets
- Lightly steamed vegetables
- Stir-fried vegetables
- Fish
- Salmon
- Organic beef

Bladder Problems

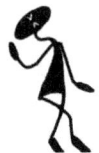

Troubled Mindset

- You feel powerless yet angry.
- Your cries for help are unheard, even by yourself.
- You're left "pissed" or out of control inside.
- You are trying to control the external environment to compensate for feeling out of control.
- Your upsets and frustrations are deeply rooted to the extent that you may have forgotten that emotional chaos doesn't resolve; instead, it dissolves your personal integrity and encroaches upon your personal space.
- You yearn to escape.
- Getting up again and trying to move through life with less pain and upset requires a force that is beyond forced will power.

Bladder Problems

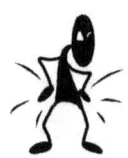

Healing Mindset

Take the time to step through every part of your life.

- Find the areas of life where you are a victim and turn those areas into discovery.
- Find the parts that you have become angry and upset with and turn that area into leading your heart and mind to new clarity and function.
- Find the parts of yourself where the sadness makes you wish too much and try to manage others so that you can be okay.

You don't have to be a victim. You have control of your mind. You can do this. Stop, back up, let the blame and shame go. You are a wonderful soul, just step into your power gradually with less wishes, fears, and upsets.

Bladder Problems

Affirmations:

- I am free.
- I am safe to let go of the past.
- I am in control of my body and life.
- I release my resentments.
- I am self-responsible.
- I make conscious choices for my life.
- I forgive.
- Be me today.
- I don't listen to clutter. I listen to clarity.
- I let the afflicted parts of me be healed by love, divine power, and justice.
- The grace of life is my friend.
- I let it heal my heart, my lung, my spleen, my pancreas, my kidney, my colon, and my liver.
- I am sure that I can clear the toxins and change my life into a simple functioning organ of living, loving, and experiencing.
- Let the pain change my heart.
- My philosophy of life is simple: Touch the moment, Feel the oneness, Smell the roses, Taste the joy, Hear the song, See the clarity and light.

Supporting Foods:

- Greens
- Beetroot
- Celery
- Cranberries
- Cucumber
- Parsley
- Pomegranate
- Watermelon

Bleeding Gums

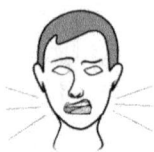

Troubled Mindset

- You have let yourself get into too many situations that are gradually bleeding you. They are pulling your attention, draining your energy, and causing you to have silent suffering.
- It feels unfair that you can't just 'fix' it or get it 'right.'
- You push forward, but it feels joyless as you subtly drain away your life force.
- Your body is begging you to take care of yourself, but you have been refusing to listen honestly. Why? Because you have so many other thoughts, responsibilities, quests, goals, and fears of stopping.
- You have been unwilling to challenge your course in life.

Bleeding Gums

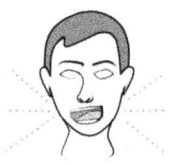

Healing Mindset

Take time right now and consider that which you have been avoiding. You may hurt yourself or hurt the feelings of someone else. You may have to let go of some crazy addiction to your ideas and goals. But if you don't reanalyze your actions, your goals, and your intentions, you will be slowly bleeding yourself to nothing.

Take the moment to do the little things to take care of yourself; this is more important than the major goal. Your major goals have become like shadows covering what is wearing you down to the point of subtly bleeding you of your life force. It is time to stop, pause, and look at yourself and all that you want to do. Look at what is possible and all that you resist. Listen and act on what is truth, and not the personal denials.

Bleeding Gums

Affirmations:

- I choose time every day to look at the real me.
- I find and center my life on me - the core self me.
- I choose to transform the need to please into being okay with being myself when I stand up with courage.
- I communicate clearly and beneficially to my cause and my health.
- I care, and I share that which honors my body and soul.
- I easily detect my self-deception and quickly adjust my awareness, communication, and actions.

Supporting Foods:

- Bell peppers
- Oranges
- Lemons
- Grapefruit
- Spinach
- Spicy peppers
- Green leafy vegetables
- Black beans
- Whole grains
- Sprouted almonds
- Garbanzo beans
- Pumpkin seeds
- Salmon
- Jicama
- Lentils
- Millet
- Tofu

Blisters

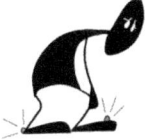

Troubled Mindset

- Anger and upsets caused by perceived insults and betrayals of others are causing you inner turmoil and resentment.
- You retaliate by assuming a defensive posture founded on the justification that they harmed you first (e.g. "You did this, so I'll show you."). In reality, you are subconsciously seeking to protect yourself and your emotions so you don't feel vulnerable.
- Blame is not a game that you win; everyone loses.

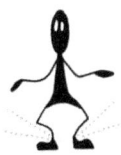

Healing Mindset

Let it go. You are hurting yourself and not letting life work itself out. Be true to your mature self and let it be. Learn that irritations are only indicators of self-suffering and things that you are going through with deep pain. Now you can change it into self-love for what you can be and do. Instead of burning everything away, value the many parts of your life and yourself. Slow down when cleansing your frustrations. One step at a time, clear out the negative emotions.

Blisters

Affirmations:
- I recognize when I persist in my resistance.
- I am first generous with myself, and then I use my willpower to go forward.
- As I root into my core values, my will is indeed my friend.
- My agitation is only a sign that I want support.
- I readily accept the support of those who care and are willing to be there for me.
- I give my heart time, my mind peace, and my body energy.

Supporting Foods:

- Berries
- Citrus fruits
- Broccoli
- Spinach
- Bell peppers
- Onions
- Tomatoes
- Apricots
- Asparagus
- Carrots
- Fish liver oils
- Brown rice
- Eggs
- Liver
- Milk
- Oatmeal
- Organic soybeans
- Sweet potatoes
- Wheat germ
- Whole wheat
- Eat a well-balanced diet including foods high in Vit. C, Vit. A, and Vit. E.

Bloated
(Body Wide Water Retention)

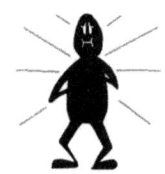

Troubled Mindset

- The messages of life, the messages from your mind, and your relationships are in conflict and confusion.
- Your body is trying to protect you from all forms of attack, including your personal negative thinking.
- You are ultra-sensitive internally, so you try to keep going by coping with foods, words, or actions. But the inflammation continues because your internal mode of defense is too hurt inside.
- You pretend on the outside to protect yourself in all situations.

Bloated
(Body Wide Water Retention)

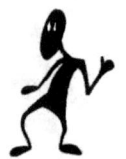

Healing Mindset

You need to trust, but what and who? So, before trusting, find the simplest things in life to connect with. Immerse yourself in nature, breathing, and eating simply. Be true to this, and then start to trust that there is purpose in relationships, purpose in challenges, and purpose in pausing life to reassess and release.

Life may not be exactly what you want; the other person may not be nice, but that is not the purpose of life. Reconsider what is most important. If it is outside of yourself, then you may experience the same underlying inflammation, suppressed resentments, depressing sadness, and false assumptions that have led to bloating. Release your misgivings and denials. Be at peace with the unpredictable winds of life, and watch the bloating reduce with ease.

You are sensitive to foods, sensitive to others, and you fear the possible and the impossible. It's time to consider real courage and real faith. Hope is not a wish; hope is having courage in what is, not what can't be. Hope is a value and virtue that is not watered down with pain and suffering. Pain and suffering help you to develop hope when you take life as a wonderful challenge to embrace so that you can develop your individual spiritual character.

Bloated
(Body Wide Water Retention)

Affirmations:
- I hope in my ability to face another day without fear or resentment.
- I have hope for things that are possible.
- I have hope in my joy in living the experience of life with courage, gratitude, and depth of insight.
- I can catch myself going into a personal defense of negative self-talk, blaming others, or fear of relationships with others or with food.
- Once aware, I choose to not make daily events so important.
- I choose life over self-defense.
- I choose life and joy over the need to harbor emotions of sadness, resentment, or pain.
- I am so grateful for life and all its amazing experiences.
- I heal the internal frequencies that fear too much.
- I choose faith, hope, and love.

Supporting Foods:
- Lettuce
- Celery
- Turnip
- Kohlrabi
- Rye
- Amaranth
- Adzuki beans
- Asparagus
- Alfalfa
- Pumpkin
- Papaya

Blood

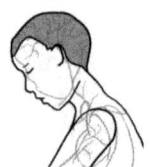

Troubled Mindset

- You want to live fully, but your body holds and harbors emotions of anger, fear, and sadness.
- You can't feed your fears and live fully.
- You are lacking an important and healthy level of self-love.
- The blood is moving quickly and ready to offer some nourishment, but if you are angry or resentful, you block your own self-nourishment.
- The body will build up substances that reflect your mental state.
- Your diet reflects your personal needs to suppress your feelings and problems.

Blood

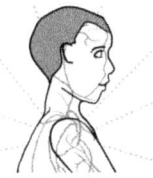

Healing Mindset

Gradually change your diet to reflect a life of nourishing your body, mind, and soul. You can only care for yourself as much as you truly love yourself. If you love harmful diet habits, that is what your body will reflect back to you. If you care little, except for living in denial and blame, your blood is a mirror of that in substance, form, and action.

Truly live by living what is supportive to all parts of you. The river of denial has too much sludge. The stream of emotional consciousness carries whatever you think and feel. Choose the day of living joy, happiness, and sharing what really cares for you and others. Turn anger into action, fear into love, and sadness into change.

Blood

Affirmations:

- I choose to care for myself with kindness and strength.
- I have little to gain with excess negative frustration.
- I choose this day to live in joy, happiness, gratitude and sharing my beautiful day with others that care.
- I turn anger into action, fear into love, and sadness into change.
- Thank you, God, for this day that I am fed with the nourishment of body, mind, heart, and soul.
- I open my cells to the fullness of self-nourishment and divine support.

Supporting foods:

- Chew your food slowly
- Apples
- Carrots
- Celery
- Cucumber
- Raspberry
- Tomato
- Watercress
- Lemon
- Lime
- Garlic
- Grapes
- Red beets
- Watermelon
- Black beans

Blood Clots

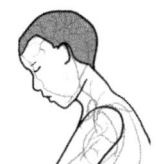

Troubled Mindset

- You are filled with a deep resentment that has developed into a suffering.
- You can't get your anger out because you don't know what the consequence will be.
- Instead, you harbor it in many different places and spaces in your body, memory, and life.
- You allow your unhealthy thoughts, food, and lifestyle to materialize in your blood because, over time, you felt helpless in dealing with the controlling nature of others.

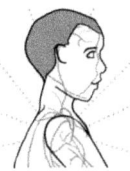

Healing Mindset

You can be free of the deep-seated hatred, resentment, and fear of actualizing peace. Your fear of peace was only your fear of lacking control of the situation. You were afraid that if you were happy, they would control you more.

It is time to gradually and progressively move through, part by part, and piece by piece, your long-held dark feelings about what has happened. Trust that your gradual healing can bring peace and joy. Step daily with confidence and hope and start dissolving the false beliefs, and move into faith, hope, and courage.

Blood Clots

Affirmations:
- I am grateful for how life shows up.
- I concern myself first with enjoying my relationships before trying to change them.
- I support myself with healthy thoughts and foods before taking care of others.
- I let the recycling of problems be dissolved, released, and let go to mother earth.
- I let the angels and nature be my buffer against the darkness of others.
- I know that they support me through my experiences.
- I am not hate, nor fear.
- I am filled with love, courage, safety, and a natural flowing of life force energy.

Supporting Foods:
- Chew your food slowly
- Apples
- Carrots
- Celery
- Garlic
- Grapes
- Red beets
- Watermelon
- Black beans
- Onions
- Lemon
- Lime
- Kelp

Blood Pressure: High

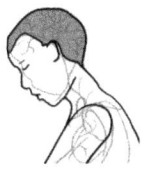

Troubled Mindset

- You feel angry with those who have control over your life or over the lives of the ones you care about.
- You wish it would be different, but there is nothing you can do about it.
- You may harden your heart towards them or yourself.
- You may think that by putting pressure on yourself, you can prevent something from happening. Unfortunately, this is impossible because you have little control over other people's lives.
- You are in a lie when you think that others make you angry and upset.
- You feel the pressure of the day, and your life, and you have no idea how to change it, but you apply the internal pressure anyway.
- You are angry and overwhelmed with your body, life, and relationships.
- Your need for them to change is preventing you from living and moving to your own beat and rhythm.

Blood Pressure: High

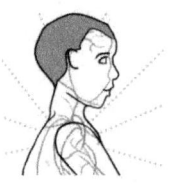

Healing Mindset

Learn to be real with what you can do. Learn to be real with what is actually going on. Study healthy boundaries and apply them in your life. Learn to recognize your anger as a signal to stop recycling negative thoughts about others. Stop those thoughts so you can stop pushing them to feelings of resentment.

Let your pressured thoughts be released with breathing, stretching, and simple actions that simplify your way of living. Your body is amazing, so live your life that way. Live like nature: moving the clutter, expressing your anger and pain, and refreshing your mind and heart with new possibilities of living. Stop forcing life, start encouraging yourself to live in an organic way.

Blood Pressure: High

Affirmations:

- Wow, life is amazing!
- I feel alive and refreshed every day.
- I am here now, and I will step into the future with curiosity and encouragement.
- Life is an experience, and I will live it while enjoying the daily challenges.
- I turn anger into opportunities to move through my frustrations.
- I am so glad that I can't change them because I can transition and transform my immature self into a responsible, intriguing, strong individual with goals, actions, and positive, exhilarating learnings.

Supporting Foods:

- Water/Get hydrated
- Sweet potatoes
- Green leafy vegetables
- Fresh juices of beet, carrot & celery
- Apples
- Asparagus
- Onion
- Garlic
- Bananas
- Cabbage
- Oat bran
- Citrus fruits
- Lemon
- Parsley
- Spinach
- Quinoa
- Watermelon
- Brown rice
- Buckwheat
- Millet
- Soaked flaxseed
- Dragonfruit
- Tofu
- Figs
- Salmon
- Walnuts

Blood Pressure: Low

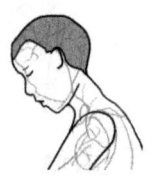

Troubled Mindset

- You've lost hope in your ability to control a situation or person in your life.
- Your feelings of helplessness are leading you down a path of defeatism.
- The pressure of life became too much to deal with, so your body flipped.
- It is keeping the pressure low physically to prevent you from overdoing it.
- Your burden and worry is just too much to imagine materializing.
- You have ignored your own needs, and, at some level, believe that 'there is no purpose or meaning anyway.'
- You commit and recommit to the needs of another while feigning that your needs don't matter, but you can't stop the resentment from rising against your injustice towards yourself.

Blood Pressure: Low

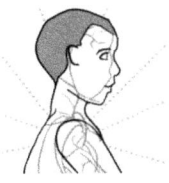

Healing Mindset

Losing hope about your situation is not the end but the beginning of surrender to a higher source and a more divine way of living. You have thought you were being connected to the true source, but you have actually been connecting to God through your worries and fears.

Find ways to connect to the divine independent of your worries and fears. Then, when you feel calmer, ask the divine for assistance. Love yourself enough that you will trust God to support you. Breathe in the strength that is all around you instead of thinking you are the only one who can do it.

Blood Pressure: Low

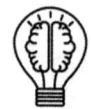

Affirmations:

- I enjoy the simple things, the interesting thoughts, the tender feelings, the peaceful inspirations, the intriguing insights, and the interactions of others.
- I trust God first and then seek answers.
- I don't have to carry all the burdens; in fact, I let the divine carry my worries and concerns, and I breathe and live with hope and strength, knowing that life has many purposes.
- Most of all, I let my body do its job.
- I can start letting go of one worry a day until each day
- I live in gratitude, courage, curiosity, and sincere expressions of love.
- I now refocus on what I can do, and I hope in what is possible.

Supporting Foods:

- Water/Get Hydrated
- Oat bran
- Apples
- Asparagus
- Bananas
- Cabbage
- Onion
- Garlic
- Green leafy vegetables
- Sweet potatoes
- Fresh juices of beet, carrot & celery
- Citrus fruits
- Lemon
- Parsley
- Spinach
- Quinoa
- Watermelon
- Brown rice
- Buckwheat
- Millet
- Soaked flaxseed
- Dragonfruit
- Tofu
- Figs
- Salmon
- Walnuts

Body Odor

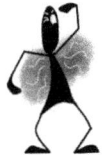

Troubled Mindset

- You're not honoring how you actually feel about what you are doing.
- There is fear of being embarrassed, of shock, fear of rejection, and/or fear of overwhelm.
- You are concerned about others' thoughts, but you are your own biggest critic.
- You are suppressing frustration about having too much at stake.
- You just want to enjoy the experience, but can't because of all the factors involved.
- So, because of the inner conflict, you have some deep-seated self-criticism and need to control the outcome, which is not working anyway.

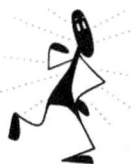

Healing Mindset

Practice recognizing what is really happening. Recognize your abilities and that life is to experience the progression, not the perfection. Laugh with yourself, and start acclimating your mind and body to being calm with people and situations. Note your talents, capacities, and honest interests. Catch your self-criticism and turn it into positive self-motivation.

Body Odor

Affirmations:
- I recognize my uneasiness about what is happening and turn it into enjoyment.
- I like the daily and life challenges.
- I enjoy the opportunity to be me.
- I observe my body calming and relaxing.
- Life is a breeze.
- I realize judgments to me and from me are just reminders to be true to the core me (self).
- I forgive and release, so I live in clarity.
- I breathe in clean air and breathe out clutter.
- I am on a journey of continual and balanced growth.
- I embrace the journey.

Supporting Foods:

- Green foods
- Celery
- Red beets
- Okra

Boils, Cuts, Fevers, Sores, Inflammations

Troubled Mindset

- 'Why don't I get to be loved?!'
- You pay little attention to your body until you have a sore, cut, or other issue.
- You have too much worry and concern on your mind.
- You hate certain events and reactions of others.
- You're hurt and angry about what has happened, and you feel it's all 'their' fault.
- You spend too much time elsewhere in your thoughts of what should be, could be, or would be.
- Blame has a place, but not in your cyclic mind.

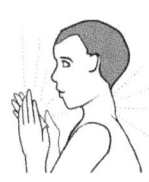

Healing Mindset

The answer is inside of you. Be aware of your body. Love your body. Appreciate your body for all that it gives to you. Complaining about your body or blaming others will not solve your problems. It will divert you from what is important. You have little to change in others because they don't change anyway. Even your body feels like a third person to you. Be respectful to your body and take care of your precious commodity that has a life to live instead of a mechanical life to give. Release any lingering feelings of discomfort or resentment that might be causing you distress through boils and cuts. Gently allow them to drift away without letting them harm your inner peace.

Boils, Cuts, Fevers, Sores, Inflammations

Affirmations:
- I love my body, my mind, and my heart.
- I realize the precious gift that this body is.
- I choose to take moments today to let go of the self-destructive denials, and harmful blaming of others.
- I want to be true to my needs.
- I am true to my need for self-reflection and self-care.
- My angry regrets that feed my negative mind are in the past.
- I replace them with thoughts of appreciation of all that I am learning and developing.
- I am aware of my body, where I am, what I am thinking, and how I am feeling.
- I am full of gratitude and feel love for all of God's creations, including the other person and myself.

Supporting Foods:

- Water/Get hydrated
- Kelp
- Garlic
- Citrus fruits
- Berries
- Carrots
- Chlorophyll
- Black beans
- Seaweeds
- Radishes
- Sprouts
- Buckwheat
- Mung bean

Bones

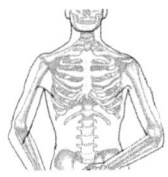

Troubled Mindset

- You have been on the breaking point for a while, but you have to keep managing to get by.
- You hold onto the feeling of resentment about being controlled, and you might even feel out of control.
- You tend to punish yourself or resist anything/anyone that you feel puts pressure on you.
- The pressure and reactive resistance inside you are contributing to your deteriorating, hardening, or weakening bones.
- Don't let this moment slip by with feelings of frustration that lead to accidents and broken bones. Is anything so seriously wrong that you are willing to break yourself over it?
- If your bones are deteriorating, you have been giving your support with little in return.
- Wishing life would be different isn't making you stronger.

Bones

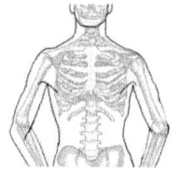

Healing Mindset

True strength and real immune protection do not come from pleasing nor fighting. They come with calm and neutral confidence. It is time to reflect and define your boundaries.

See this as your body's plea for positive change with flexibility. Look inward and discover your own inappropriately placed limits and rigidity. Define what it is you want to be and do before making decisions about how you are going to negotiate situations with others.

Regardless of your situation, your body and mind need more personal heart care. Be strong, by honoring and respecting your real needs and desires.

Refer to the body area for more information.

Bones

Affirmations:

- My bones are alive and well.
- They enjoy the nutrition of life and glory in the strength of character and strength of structure.
- My bones want to communicate strength, courage, and protection.
- My immunity starts with being true to my core intention of taking care of my inner self with strong structure, proactive immunity, and intriguing communication.
- I function freely when my structure is safe and strong.

Supporting Foods:

- Fermented foods
- Bone broth
- Kale
- Spinach
- Arugula
- Grapes
- Crab
- Pineapple
- Yogurt or kefir
- Raw milk
- Dark green leafy vegetables
- Fermented raw dairy products
- Sardines
- Flax seed
- Chia seed
- Pumpkin seeds
- Grass-fed beef
- Swiss chard
- Almonds
- Avocados
- Black beans
- Broccoli
- Clams
- Oysters
- Salmon
- Kelp
- Soybeans
- Wheat germ
- Hazelnuts
- Oats
- Molasses
- Garlic
- Onion
- Farm fresh eggs

Bowels

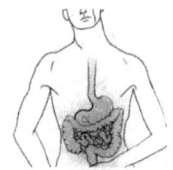

Troubled Mindset

- You may be holding your tongue when it comes to saying hard truths, or you may be holding on to experiences and beliefs from the past that do not serve you.
- You tighten up to control your internal environment because you don't feel you can control what's going on around you.
- You see your perspective as the only true perspective, and from that space, you are conflicted because if you speak out, it will cause discomfort for those around you.
- Ascending Colon: You may have often been charitable with others in their time of difficulty, but you aren't offering this to yourself. Instead of kindness towards yourself in hard circumstances or deep feelings, you've abandoned your sense of value. You have believed you are too flawed to get it right. Lovingly acknowledge your innate worth and nurture yourself during the dark times.
- Transverse Colon: You may be hiding from the world, including yourself. You've believed no one can understand or appreciate your true self when you try to share. When you are clear and honest with yourself, it will be natural to be open and understood by others.

Bowels

Troubled Mindset (continued)

- Descending Colon: You tense up and control your inner self to compensate for what feels out of control externally. You've been defending yourself with others without really seeking the truth. You feel extra sensitive to the possible 'blow' of a new perspective. Relax. Breathe and release any need for control. Trust in the highest and best for all so you can flow with life and others.

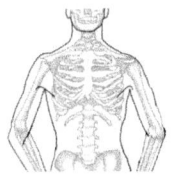

Healing Mindset

Adopting a 'live and let live" attitude will help as you deeply accept the agency of all. There may be more to the 'big picture' than what you have personally observed. There is a higher way to connect to others. It involves a deeper respect and honor for the vast perspectives and experiences of all. Release the need for control, return to trust, and let go of the past to make room for positive change.

See Colon Problems.

Bowels

Affirmations:
- I release the need to be right.
- I breathe in peace and breathe out the need for control.
- I offer love to myself, even in my dark and painful moments.
- I open myself to a higher way of relating to others.
- I deeply accept the agency of all, including those in my close relationships.
- I release the old and allow space and room for positive growth.
- I am clear and honest with myself.
- Sharing my authentic, honest self is natural and fun.
- I open up pathways for understanding and connection.

Supporting Foods:
- Water/Get hydrated
- Apples
- Asparagus
- Bananas
- Cayenne pepper
- Romaine lettuce
- Barley
- Beans
- Beets
- Cabbage
- Citrus fruits
- Green peppers
- Carrots
- Fish
- Kale
- Millet
- Okra
- Rice
- Watermelon
- Ginger
- Fibrous foods, if safe; otherwise, steam the fibrous vegetables
- Meats (moderate amounts and not fried)

Brain Problems

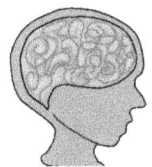

Troubled Mindset

- "Who am I anyway?" You've lost base with yourself due to conflicts between your objective and the divine purpose behind it.
- It has to do with a deep conflict around your relationship to authority.
- Processing information or experiences has been very confusing.
- Nothing seems to fit anymore.
- You may feel deserted by your divine support/authority or disillusioned by your experiences with authority figures in your life.
- Your lack of trust leads to high anxiety and proud resistance.
- Your negative thoughts fly chaotically.
- You may battle with yourself to keep from blurting this negativity out, or you may become disinterested and depressed.
- You've been in your head a lot.
- You may have thought you had all the answers.
- Those answers might have been technically accurate, but you've forgotten to keep your heart and soul a part of the big picture.

Brain Problems

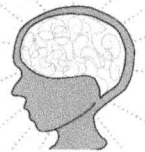

Healing Mindset

Engage with your heart. Connect to your soul. Tune into who you really are, and remember to do all things with a deep love and caring for all.

Use humility as you find a new, appropriate balance with your relationship to authority. As you settle into an appropriate understanding of your purpose and value in relation to the authority in your life, including divine authority, things will begin to fit together again.

Brain Problems

Affirmations:
- My mind is strong and capable.
- I appreciate the thoughts that I do have; for even thought is a gift of nature.
- I respect any confusion as a sign that I have too many masters demanding my attention.
- I will now bring back what is me and let go of what is not me.
- My real self is respectful to my core values.
- I am courageous enough to be true to my needs first, and then the needs of others.
- I enjoy challenging thoughts and let go of conflicting agendas inside.
- I release negative emotions.
- My brain will follow the mind, and my mind will follow my true intentions.
- My real intention is to enjoy life fully with clarity, hope, and joy.
- I reconnect the many parts of my mind and brain to function fully and completely for the good of all my body and soul.

Supporting Foods:
- Walnuts
- Chia seeds soaked
- Soaked almonds
- Micro-greens
- Salmon
- Fermented foods

Breast Problems

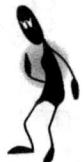

Troubled Mindset

- Part of you wants to nourish and experience love with those whom you love.
- Another part of you harbors resentment that they don't give or offer you more.
- In some cases, they are mean and attacking.
- Be careful; you may take your kindness and twist it into self-criticism and subtle hatred that will harm your breast physiology.
- Be wise to nurture no further than your capacity to do so, with real understanding and kindness.
- If you are fake in your giving because you feel obligated or do it anyway when you feel betrayed, then the consequence could be that the milk ducts for nursing will be sour, the fat cells will start to be infected, and/or the lymph nodes will become toxic.

Breast Problems

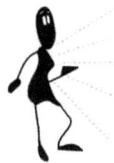

Healing Mindset

Enjoy nourishing with understanding and love as you feel is appropriate, and no more. Nourishment and love don't solve the world's problems; they just help people along.

What solves the world's problems is when an individual decides to be responsible and shares responsible love, not codependent love. Support at the level that the other person can responsibly receive and act on.

Breast Problems

Affirmations:

- I am freely able to nurture myself and the people around me.
- I love to nourish those who responsibly receive my offerings.
- I let the demands of others be interesting requests that go through my filter of awareness, curiosity, and intrigue.
- I nourish others from my balanced self.
- I feel blessed to offer my heart.
- I am blessed to see, hear, and understand the level of caring that is truly best for them and for me.
- It is good to be patient.
- Sharing is caring, and caring with what is appropriate to share is lovely and rewarding.

Supporting Foods:

- Alfalfa
- Avocados
- Fish
- Meats (not fried)
- Parsley
- Safflower
- Onion
- Garlic
- Brown rice
- Millet
- Oats
- Broccoli
- Brussel sprouts
- Orange bell pepper
- Chia seeds, sprouted
- Flax seeds, sprouted
- Papaya
- Pineapple
- Salmon
- Cauliflower
- Oranges
- Jicama
- Carrots

Bronchitis

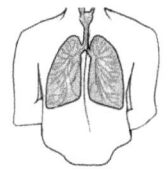

Troubled Mindset

- You feel irritated because you find it challenging to express your thoughts, and this irritation is aggravated by the person you hold responsible for this difficulty.
- You dislike feeling unable to take control and bring about change.
- You are hiding some truth from yourself and/or others.
- You've held back things you wanted to say, or you feel you said too much.
- You need safety and security in the idea that you will be okay if you express yourself.
- You may be targeting past resentments at yourself.
- Not being able to fix the problems, and feeling responsible somehow to fix them, leaves a depressing sadness and upsetting anger for things as they are.
- There is a coldness trapped in your lower body that makes you sluggish in moving forward.

Bronchitis

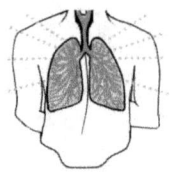

Healing Mindset

Your power is to change you. Be willing to be okay with making mistakes, being embarrassed, and being upset with others. Be okay with not being able to express everything you feel, because sometimes they can't hear or understand what you want to say. Be okay with finding your real need, your real peace, your real truth. And your real truth is never that the other person change, that is a false belief. The real truth is connecting to the inner self, inner insights, and core values.

Bronchitis

Affirmations:
- I release any and all resentments and upsets towards others and myself.
- I release the coldness within and find warmth in my true self and core values.
- I am an awesome being of love, warmth, and consideration.
- I no longer hold the sharp conflicts that keep me away from being me. What others may misunderstand is only a signal of what they can't embrace yet.
- I am ready and willing to release and enjoy, move and stretch, breathe and live.
- I move my self-doubt, my self-judgment, my self-pain, into quiet vibrations of experience.
- My time is living the frequency of expressing joy, sharing, lots of energy, and fun.
- I am warm and engaging with others and life.

Supporting Foods:
- Drink water
- Herbal teas
- Soups
- Garlic
- Onions
- Pure water
- Soup broths
- Acorn squash
- Banana squash
- Steamed zucchini
- Celery juice
- Watercress
- Apricot
- Anise
- Soaked flaxseed
- Soaked chia seed
- Pineapple
- Papaya
- Shiitake mushroom

Bruises

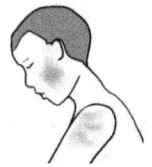

Troubled Mindset

- You've "beaten yourself up" because you disapprove of something you've done.
- With irritation or emotional aggression, you mentally/emotionally punish yourself.
- That self-punishment is physically manifesting.

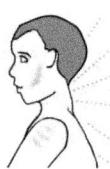

Healing Mindset

Use gentle kindness toward yourself through any blunder. Everyone makes mistakes. Learn from them, change your approach or perspective and forgive yourself. Look inward to discover the resolution to your conflict.

Check the body area for more details.

Bruises

Affirmations:
- My true strength is both in the boundary and my intention.
- I am strong because of who I really am and the firmness to be true to my core values and love.
- I love myself.
- I protect myself.
- I live in the adventure without needing to bruise and bump into everything that I am not.
- I am noticed for me as me.

Supporting Foods:
- Dark green leafy vegetables
- Buckwheat
- Pineapple
- Papaya
- Kale
- Garbanzo beans
- Lentils
- Millet
- Pumpkin seeds
- Tofu
- Collard greens
- Oats
- Almonds sprouted

Bulimia

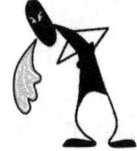

Troubled Mindset

- You have had difficulty facing the anger and judgment of your dad or parent.
- You fear the villain in others but mostly in yourself.
- You fear the lack of control of life and losing control of your body.
- Fear of being rejected is overwhelming your sense of reality.
- You are harboring feelings of self-contempt and believe you need to be punished.
- Hunger for growth and self-love are driving you to overeat.
- Your body rejects the food, knowing it's not what you need.

Bulimia

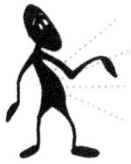

Healing Mindset

Take a moment and see the future. Do you fear the consequences you are offering your gut and body? Or do you fear the consequences of the present moment? Both are fears. Fear is not truth and joy. Transform your fears by seeing that your enemy started with fear and moved to anger. Remember, your enemy has more fear than you do; see them as a little child trying to be a bully.

That is also what is happening inside of you; you are being a bully to yourself. Don't fear to listen to your inner child. He/she needs tender care and tender love. The energy is reversed right now, and you are scared of feeling life and feeling real. You are afraid of feeling shame. Shame is not the problem, but a sign of a problem.

Take a deep breath every time you want to physically act out, then take a walk and breathe. Walk slow and fast to help your physical body progress through the fear with the movement of body, breath, mind, and soul. You are awesome, now step into that slowly and gradually every day.

Bulimia

Affirmations:
- I am free to go about life without the worry of body and mind.
- I am not afraid of the bullying or shaming of others.
- I am not afraid of their words and actions.
- I am strong and choose this day to serve my inner true self.
- I find and live my true core values.
- I look, find, and live real love, real sharing, real caring, real joy, and real life.
- I love my gut; I gradually and slowly coach it to handle the energy to move it gradually down to my feet and then on to the earth.
- When scared, I visualize a candle warming my toes and then my feet and then my legs and then my lower belly.
- I am part of the warmth of nature because nature loves me, and I love divine nature.
- I am free to be me.

Supporting Foods:
- Acorn squash
- Banana squash
- Watercress
- Ginger tea
- Grapefruit
- Celery
- Eggplant
- Jicama
- A little salt water
- Spaghetti squash
- Home-cooked soups
- Lightly steamed carrots
- Black beans & Brown rice
- Dark green leafy vegetables
- Home-cooked chicken soup
- Organic omega-3 egg & brown rice

Burn

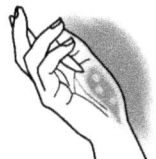

Troubled Mindset

- You are not paying attention to what is happening around you.
- You may be so engrossed in your agenda that you need to start paying attention.
- Your emotions are in excess: is there too much anger, too much resentment, too much complaining, too much sadness, too much overwhelm?
- If you don't manage your internal world, the external one will start abruptly waking you up.
- Life is not fair, it hurts, it is tough.
- Everything you touch or experience might be too much right now and you need to pause and listen to yourself.
- Is the magnitude of your suffering such an issue that you're willing to distance yourself from the joy of living to so easily be burned by life?
- You might consider waking up to smell some roses instead of always focusing on the thorns.

Burn

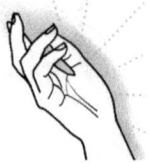

Healing Mindset

What will it take to change the beliefs, self-talk, and emotions that are burning you up inside? If you don't change your inner negative demands, they will crush and outweigh any positive reasons and efforts.

When you feel too sensitive to everyone and everything around you, create a positive, quiet space around you and in you. You need to give the body and the mind time to pull in deep resources for healing. If you ignore the essentials of taking care of your personal healing you will feel scared and carry an injurious feeling of resentment.

Many thoughts and negative emotions can harm your life and the lives around you. So, when you feel resentment, it is a sign and signal to stop and take care of yourself and your heart. Let the messages from within your body lead you to self-care.

Burn

Affirmations:

- I am ready to take a breath and be alive.
- I can deal with life reasonably and calmly.
- I pause to calm the drama and deal with life sensible.
- I am ready to change my thoughts and heal my heart.
- I honor and respect my body.
- It is not worth the pain to have to be right.
- In peace and gratitude, I accept what is.
- I am grateful that something stopped me in my tracks so that I can see what is going on.

Supporting Foods:

- Acorn squash
- Avocados
- Banana
- Celery
- Celery juice
- Cilantro
- Cucumber
- Jicama
- Kiwi
- Lentils with turmeric and cucumbers
- Melons
- Nutritional yeast (non-fortified)
- Pumpkin
- Quinoa
- Salmon
- Sprouts
- Squash soup
- Watermelon
- Yellow squash
- Zucchini

Burning Tears

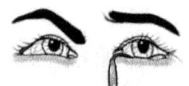

Troubled Mindset

- You hate what has happened, but the burning is being held deep in your heart.
- Each day you wish that it would be different, but you feel helpless.
- It feels like you can do nothing to change today's outcome, including your own hidden bitter feelings.
- You felt betrayed and injured.
- You have felt so sad; now your body is hurting too.
- The body is pushing to release the sharp objects that keep jabbing your thoughts and the back of your heart.

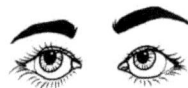

Healing Mindset

It takes courage to embrace losing someone, something, or a dream that is not replaceable. Life has many times and experiences when the path is interrupted in a way that makes a person choose. It is a choice whether to hold onto the past dream, or to allow that dream or that someone go. You could release them to the earth to be transformed into a new life experience that is full of the gifts of the past.

Pain is only a gift when it is buried with the intention of growing something new and different. Metamorphosis gives us the moth or the butterfly; it is your choice.

Burning Tears

Affirmations:
- The sun is never brighter than when it shines through a billowing cloud.
- I take this opportunity to find the color, the light, and the joy in finding the healing of my deepest of pains.
- God, whatever you give me today, I am willing and ready for the adventure.
- I am grateful for the experience of the bitter because I am able to discern real sweetness much better.
- Thank you to everyone that has been an instrument in my life growth and experience.

Supporting Foods:

- Beets
- Berries
- Cantaloupe
- Carrots
- Celery
- Corn
- Crenshaw melon
- Cucumbers
- Grapefruit
- Honeydew
- Lentils
- Lettuce
- Micro-greens
- Oranges
- Papaya
- Peaches
- Peas
- Pineapple
- Quinoa
- Sauerkraut
- Sprouts
- Water
- Watermelon
- Yam
- Zucchini

Burnout

Troubled Mindset

- "When you chance to hit a wall, do not let it stay. Quickly turn the pain away and get back your pace today." This is not good advice, but that is what most burnouts do. They go and go until they hit the wall one too many times, and then the body goes into compensation mode.
- Not allowing anymore overwhelming, 'pushing through life.' The adrenal glands do have a limit, even with all the artificial stimulants.
- When the body is being forced, it will eventually rebel so that you won't kill yourself. Also, burnout comes from avoiding conflicts and doing the difficult.
- In avoidance, it takes more energy to accomplish anything. Then in burnout, it is even that much more difficult.
- You are fighting your own uphill battle.
- You view life that you are carrying even burdens you, like you are going uphill in a snowstorm with the wind blowing in your face.
- If suffering were an art form it would look dark, heavy, hopeless, frustrating, and endless.

Burnout

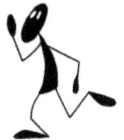

Healing Mindset

It is time to take out the trash and burn it properly. Your body is trying to get rid of all the emotional and mental burdens you justify carrying around. You only have two options: keep enslaving yourself to the current behavior of overwhelming yourself, or take a new view and a new heart.

The new view is to get behind and underneath the drive that you have to do what you do, to think what you think, and to feel what you feel. The driver is holding the key, and if you fight the driver, you will exhaust yourself and be left standing in the fumes.

The driver of burnout is afraid of something or someone or some possible outcome. The driver inside may be too perfectionistic, or too competitive, or too worried, or too confused. No matter what the problem is, stop and get a handle on your core needs and values, and compare them to what you are doing. If your core values don't match your thoughts and actions, then take the time to clean up your thoughts, emotions, and actions.

Simply, simply and oh yeah, simply. Come back home to yourself. Find some peaceful grace right in front of your face.

Burnout

Affirmations:
- I have passed the test, I am simply the best at being me.
- I love myself enough to take a walk, enjoy a laugh, and give a hug.
- I am looking for one smile an hour today.
- I turn my burnouts into physical warm-ups every morning.
- I laugh at danger and smile at strangers.
- I ask God for strength to do His will as I let go of mine.
- I feel the grace of truth fill my soul with peace, insight, and wisdom.
- I appreciate the simplicity of life.

Supporting Foods:

- Brewer's yeast
- Fermented foods
- Greens
- Sprouts
- Microgreens
- Fresh vegetables
- Fish
- Sprouted beans
- Fresh herbs
- Fresh fruit
- Small meals eaten slowly
- Soaked chia seeds
- Sprouted seeds

Buttocks Problems

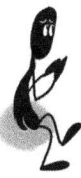

Troubled Mindset

- You're hanging on to old guilt.
- You haven't thought very highly of yourself, and you struggle to trust others.
- You're ticked about what has happened, and you feel like throwing it back at the world.
- You don't feel you know enough or have the power to stay safe, so you hang on to the negativity of the past to remember what not to do or who not to trust.
- You have a poor relationship with your sexuality or intimacy.

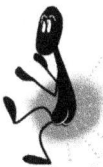

Healing Mindset

Life can be messy. The only way back is to learn and grow from our experiences. Keeping the pain or guilt is unnecessary. You can release the pain and remember the lessons, then open your heart once again with wisdom and renewed strength. As you do so, it will make it easier to gain confidence and forgive yourself and others.

Buttocks Problems

Affirmations:
- I have suffered enough.
- It is okay to let things change for my good.
- The past embarrassments are now humorous moments.
- I have taken life way too seriously.
- I enjoy the laughter and the humor with others and deeply with myself.
- In the quiet moments, I realize how blessed I am, and I let the old flush out.
- I move with ease, I sleep with calm, I breathe with peace, and I act with courage.

Supporting Foods:

- Pineapple
- Salmon
- Seaweed
- Spinach
- Yam
- Agar Agar
- Kohlarbi

- Asparagus
- Avocado
- Bell pepper
- Beets
- Broccoli
- Cauliflower
- Chili pepper

- Cucumber
- Dragonfruit
- Garlic
- Jicama
- Kelp
- Kiwi
- Onion
- Papaya

Cancer

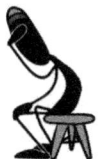

Troubled Mindset

- There are many intense and negative emotions flooding through your system.
- This could be from one big traumatic incident or years of unresolved inner conflict.
- The drama that turned into a trauma that overwhelmed your senses, thoughts, and feelings has taken over.
- It is a part of yourself gone wild and is not listening to your central core command center.
- The resentments that have risen, the hatreds that smolder, and the deep regrets that snake along inside, is causing you to hold onto to destructive thought patterns and negative emotions that are feeding the monster.
- Thinking that you are the cause of your problems is triggering beliefs that you are trapped in a world of hopelessness and hidden regrets.
- What heavy emotional burden is more important than your health?
- Anger or regret will not get you well.
- Determination and caring for yourself will help your immune system do its job.
- Check a specific area of the body for more information.

Cancer

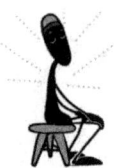

Healing Mindset

This obstacle is pushing you to stop, look, and listen. Intense moments of drama/trauma get embedded in the brain/mind and connects to responses in the body/mind. It can cause the cells of the body to have multiple messages leading to problems of disease and illness. While you seek medical advice and treatment, open your brain/mind and body/mind to the authentic inner healing of releasing all hatred, all blame, all regret, fear, and anger. Past burdens and struggles could be your ruin unless you let them make you strong. Be sure to make every moment count. Learn to experience joy with your relationships.

You can't find the resolution with your head down, and your eyes fixed on the doom and gloom. Wake up to living daily, becoming alive with breath, discovery, sharing your smile, feeling the sunshine, and the caring of others in simple ways. Open yourself to receiving help from others and the divine. Have faith in the goodness of others and the goodness of your body. Be grateful for every moment. It is a gift.

Remember, regret and resentment block forgiveness of self and others. Lack of forgiveness of others, or self, blocks true healing. Healing is organic, and so is genuine love and forgiveness. Become authentic and look at your life and change today.

Cancer

Affirmations:
- I really love life and live it fully now.
- I forgive. I let go of all pain and judgment.
- I really love life and live it fully now.
- I have fun.
- I trust in a higher purpose.
- I choose the highest and best for all.
- Today I embrace the moment.
- I value the experience of breath, of touch, of feelings.
- I enjoy the smile of a child, the warm embrace of a friend, the caring of family.
- I choose to deeply understand my role in my healing.
- I choose to encourage myself daily to find the positive repetitive rituals that keep my mind focused and ready.
- I breathe new life and release the old.
- I really do enjoy living, and my cells are ready to stand up for me.
- I am the good fighter for my daily cause of healing.
- My immune system is my friend and support.
- I trust in my purpose in sharing my life with others, and I trust in a higher purpose.
- I choose the highest and best for all.
- I let go of the hatred and regret and transform them into progressive beliefs and positive emotions that bring joy, healing, and strength.
- I thank the divine nature within me, and I align my soul to the healing powers and love of God.
- I am now ready to face life and enjoy the process of living my path.

Cancer

Supporting Foods:

- Kale
- Collard greens
- Broccoli
- Cauliflower
- Brussel sprouts
- Kelp
- Sea vegetables
- Shiitake mushrooms
- Swiss chard
- Spinach
- Asparagus
- Bell peppers
- Celery
- Cabbage
- Crimini mushroom
- Extra virgin
- Olive oil
- Turmeric
- Ginger
- Non-GMO organic Strawberries
- Black beans
- Eggplant
- Garlic
- Pineapple
- Watermelon
- Grapefruit
- Organic grapes
- Organic raspberries
- Organic blueberries
- Fiber from vegetables and organic fruit
- Soaked flaxseed
- Soaked chia seeds
- Walnuts
- Soaked almonds
- Winter squash
- Beets
- Beet greens
- Onions
- Avocado

Candida

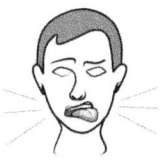

Troubled Mindset

- You doubt your capacity, intelligence, understanding, or performance a lot.
- You resent that you can't seem to find your personal power.
- These are very old concepts, patterns, and negativity that you are holding on to.
- You blame others instead of grounding in and rising to the occasion.
- Fear and feelings of powerlessness justified your belief that you need to keep some things secret.
- This has led to a reminder that your unresolved emotions and pain are still bugging you, and they want out.
- You will often do things to sabotage your health, which may be an unconscious urge to get you to move out of your way and let go of the fear, regret, secrets, denials, and half-truths that you have been telling yourself.
- Of course, you may think that is what everyone else does. Think again, human. It's time to change.

Candida

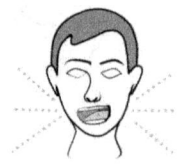

Healing Mindset

Be ready to be real. "Be not afraid" to be you, yourself, the authentic you! This means you need to figure out who that is. While you are secretly wishing things to be different, you are sending mixed messages to your brain, your body, and your heart. Get your act together by writing down what you feel, what you believe, what you hold as deep values and truths.

Test yourself; are you living your core values? Or are you just pretending to, and telling yourself and others your pretending thoughts? Be true to you and what you believe. Let go of the fear and be one with your real self. Listen carefully to understand how to make the appropriate changes and see obstacles as opportunities for growth. Deeply nourish your body with healing foods.

Candida

Affirmations:

- I find energy in living in the moment.
- Instead of hiding my feelings and thoughts, I share them with those who care, with God, and journal.
- When weak, I turn to breath and hope.
- When in pain, I turn to clarity, focus, and movement.
- When in confusion, I turn to simple thoughts, simple walk, simple talk.
- When in frustration, I turn to faith and defining the real meaning of life.
- I take the opportunity to honor and respect my body before any fungus can take advantage of me.
- I am worth so much.
- I am beautiful inside and out.
- I love myself and express myself freely.

Supporting Foods:

- Vegetables
- Celery
- Jicama
- Zucchini squash
- Yellow squash
- Red bell pepper
- Salmon
- Brown rice
- Millet
- Quinoa
- Oat bran
- Garlic
- Dark greens
- Chlorella
- Spirulina
- Plain yogurt

Canker Sores

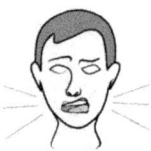

Troubled Mindset

- You blame those who you let manipulate you.
- You can't state your frustrations, so you bite your lip.
- You build up physical sensitivities to pathogens and certain foods because you are emotionally sensitive to too many people, judgments, and foods.
- You regret what you can't control and harbor the deep resentments in your mouth sores as a reminder from the body that you lack control of.

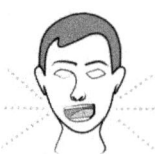

Healing Mindset

Getting the negativity 'out' or stuffing it back 'in' aren't great options. You need to see life for what it is. If there are people that judge you as if "it is all your fault," then realize today that they are reflecting their lack of control onto you. Stop the self-blame that attracts their judgments. Exchange it with honest responsibility and personal power. Pause your thinking, breathe, move and begin releasing the pain in other ways. Acknowledge what your conflict is, release the feelings of anger and regret, and begin the processing of positive change.

Canker Sores

Affirmations:

- I "lesser" the fester inside with positive encouragement to be safe.
- I encourage myself and feel safe.
- I am capable to express my feelings with confidence, and I feel strong when wronged.
- I value each experience in a way that I always have options.
- I always have a choice of a positive attitude when confronted with feelings of being trapped.
- I am free to release blame.
- I desire the moments of being cherished and honored.
- I am open to a life of positive expression of love.

Supporting Foods:

- Onion
- Garlic
- Plain yogurt
- Green leafy vegetables
- Sauerkraut
- Kimchi
- Kefir

Carpal Tunnel Syndrome

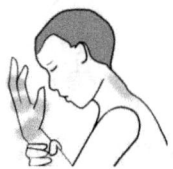

Troubled Mindset

- "Why is everything so unfair?!"
- Hands and wrists have to do with what you are 'doing' in your life.
- You may feel like you are doing it all wrong, or you really just don't like whatever it is you do.
- You may feel like it is too much, or you simply don't believe in your ability to be successful.
- Even if something did work out, you don't trust it to last. This is once again reinforced by the encompassing belief that everything is unfair.
- You lack the support that you need to be able to do everything you have to do.
- You are concerned with the opinion of others, but you still need to stay on task.
- You feel manipulated, so you try to control your situation, but it is getting more and more difficult.

Carpal Tunnel Syndrome

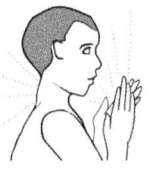

Healing Mindset

Believe in your abilities. Believe in your possibilities. Stop listening to the voices of guilt, blame, frustration, and fear. Your muscles in your wrists are fatiguing because they are trying to hold the thoughts of the mind and the emotions of the heart together on the same team.

Become congruent in your head and heart first, and then do your tasks. Doing is a reflection of what is intended from within, so take care of your inner fears and judgments first.

Carpal Tunnel Syndrome

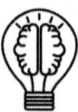

Affirmations:
- I make sure I am grounded before I do my tasks for the day.
- I can do this.
- I breathe. I stretch. I move with ease.
- I support my bones and muscles with healthy nutrition, supportive clothing, releasing stretches, and positive thoughts.
- I enjoy working and doing tasks.
- I listen to my inner voice of courage whenever the other voices try to drown out any good.
- I feel light and strong.
- I enjoy the challenges that I am facing and confidently coach myself through the changes to be made.

Supporting Foods:
- Swiss chard
- Spinach
- Summer squash
- Pumpkin seeds
- Broccoli
- Basil
- Cucumbers
- Green beans
- Flaxseed (soaked)
- Romaine lettuce
- Celery
- Tomatoes
- Collard greens
- Asparagus
- Cremini mushrooms
- Shiitake mushroom
- Farm-fresh eggs
- Eggplant
- Cod
- Salmon
- Sardines
- Scallops
- Lamb
- Grass-fed beef
- Roasted turkey

Cervix

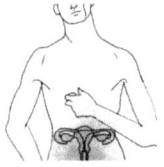

Troubled Mindset

- You struggle to appreciate your femininity, and you hold onto conflict with patriarchal attitudes that have contributed to this negative perception of yourself.
- You fight with the part of yourself that accepted these attitudes.
- You may have been sexually suppressed, abused, or exploited and have not yet found inner resolution for the event(s) or struggle of what has happened.
- You may have really tried letting go of any old way of being but can't seem to deliver new experiences.

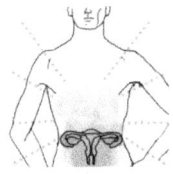

Healing Mindset

Don't quit. Change may happen right when you feel the desire to quit the strongest. You can't change what has happened or control others, but you can choose to be a friend to all of you and to be a unifying force for good. As you do this, open to and accept appropriate and positive nurturing for yourself, the kind that honors every part of you. Connect with your true feminine power to bring life to your creativities and influence positive change for those around you.

Cervix

Affirmations:
- I am strong and sensitive.
- I am open to express and protect my core.
- I balance life's responsibility without sacrificing myself.
- My fears of additional betrayal are a voice that I will calm with love because it is time to release the pain of the past, grow from it, and transform it into new strengths.
- I am objective with my intentions and tasks.
- I let the energy of others pass by, and I let the warmth of mother earth empower me to be truly myself.

Supporting Foods:

- Alfalfa
- Avocados
- Fish
- Meats (not fried)
- Parsley
- Safflower

Chest Pain

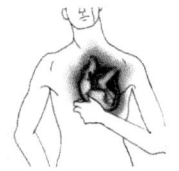

Troubled Mindset

- You feel like joy has been sucked out of life.
- You feel that you have given love, perhaps an abundance of deep or even unconditional love, but without feeling or allowing love in return.
- You block love as protection or self-preservation from possible rejection, which is what you expect.
- You have hoped that you could continue to love others without needing them. This makes loving feel heavy, leaving you exhausted rather than rejuvenated.
- You keep insisting others need to change rather than finding what needs to change within yourself.
- Being honest, and therefore vulnerable with your sadness feels too frightening and unsafe to attempt.
- Every day the inner conflicts grow deeper and stronger.
- Every day you are pushing the denial of what is really going inside of you while desiring to have things be different on the outside.
- Consider how you go forward, thinking that things might change.
- You are wishing that the other person would be different, longing for love from someone who doesn't know how to speak your love language and hoping for some outcome that is not possible, while the other person or people keep acting a certain way.
- Wishes are like fishes, swimming around without any control. If you have fear and resentment, these fishes become like sharks to your inner world, and your body can't take that anymore.

Chest Pain

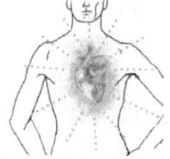

Healing Mindset

It is time to conclude that you are in conflict with yourself. You have opposing desires and conflicting needs. Find the parts of you that are afraid and start a gradual process of bringing courage to your heart and mind.

Find the parts of you that are hurt and sensitive to the destructive energy from verbal attacks. See that the bully in them is covering up their pain and fear. Have your body bury the pain and sensitivity in the earth. Listen to those who honestly care for you. Listen only to the valid respectful words of others.

Stretch, breathe, and renew your thoughts daily. It is time for you to calm your little fear side, and gradually grow into your mature self in all areas of your life. You will be fine, just take the steps to be true to you.

Chest Pain

Affirmations:

- I wonder if there is enough room in the world for all the creative things I want to do.
- I ponder the possibility that I am chosen to be myself living my passion.
- I reflect on the reactions of the past and choose a new path for my internal thoughts and feelings.
- I articulate my experience with every muscle relaxed.
- I meditate on the value of challenges and my growth of character.
- I sing a song of praise to the gift of life and my unique body.
- I choose to connect to the energy flowing from my body to the earth.
- I relax my right shoulder, then my left, then my right hip, and then my left.
- I touch someone in need and release their needs to the universe.
- I feel the comfort and warmth of someone who deeply cares.
- I find the energy of life deep within my core.
- I cherish my vital energy and spend it wisely.

 ## Supporting Foods:

- Apples
- Black beans
- Broccoli
- Brown rice
- Romaine lettuce
- Shiitake mushroom
- Wheat (if not gluten sensitive)
- Cabbage
- Cauliflower
- Corn
- Garbanzo beans
- Butter (organic)
- Kale
- Lentils
- Oats
- Fenugreek
- Fenugreek sprouts
- Red legumes

Cholesterol

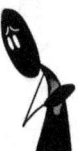

Troubled Mindset

- Your life is stalled and you are frustrated with how much effort it takes to keep moving.
- You feel desperation to keep up the pressures of life while trying to maintain some sort of happiness.
- You may believe that you aren't meant to be happy.
- Perhaps you believe there is nobility in suffering, yet you still crave to have joy.
- Your cravings lead you to hide your real thoughts, feelings, or actions.
- You secretly do 'fun' things to compensate for the insistence on living a 'no fun' lifestyle.
- You have a secret and still, wish to push your agenda.
- If you openly push your agenda, it makes you more angry that others don't cooperate.
- If you secretly push your agenda, you feel sad and sluggish inside and wish they would change.
- You are waiting for the next bad thing to happen, which can lead you into the next state of heightened awareness.
- This swing of anxiety and then sometimes feeling down and depressed makes the body store more fats and cholesterol to buffer your frustrations and upsets.

Cholesterol

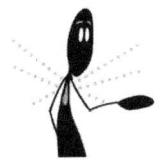

Healing Mindset

Happiness and life are not meant to be in opposition to each other, but in concert with one another. Get creative. Decide to be here, in your body, not in your worry or upset. Keeping your judgments to yourself, and then pushing an agenda (whether it is subtle or not), won't solve your problems. Dissolve those judgment with compassion and understanding.

When feeling stalled and frustrated with the extra effort it takes to move, slow down enough to go at the pace that is aligned with what is safe for your body. Respecting the body's needs will help the body respect your needs. As you pace yourself, you will feel inner support and inner strength.

Choosing to take the challenge of the day and deal with it with intrigue, opportunity, and possibility will give you energy, excitement, and eventually joy.

Cholesterol

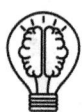

Affirmations:

- I live each moment and thrive in THIS moment to be fully present with me, myself, and I.
- I look around and appreciate the gifts and contributions of others.
- I release the self-judgment and blame towards others.
- I have nothing to escape from.
- I need no secrets, nor feelings that compel me to force my way to get along.
- I take each challenging path as an opportunity to grow.
- I calmly communicate with others in an assertive, productive manner.
- I am safe to release my inner need for a secret and transform it into healthy open conversations.
- I have enough. I am enough. I do enough.
- I enjoy the strength that my body already gives me.
- I am cleaning out the old and enjoying the new.

Cholesterol

Supporting Foods:

- Water/Get hydrated
- Apples
- Bananas
- Carrots
- Cold-water fish
- Dried beans
- Garlic
- Grapefruit
- Olive oil
- Eat in moderation - nonfat milk
- Low fat cottage cheese
- Skinless white poultry
- Water-soluble dietary fiber in barley
- Brown rice fruits
- Brown rice bran
- Drink fresh juices, especially carrot, celery, & beet
- Use only cold pressed oils such as olive oil
- Soybean oil
- Primrose oil
- Black currant oil
- Oats
- Oat bran
- Guar gum

Chronic Fatigue Syndrome

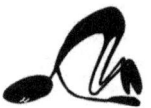

Troubled Mindset

- Your body is afraid that you will overdo it.
- You will not listen to the needs of your body, and you overwhelm it again and again. Now your body is trusting you less and less.
- You don't hold space for you.
- You let yourself be 'the burden' or 'the space' for others' needs, wants, and agendas.
- You are afraid to be yourself because of some guilt or fear.
- Sometimes you are afraid of what will happen if you do get well.
- Your body listens to the voices of pathogenic people more than your true voice.
- Or, you listen to your 'critical self' and forgot who the true and empowering self really is.

Chronic Fatigue Syndrome

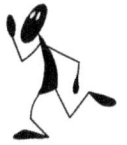

Healing Mindset

Wake up to an empowering self. See the self who is an encouraging, supportive, and understanding soul. Enter into the you who loves discovery and seeking for truth. You can do this, just live gradually for a while. Acknowledge that physical weakness will wear on your emotional states and mental acuity. So, take time to be quiet in your mind. Let some of the energy be used to heal the inner parts of your body and mind.

Open your heart to receive caring from others, but it is not your friend when they are critical, so let that energy pass by quickly. Healing only happens in supportive and caring states. You, too, share when you care. And when you can't reserve the energy for your own inner health.

Chronic Fatigue Syndrome

Affirmations:
- I am not the fatigue.
- I am living, breathing, feeling, sensing the gifts of life.
- What an opportunity it is to live, to breathe, to taste, to touch, to care, to share!
- There is more than enough energy in the universe; in fact, I am using enough now.
- I make each day simpler.
- All worries are draining to the earth.
- I receive the love and life force from the heavens and mother earth each and every moment.
- I have clear paths of energy throughout my body.
- Any obstacle is for teaching and growth.
- The paths of energy are strengthened with each challenge.

Supporting Foods:
- Drink plenty of water at least eight 8oz glasses a day.
- Eat a well-balanced diet including raw fruits, vegetables, and fresh raw juices.
- Whole grains
- Raw nuts
- Seeds
- Skinless turkey
- Deep water fish
- Yogurt
- Kefir
- Green leafy vegetables
- Wheatgrass

Chronic Illnesses

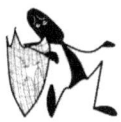

Troubled Mindset

- You have to choose to follow your role as "someone who is sick" or "someone learning about the challenges of life in a productive way."
- There is confusion from the inner fight within. Who is the real enemy? And what should be done about it?
- You have multiple agendas inside, and each and every one of these, the body thinks is necessary.
- You fear the future, worry about things worsening, and have concerns that if you recover, your loved ones might leave you. These fears and others keep you on the sidelines of life.
- All your fears together are draining your energy and keeping the immune system confused and overworked.
- You've been emotionally hurt, but holding onto regret or blame keeps the vicious cycle going.
- It's not your fault that you're dealing with an illness. However, it is within your responsibility to gradually and methodically shift your mindset towards your body, fostering a sense of gratitude, providing caring support, and taking positive actions.

Chronic Illnesses

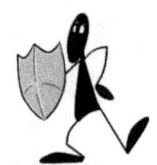

Healing Mindset

Enjoy each moment that life gives you. Focus on the little progress and cultivate gratitude for the little joys.

Start in the moment by focusing on the positive around you. You have a lot of energy, but it is being used to keep you going. Take the energy you have and carefully allocate your day to tasks that don't overwhelm you.

Take your thoughts and positively organize them, use them, and share them. You are a good person. You are a light. You are a gift to others, so let it be so.

Chronic Illnesses

Affirmations:
- I feel a calming energy flowing down my body to the earth.
- I let the confusion settle into the brightness of one clear moment of insight.
- I know my inner fight is mostly my body trying to figure it all out and trying a bit too much.
- So I settle it down for positive healing.
- I appreciate all that my body does for me.
- I appreciate the alarms because they indicate there is something that needs attention.
- I release the need to overreact.
- I listen to my body with caring understanding.
- It is wonderful to have information that can lead me to a path of healing.
- I enjoy the path of healing and insights.

Supporting Foods:
- Apple
- Micro greens
- Celery juice
- Celery
- Avocado
- Sprouts
- Squash
- Congee rice (cooked for 2 hours)
- Slowed cooked soups
- Long and slow cooked organic meat
- Farm fresh eggs
- Steamed vegetables on rice
- Soaked sunflower seeds
- Soaked chia seeds
- Roasted garlic
- Carrot steamed
- Red beets steamed
- Romaine lettuce

Claustrophobia

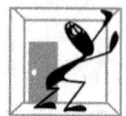

Troubled Mindset

- Oh where, oh where, did you go? You are focusing on the possible future and the fears that have been passed on to you.
- It started long ago when you lost a deep connection to your mother or father.
- It could have been in the womb or from a major physical or emotional trauma.
- Your perspective is orbiting around fear like a gravitational pull.
- The body and neurological system have got stuck in the fear of doom.
- The fear of control, loss of freedom, manipulation, death, and being trapped with no escape are recycled regularly.
- The trauma is coming from the recycling of possibility, not reality.

Claustrophobia

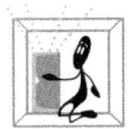

Healing Mindset

The depth of your primal fears is making you run from your tender self. Find and embrace the innocent self that needs calm breathing, loving moments, and strength that comes from the courage to face life just one simple step at a time; breathe at this moment, release it, and breathe in again as you embrace the next moment.

Take it slowly and build inner trust one little piece at a time. You can do this. Breathe, and discover the possibility of the simple challenges. Orient, then reorient yourself around trust, hope, and the personal power found within. Calm the body, mind, and heart each step on the way.

Claustrophobia

Affirmations:
- I see now that I have let a fear of looking inside push me to close up, and so I have been resisting looking inside.
- I am ready to take the chance to see my inner self.
- I trust to look inside first and breathe, then gradually build my space outwards to beyond my fearful place.
- There is plenty of air; it is time to let some of it through my lungs.
- There is plenty of love; it is time to let some of it through my heart.
- There is plenty of hope; it is time to let some of it through my mind.

Supporting Foods:

- Bananas
- Soups
- Cucumbers
- Carrots
- Salmon
- Micro-greens
- Lightly steamed vegetables
- Boiled egg over brown rice
- Feta or high quality cheese
- Watermelon
- Jicama
- Papaya
- Sprouted cereals
- Romaine lettuce
- Quinoa
- Amaranth

Cold

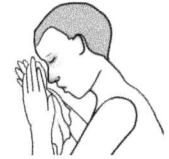

Troubled Mindset

- You are trying to do too much.
- You became confused or scattered, and you forgot to take care of your true needs.
- Your responsibilities feel overwhelming.
- You have been fearing that it all won't work out, so you overdo yourself.
- Your body is telling you to relax and calm down, but you're not being attentive to your physical needs.

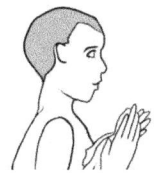

Healing Mindset

Take time to recenter and return to your divine path with deeper roots. Of course, there is no way to be everything to everyone. Set aside your hyper concerns. Be what you truly are. In other words, enjoy the day first, and then do what you need to do, because there is no way you can do it all.

If your fears materialize, that is the time to see how mature your emotional world is. The mature person learns how to take the waves of too cold and too hot and discovers the magnificent within the mundane, and the growth within the conflict. Relax and embrace the idea of everything working out for the highest and best. Ground yourself, rest up, and move forward.

Cold

Affirmations:
- I am positive that I was doing just fine.
- I am sure that this is just a momentary setback.
- I am using this moment to reflect, release, and recharge my body and my mind.
- My body needed a reset and detox, so I am using it for my good.
- I love giving myself warm and caring time.
- I am so ready to renew and build up my strength once again.
- I thank the body for reminding me to be good to myself by eating good foods, feeling good moods, and think positive thoughts.
- I am positive that I am warmer than it seems.
- I breathe and calm my body.
- I send warm energy to my core and bring that warmth to the surface.
- I find and release my upset that cracked into the immune system and made me weak.
- I heal it with love and acceptance for myself.
- The upset was only temporary and not permanent.
- I can find my truth.

Cold

Supporting Foods:

- Water/Get hydrated
- Cayenne pepper
- Fermented foods
- Jicama
- Celery juice
- Carrot juice
- Steamed broccoli
- Steamed cauliflower
- Steamed red beets
- Warm broth soups
- Congee (Extra slow cooked rice)
- Turkey soup with healing spices
- Micro-greens
- Squash
- Watermelon
- Asparagus
- Chicken soup
- Green onions
- Ginger
- Lemon
- Garlic
- Warm teas
- Parsley
- Cinnamon spice
- Clove spice
- Thyme spice

Cold Extremities

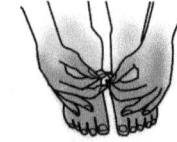

Troubled Mindset

- You want to be safe, and you want to be active, so you move forward, but you keep a part of yourself behind.
- You know you can do it, but then again, you subtly question, "can I?"
- Why have any fears anyway? Because you try to cover your tracks and prepare.
- The funny thing is that you still miss some big, key things when it comes to life's risks. So, you choose to stay warm in your middle and cold on the extremities.

Healing Mindset

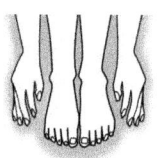

You can take the day and seize it. Why wait for another day to be strong and true to your core values? It's time to embrace the strength of your hope, capacity, and capability. But, before that, check in with your real intentions and align them with what is realistically possible. You have feared being honest with yourself about life. Positive observation is beneficial and productive. Your fear of taking the steps comes from your childhood. Slow down a bit and then speed up. Take a moment to be safe, to be loved, to be real with what is. Give yourself a good pat on the back and let the perfectionism go right out the window.

Cold Extremities

Affirmations:

- I am true to my heart and honest with my mind.
- I stop the fear, turn it around, and send it back where it came from.
- I feel the earth move under my feet and the sky all around me.
- The grass is greener because the sky is bluer and my heart is warmer.
- I discover the magic in the path of discovery while keeping my feet on a steady path.

Supporting Foods:

- Cayenne
- Sauerkraut
- Warm soups
- Cauliflower
- Red potatoes
- Onions
- Garlic
- Squash
- Root vegetables

Cold Sores

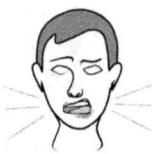

Troubled Mindset

- You are upset at someone.
- You hate what has happened to you.
- You resent the heavy load you carry.
- You wish things would have been different, but it is out of your control.
- The conflict between what you do and how you feel about it makes it harder to cope with the demands of life.
- You go along with what you're told, to get acceptance or approval, but end up feeling dominated, manipulated, or deceived.
- If you let the other person know what you are really feeling, then you think they will overreact. Thus, you let your feelings and emotions fester inside. But these grow into a sore that is visible to all.

Cold Sores

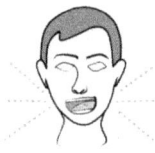

Healing Mindset

The pain and upset you feel is not the problem. The issue is how you handle it. Everyone has conflict. It is how you deal with the conflict that determines your experience.

Choose to work through your conflict to understand that you are conflicted inside. Your memories betray you. Your memories are demanding conflicting needs.

Start simply and honor one need at a time. See that your enemy needs the same. Hate and anger is hurting you. See that the other person has needs that are immature and start there to understand them. Understanding can open the door to letting go of pain and festering emotions. Write every day your blame, then write what you are growing positively in your life due to the problem, then write what you plan to do with what you are learning. Release the need to be angry and transform it into the drive to take action to change your inner and outer world.

Cold Sores

Affirmations:

- I choose to find comfort in what really matters.
- I let the petty things go and realize that my well being and life is more important than past regrets and past conflicts.
- I am growing a new understanding and gifts every day.
- I enjoy the discovery of expressing my true feelings without fearing the reaction.
- I can do this, express without all the stress.

Supporting Foods:

- Green leafy vegetables
- Onion
- Garlic
- Plain yogurt
- Sauerkraut
- Kimchi
- Kefir
- Lima beans
- Salmon
- Soaked sunflower seeds
- High quality cheese
- Brewer's yeast
- Carrots
- Chicken
- Farm fresh eggs
- Fish
- Peas
- Spinach
- Small red potato
- Jicama

Colon Problems: Large Intestine

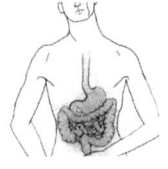

Troubled Mindset

- Colon problems are worry in action. In other words, your anxiety, and constantly thinking about what should have been, what could have been, or what might happen, is bugging you so much, that you try to ignore what actually is happening. Instead, you push yourself forward.
- You tend to be critical as you hold onto the past and withhold your love from life.
- You're blaming and hating others for your emotional pain.
- You feel confused, irritated, embarrassed, and frustrated about what has happened and can't see past the dark clouds of the past to enjoy the light of possibility.
- You insist that your mistakes or flaws make you unlovable and create 'self-fulfilling prophecies' to reinforce that belief.
- You'd rather just 'through it all out' than to face it.
- Guilt and self-blame leads to a subtle shame that no one can fix because your inner dialogue is assuring you that you are "bad" or the "problem."
- Rarely are the constipated thoughts and feelings of an individual true. For if they were true, the problem would show up in another way and not constipation.
- Yes, you have made mistakes, and you are not perfect.
- You are constantly thinking of ways to be more perfect or be better. And sometimes you wish you could be somewhere else or be someone else, but oddly enough, you are not even you when you do that.

Colon Problems: Large Intestine

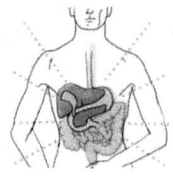

Healing Mindset

You can come to the realization that you are not your shame. You are not that awful. Maybe a little bit; meaning, you do make mistakes and have created issues around you, but so does everyone else. The problem is not that you made mistakes. The problem is that you won't let go of the self-criticism that you made a mistake. The energy of shame is worse than the mistake that you made.

You can build the courage and fortitude it takes to be true to your human side and your divine side. You must have wanted to experiment with life, so now do it. Experiment with the idea of learning to live life with the intention of making mistakes so you can learn from them. Live now, be you, be happy, be in truth. See specific colon area.

Colon Problems: Large Intestine

Affirmations:

- I gladly let go of the past and make room for beneficial change.
- I learn from the past.
- I am clear.
- I am for insight.
- I lovingly approve of myself.
- I am doing my best.
- I calmly rest into peace.
- I make room for beneficial change by letting go of the past and my self-criticism.
- Judgment is a sign that my mind got ahead of my heart and my body.
- I give myself permission to be an experimenter of life.
- I give myself permission to make a few mistakes every day.
- I give myself permission to laugh at the silliness of self-judgment.
- I am insightful.
- I lovingly approve of myself, my heart, and my life.
- I am doing my best.
- I calmly rest my worries and enjoy the rest of my life with positive action and peaceful intentions.

Colon Problems: Large Intestine

Supporting Foods:

- Water/Get hydrated
- Eat plenty of raw foods and vegetables
- Whole grains
- Brown rice
- Fish
- Small amount of meat
- Raw nuts and seeds
- Legumes
- Apples
- Asparagus
- Bananas
- Beets
- Cabbage
- Carrots
- Celery
- Citrus fruits
- Green leafy vegetables
- Peppers
- Watermelon
- Millet
- Oats
- Barley

Colon Problems: Small Intestine

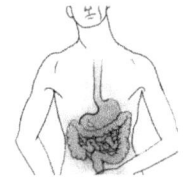

Troubled Mindset

- You are struggling to assimilate and learn from your life experiences.
- You are facing a challenge and can't figure it out. It is difficult to discern what is best for you and what is not.
- You wish you could just escape being responsible for determining what you really need emotionally and physically.
- Because of the traumas of the past, you sabotage your thinking when it comes to nourishing your body.
- You even forget sometimes your personal commitments to yourself and go back to foods and thoughts that are harmful in the long run.
- It stems from having felt victimized, misunderstood, betrayed, and not trusted.
- You lack the understanding of why you were hurt, and your gut reminds you through pain or discomfort.
- Now you hold onto your low self-value, fear, and low self-confidence.
- You carry excess guilt and worry for any mistakes.
- You hate your vulnerability.
- You repress your anger and troubling memories.
- You worry and fear that you might be dealing with abandonment once again.

Colon Problems: Small Intestine

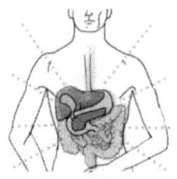

Healing Mindset

You need to organize your thoughts and logic. But to do that, you need to deal with your fears and pains that have led you to be mentally scattered. Your mind will be diverted by the sufferings of the past because the subconscious is trying to protect you from any perceived trouble.

As you balance your heart pain and past memories, you will grow empathy for others, and for your inner self. Be kind to yourself and others. Offer yourself gratitude, love, and understanding. Look and see if you have room and space for new learning, acceptance for life experiences, and the gifts of dealing with life logically and emotionally. As you mature your abilities of communication and learning, gather facts and details that build truth, and not stubbornness. Responsible recentering of your mind and body will easily bring comfort to your digestion and body. Meditate with focused breath to distinguish between what is positive and useful for your growth and what is not.

Colon Problems: Small Intestine

Affirmations:
- I am positively open to learning from all situations and all people.
- I respect myself today, yesterday, and tomorrow.
- I am teachable.
- I am a likable person.
- I treat others as my equal.
- I am courteous, respectful, and friendly.
- I am patient and joyful.
- I give equally and accept freely.
- I filter what is necessary and good for my body and soul and let the rest go.
- I am alive with life, fun, experience, and adventure.
- I am organized and flexible.
- I appreciate the kindness of others.
- Every step I take, I move with clarity, fluidity, courage, and discovery.

Supporting Foods:
- Alfalfa sprouts
- Fenugreek sprouts
- Mung bean sprouts
- Banana
- Broccoli
- Brussel sprouts (with minimal butter)
- Brown rice
- Cayenne
- Celery
- Cucumber
- Fenugreek
- Kelp
- Lettuce
- Mango
- Garlic
- Papaya
- Pineapple
- Sauerkraut
- Sprouts
- Turkey

Constipation

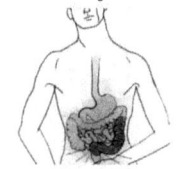

Troubled Mindset

- "I just can't let go."
- You are stuck with holding onto an idea, a belief, or an emotion that is more important to you than being healthy and happy.
- You are holding on because it is scary or uncomfortable to change.
- In part, you may feel you're missing an important detail, so you hold onto the waste. Simultaneously, listening to and understanding other perspectives and possibilities is burdensome to you. This double-bind sabotages your growth, leaving you feeling twisted inside and backed up emotionally.
- You fear yourself in new arenas.
- You fear what others may think or do.
- You fear letting go of past patterns and feelings.
- You hate your situation or another person.
- The pressure is mounting, and you are not clear on which direction to go.
- You feel there is a need, but you are not sure what it is.
- You try to save the day and 'make it stop' without truly relating to or understanding the nature of the issue.
- The problem is exacerbated when you use control, possessiveness, or anger to push your will.

Constipation

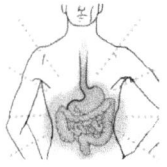

Healing Mindset

Honor and nourish yourself past all the negative self-talk and the negative regret. The subtle blame and hatred are harmful. Replace them with gratitude for the learning and the opportunity to plan and take action in a new way. Nourish your body with vital minerals. Relax the need to 'fix it' and put your trust in a higher way.

Seek resolution with your mind and your heart. When they are aligned, it will help your body calm down. Let spring arrive and let go of the winter. Submitting your control and choosing joy in the process of life will reap great rewards.

Constipation

Affirmations:

- I trust in my body.
- I trust in the process of letting go to let God.
- I am safe to open to new perspectives.
- I don't need the fears and blame that block my progress in life.
- I am ready to live fully and passionately.
- I want to be fully engaged in life.
- I embrace the ups and downs of living with gratitude, resilience, and drive to take the next step with courage and love.

Supporting Foods:

- Water/Get hydrated
- Apples
- Asparagus
- Bananas
- Barley
- Beans
- Beets
- Cabbage
- Carrots
- Fish
- Kale
- Millet
- Okra
- Rice
- Citrus fruits
- Green peppers
- Romaine lettuce
- Watermelon
- Cayenne pepper
- Ginger
- Fibrous foods if safe, otherwise steam the fibrous vegetables
- Meats (moderate amounts and not fried)

COPD
(Chronic Obstructive Pulmonary Disease)

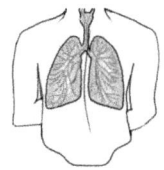

Troubled Mindset

- The overwhelming feeling of desperation for breath and life has caught up to you.
- Why did you wait so long to face some of the feelings that you have been suppressing?
- You have held back fear and anger and turned them into anxiety and emotional discomfort.
- What happened to the dreams and the wishes that life could or should have been better?
- Whatever happened to the goal of something better?
- If only you could go back and change this, or that, or everything.
- Regret doesn't heal it; it just makes the suffering last a little longer and go a little deeper.

COPD
(Chronic Obstructive Pulmonary Disease)

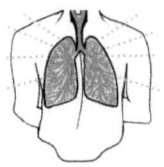

Healing Mindset

Wake up to 'make up' with the small parts of yourself that need some love and attention... but maybe they need some tough love. The kind of love that doesn't allow your fear to take over. The kind that coaches your worry or fearful side into taking action and being proactive. The type of tough love that takes suppressed resentments and changes them into letting go of that which can't change, and allowing the best out of life.

A garden grows beautifully when you take the weeds and till them in. Take your weeds and turn them into emotional and spiritual fertilizer. Let your sadness and grief leak out with your tears, fears, and breath. Catch those doubts before you second guess yourself into another problem.

Let yourself grow with positive emotional maturity; you have it within you. Pay attention to the moment and learn to breathe with little effort by starting slowly and consistently. Trust your body, don't fight it, and listen to an inner voice of care, strength, and courage.

COPD
(Chronic Obstructive Pulmonary Disease)

Affirmations:
- I am appreciative of each and every moment.
- I love the opportunity to live this day.
- I cherish love and relish in sincere appreciation.
- I take my grief, make it brief, and lose it to a brighter hope and a better future.
- I hope, I pray, I sing, I love.
- May my heart be as joyous as a child on a summer morning at the park.
- I release the past and make room for many amazing moments.

Supporting Foods:
- Turmeric
- Cucumbers
- Celery
- Thyme
- Fennel
- Salmon
- Pineapple
- Papaya

Corns

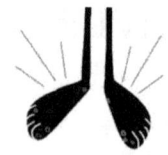

Troubled Mindset

- You fear things won't work out.
- You wish every day for a different outcome, and you push inside as if it will change.
- Your desires are resisting reality.
- You have deep judgments toward those who have got in your way or have hurt someone you care about.
- Hardening a part of your heart is not the answer, but the indicator that you have been stuck in the past.
- You got lost in your need to force things to be different.
- You end up feeling apprehensive about the future with fear of failing amidst a lost sense of direction in life.

Healing Mindset

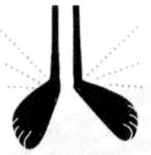

You can "take each moment and live each moment." Find the stony heart; it has become your own obstacle. It started as a protection, but that time has now passed. Notice the resilient strength you have created; it has kept you going. See this positive outcome of your experience, then let go of your need to please on the outside and the need to be so upset that others are not different. Learning to dissolve your frustration will help you dissolve your obstacles.

Corns

Affirmations:
- I resolve to dissolve my hardened frustrations with people and my life.
- I approve of the actions of others because they are learning, and so am I.
- I am grateful for the strength of character that I am maturing each and every day.
- I am free to be expressive and open.
- I appropriately share my truth and enjoy the insights of others.

Supporting Foods:
- Raw vegetables and juices to balance ph
- Japanese salt plum (umeboshi)

Cough

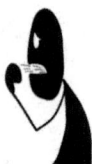

Troubled Mindset

- You are uncomfortable with your situation.
- You want to be responsible, but you fail to realize what your true responsibility is.
- You secretly blame others while wishing you could be different as well.
- Both your self-criticism and your blame are a defensive strategy against change.
- The burden of this conflict makes you easily affected by others' thoughts or opinions, hence the defensiveness.
- You have an underlying irritation that life is not what it was supposed to be.
- You feel guilt, shame, and anger for what you cannot control and for being challenged on things that you can't imagine how to change.
- You wish to be nice and to be strong, but fear takes over instead.

Cough

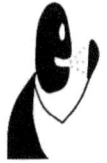

Healing Mindset

You need to face your expectations. See how they don't match reality. You need to be honest with those things that irritate you. Are you going to give away your power to the irritating feelings? You're thinking that the problem is their behavior or your weakness has become a problem. Stop focusing on the irritation and your inability to move through your emotional constipation.

Start focusing on breathing through each negative thought, each negative feeling, with simple awareness and action. The body is reacting to your worry and doesn't want you to internally express it anymore. So, appreciate the irritation for what it is, only an indication to be free of self-judgment. You are a child of the earth and the sky. Your real self is a beautiful being. Start there and gradually build your confidence up once again.

Cough

Affirmations:
- I am a child of truth, light, hope, and love.
- I calmly deal with the irritations of life with understanding and reality.
- I am simply going to take each moment and have the faith to breathe through it with courage and self-love.
- I am confident now.
- I calm my body to accept the momentary problem and move it through to the earth.
- I appreciate the signals of my immune system.
- I take care of my body, my heart, and my mind with equal amounts of care.

Supporting Foods:
- Water/Get hydrated
- Bone broth
- Raw garlic
- Ginger
- Fermented foods
- Apple cider vinegar
- Raw honey
- (See bacteria / virus / parasite)

Cramps

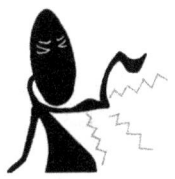

Troubled Mindset

- You have two worlds inside.
- There is a part of you that has these subtle fantasy beliefs like: "You are so amazing. You are so phenomenal. You have no problems. Everyone loves you."
- Then you have this other world of false beliefs like: "You are not going to make it. You will be found out. You are in trouble."
- These conflicting areas of the mind cause your muscles or abdomen to react when you least expect it.
- Your body only does what it is told to do, so when there is conflict, the body tries to satisfy both sides.
- In this gap comes the inner tug-of-war with self where you "grab on tight!"
- In a panic, you cling to the old beliefs, emotions, or circumstances, fearing that a change could only be disastrous.
- Check the specific muscle or area for more information.

Cramps

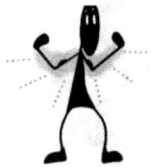

Healing Mindset

You can deal with your inner tug-of-war by first realizing you are fighting yourself. Then laugh at the possibility that you think more about what other people are thinking about you than they can actually deal with or even want to! You are simply creating an inner circus of conflict that no one cares to see.

Let the hidden monsters that you feed daily come out into the sunshine. Hidden or silenced, the problem often seems much larger. Let the problem be seen for what it is. Be happy that you care. But care about what you truly can share with those around you. Be true to yourself by letting go of the constant conflicting worries.

Cramps

Affirmations:
- I am ready to be.
- I am safe in my environment.
- My relationships reflect my moods, and I am happy to bring clarity and courage to my everyday experience.
- I have all that I need, and I am safe to express my feelings.
- I enjoy taking action in life.
- The winds of change will move quietly by.

Supporting Foods:

- Water/Get hydrated
- Lemons
- Limes
- Alfalfa
- Brewer's yeast
- Dark green and leafy vegetables
- Cornmeal
- Kelp
- Bananas
- Dairy products
- Salmon
- Chicken
- Legumes
- Almond
- Asparagus
- Broccoli
- Apricots
- Avocados
- Brown rice
- Garlic
- Yams
- Soybeans
- Tofu

Craving: Breads

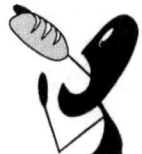

Troubled Mindset

- You are full of it and then you want more.
- Your body is wanting more and more because it feels like it tastes so good. But the amount of baked goods and bread doesn't solve anything it just makes you larger, but not larger than life - the life of your physical body.
- Everything you stuff in there will become the sponge of your conflict, making room for more stuff to stuff.
- You can't run but you can hide, which means you use the bread and baked goods because life is too much to deal with it all so you sponge and stuff.
- Consider your fears and sadness.
- You feel like a victim to your circumstances, so you find flavor in something that you think that you can control. But the flavor is not in your favor.
- The digestive tract can only deal with the internal biochemical problems that your actions create.
- Why let your frustrations lead you to false joy?
- Eating is really enjoyable when you show some respect to your body and your life.

Craving: Breads

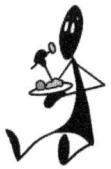

Healing Mindset

The amount of baked goods and bread doesn't solve anything it just makes you larger, but not larger than life. What if you took the time to listen to yourself every time you reach for a piece of bread? What if you took the moment when you put a cracker or baked good in your mouth and realized that this is not an escape hatch, or a pillow, or a sponge.

Face the sadness and fear of your heart. If you can't deal with it today, then gradual and consistently take time to do something cool and awesome for yourself that doesn't involve your mouth or your appetite. Become involved with walking, talking, writing, conversing, reading, and most of all creating. Find comfort in sharing with people who are encouraging you to be your best. Find love and comfort in sharing your smile and your thoughts.

Craving: Breads

Affirmations:
- I enjoy eating slowly with a smile and a refreshing breath.
- I enjoy taking a walk every time I crave, because an active life is made just for me.
- I seek wisdom and understanding from everyone I see.
- I seek to understand myself so that I can be responsible in the moment that I need the real me.
- I am full of purpose and enjoy sharing it.
- I am safe and when I'm not, I find my safety with breathing, walking, and expressing my real self.
- I am hope, truth, and joy.
- Today, I have an opportunity to be me—the me that has a choice in every action and thought.
- Thank you, God, for today's opportunities and gifts.
- I hope and seek to connect to an inner voice that supports my body's health and wellness.

Supporting Foods:
- Peppers
- Jicama
- Red beets
- Asparagus
- Lemons
- Limes
- Celery
- Cauliflower
- Apricots
- Green beans
- Corn
- Peas
- Oranges
- Orange squash
- Sprouted Almonds
- Lightly steamed or raw broccoli
- White fish
  - Tilapia
  - Halibut
- Buffalo

Craving: Chocolate

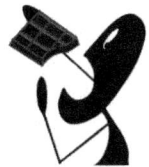

Troubled Mindset

- The secret is out: chocolate is divine; it makes everything "okay," simple, and easy for those moments when I can't deal with it anymore.
- "Oh, the delight to be released from my plight."
- To take the edge and smooth it with chocolate seems to be so great. However, it is covering up the deeper needs of safe connection.
- You have a passion that needs connection and direction, but it is not safe to share it with most.
- There is a challenge to my immune system, both physically and emotionally, but I fear dealing with my conflicts. So, chocolate covers it with a smooth filling.
- You hurt inside, but you don't want to talk about it. At least not today.

Craving: Chocolate

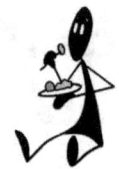

Healing Mindset

Pleasure and passion are natural, but if they are used to drown the suffering of the past and/or the fear of the future, then they will add pounds to your body and burden to your heart. Frosting over the discomforts with false beliefs and short-lived pleasures only adds to long-term upsets and disappointments.

Take these disappointments and start the path of putting a new address on them. One that will take you to find your core needs based on your core values. Be real with having authentic fun instead of quick coverups with food. Be honest with what is truly important.

Let go of the past judgments of yourself and the criticism of others. Who you are is more important than what you have done or what others have done. Take today and do something special that isn't based on food or sex. Connect your soul to nature, AND to the true nature of others.

Craving: Chocolate

Affirmations:

- I am true to myself, and my inner core values.
- I enjoy sharing my laughter.
- I delight in the sight of the playful smiles of others.
- I appreciate the calm nature of peaceful moments.
- I feel alive with my deepest breath.
- Life is a dessert full of opportunities to share my discoveries of joy and awareness.
- I am honest with my thoughts and feelings.
- I enjoy the light of day shining away the shadows of any inner cave.

Supporting Foods:

- Almond butter
- Avocado
- Cottage cheese
- Eggs
- Greek yogurt
- Lentils
- Millet
- Papaya
- Pineapple
- Quinoa
- Salmon
- Tuna
- Watermelon

Craving: Cold Dairy

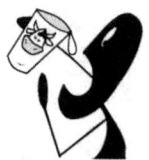

Troubled Mindset

- You use the cold dairy to freeze the pain or conflict and to make your body warm up the scared parts of yourself.
- How often have you escaped life with justifications of eating.
- Dairy targets your physical opiates, and your emotional pain killers. It works for a moment. But the temporary love is leading you to desire it more and giving you more problems of self-loathing in your future.
- When dairy is used as shield, your shield will take on the sluggish, heavy nature of where the product came from. And you will be less and less your real self and more like the source of the conflict and/or the animal that gave it to you.
- The additives in the food can also cause your body to store the substance thus locking in the physical and the tied-in emotions into your body.
- Using the fake to run from the truth makes life a difficult illusion to recover from.

Craving: Cold Dairy

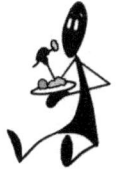

Healing Mindset

A glass of milk is healthy if you can digest it and it is not being used as a way to push every emotion deep inside. Before grabbing that next glass of cold dairy refreshment, stop and take a walk around the room, the house, or the neighborhood. Breath in some the refreshing parts of nature or of your creative mind.

"Take five to be alive before you nourish yourself with something that might put your emotions into a deep dive."

You are so worthy and capable of taking the time to take care of yourself. Your negative thoughts are not the truth. They are there just to make sure you don't make another mistake, but this self-critical process is counterproductive given your human nature.

Turn your negative thoughts and feelings into emotional and mental alarms and then turn the alarm off and go live with a smile, a hug, and an adventure of life that includes sharing, caring, and learning.

Craving: Cold Dairy

Affirmations:

- I am willing to try a new way of thinking with sensing and honoring my real body's needs.
- I am ready to be mature even when I am scared and bored.
- I can do something fun and exciting every time I have a problem in my life.
- I welcome life's challenges because I am becoming my true self.
- I find warmth and soothing in my breath, my connection to my heart, and to my soul.
- I find someone in need and enjoy making a moment difference in their life.

Supporting Foods:

- Celery
- Carrots
- Applesauce
- Peas
- Romaine lettuce
- Spinach
- Smoothie
- Avocados
- White pepper
- Sprouted almonds
- Sprouts
- Fermented foods
- Salmon
- Radishes
- Root vegetables

Craving: Gluten

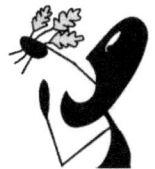

Troubled Mindset

- You are living in a crazy world around you.
- The people say one thing and often do another.
- You can't rely on their attitudes anymore because their moodiness is often painful or offensive.
- Your desire to change others is currently overshadowed by the necessity to survive, cope with physical pain, and meet nutritional needs that won't trigger stomach issues. However, you feel a strong urge to eat something containing gluten to fulfill your craving.
- You want deeper sweetness in life than what you are getting from anyone close to you.
- How many times have you been stressed and you couldn't help yourself and you grabbed some bread until you couldn't stop eating until you were full of it?
- Have you noticed that when you act out your cravings for gluten, you feel worse? This is because the body is in a vicious cycle of pain from engaging in 'pleasure.'
- The endorphins that come from eating the gluten are feeding the problem instead of solving it.
- Eating your problems away are showing you that your problems are eating you.

Craving: Gluten

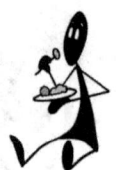

Healing Mindset

It is time to be present in time. Your craving makes you step away from your real self far too often. Being present in the here and now will help you see what you are escaping and what you are chasing. The immature self is driving you away from growing up.

It is time to embrace the fear of starvation and realize you won't. What you are running from is the thought that you will never ever be happy, get what you want, or be taken care of.

It's time to be real and authentic with yourself and slowly step into greater, genuine experience of life. Eating what is healthy and helpful first, then consider pleasure from another source, such as walking, breathing, laughing. Joyful laughter will fill your heart, so you don't have to use harmful reactive foods to harm your life. Change your view, open your eyes, open your heart to new experiences before you satisfy something that takes instead of gives.

Craving: Gluten

Affirmations:
- I am grateful for each and every moment.
- I choose this day to serve my higher good.
- I am strong and patient with my other self.
- I have so much to live for.
- I can do this.
- I turn the pain into learning and maturity.

Supporting Foods:

- Almonds (sprouted)
- Avocado
- Berries
- Black beans
- Brazil nuts
- Broccoli (steamed & raw)
- Carrots (steamed & raw)
- Cauliflower (steamed & raw)
- Celery
- Celery juice
- Fish
- Hummus
- Millet
- Mung beans
- Peas
- Quinoa
- Salmon
- Sprouts
- Squash (acorn, banana, spaghetti, yellow, etc.)
- Yam
- Walnut
- Watermelon

Craving: Ice Cream

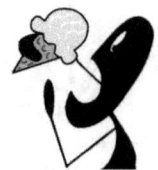

Troubled Mindset

- Your mind thinks, "Who wants to deal with all the upsets and concerns when I can grab another bowl of ice cream?"
- Avoiding upsets or concerns postpones the conflict so that your body will have sort it out. And when it can't, it stores it as weight, awaiting future processing.
- The world is full of surprises and sometimes you have chosen to take these as painful, hurtful, or scary.
- Even though some of your emotional past is deeply hidden, it pops up suddenly in daily interactions with others, and then you take it out on yourself by overeating a frozen treat.
- This is masquerading as a reward but in reality, it is harmful to your gut, body, immune system, digestion, and weight. Thus it becomes addictive because it is full of pleasure and pain.
- Your thoughts include that it is one way to create your own special surprise with what seems to be of little consequence.
- However, the problem is long term and the consequence gradually grows on you and overtakes you until you are a slave to the thoughts and actions that are mandated by the craving.

Craving: Ice Cream

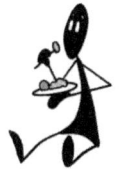

Healing Mindset

It is time to recognize that this craving is beyond your normal capacity to randomly choose to stop or change. The key is to not be random, but choose to gradually and consistently, eat less and less of the frozen treat. You will always have some upset or concern, because that is life. But life can be full of discovery when you focus on the treat of learning, growing, and sharing your heart.

You will find joy in finding those who care and appreciate it when you share yourself with them. The nice smooth creamy feeling that numbed your pain but never really took it away can now be replaced with fine foods that are creamy, but healthy, and relationships that are mutually uplifting. Last of all, start the gradual process of calming your emotional judgments and replacing them with positive encouragements.

Craving: Ice Cream

Affirmations:
- I let the fears be a gentle breeze that softly flows away.
- I choose to be free and to be the true me.
- When I need love and acceptance, I take care of myself first and then find a positive reward.
- I comfort my little one deep inside with time, understanding, and creative expression.
- I discover for myself the difference my heart feels when I comfort with making a difference in another's life.
- A generous hand and a comforting hug sweeps out the cravings from under the rug.
- I love my heart, my body, and my smile.

Supporting Foods:

- Quinoa (3 three colors mixed)
- Millet
- Spinach
- Salmon
- Cherry tomatoes
- Tangerine
- Chicken
- Broccoli
- Grass-fed beef
- Bananas
- Avocados
- Apricots
- Watermelon
- Carrots
- Celery
- Rye
- Amaranth
- Corn
- Adzuki beans
- Lettuce
- Pumpkin
- Scallion
- Alfalfa
- Kohlrabi
- White pepper
- Raw honey

Craving: Salty Foods

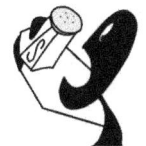

Troubled Mindset

- You think life is going pretty good and you are going to keep it that way.
- You don't try to worry but if it gets out of hand, a little seasoning helps the moment.
- You don't like to be bored and you want others to find interest in what you have to express.
- You don't think you have an attitude but you think everyone else does.
- You can keep to yourself, and you expect everyone else should.
- You like to communicate when they have something interesting to say.
- You have a deep worry that you will be alone someday, but you don't let that come to the surface.
- You have a fear others will see your tears.
- You can take care of yourself.
- You ask for what you want, take action when you need to, and find what you are searching for.
- The only path you need is an interesting one that you direct and that you can control.
- You have patience when things are working out, otherwise you put a little pressure on others to go your direction.
- The foods you eat are bland without something extra.
- You need to preserve the taste, the experience, and insights that you have and want to share.

Craving: Salty Foods

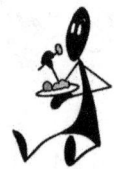

Healing Mindset

Your body needs salt and other minerals to function. It is a part of every cellular function. Your heart, your nerves, your kidneys, all need minerals to work properly. Look at your life and consider how much effort you are putting into it to function. Look how many thoughts you have that include judgments towards others. You may be pushing your blame and shame onto others so that you can go forward in your quest or work. You can stop and think about your thoughts and actions.

Take a moment and see value in your relationships. If you will do this, then you can stop and see your own emotional upsets. Judgments and emotions are signals that you can use to help yourself adjust. Forcing your words on others won't change what matters inside. Temporary control leads to more cravings and frustrations. Take a breath, take time to savor the taste of your food and life. Narrow thinking leads to bland living. Open your eyes and take a moment to see value in all things and all people.

Craving: Salty Foods

Affirmations:

- The zest of life is all around me.
- The joy of living is in every breath.
- I season my life with a vast interest in many things.
- I enjoy finding positive ways to communicate with my family, friends, and associates.
- I savor the connection with others.
- I allow my mind to be open to new ideas.
- I am safe to care when someone is lost inside.
- I notice when others are not safe and calm my thoughts to respect them.
- My mind is clear and my heart is safe.
- I am supportive and not controlling.

Supporting Foods:

- Watermelon
- Celery
- Peaches
- Pears
- Carrots
- Kohlarbi
- Jicama
- Parsnips
- Sweet potatoes
- Quinoa
- Amaranth
- Fermented cabbage
- Pineapple
- Papaya
- Seaweed

Craving: Sex

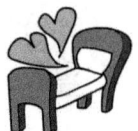

Troubled Mindset

- You are stressed in your life and you don't know who or where to turn to.
- You desperately want to enjoy living but living is not bringing you joy.
- You may be asking yourself: "What happened to the good times?" "What happened when life was simpler?" "Why can't I have what I want?" "Why is life so complicated?" "I don't understand when others refuse my need for connection and relief."
- Finding relief through sex won't satisfy the deep need for unconditional acceptance and constant bliss.
- It is as if your inner child is seeking something that never happened. As if you have separation anxiety from your mother and/or father and you are using sex to reconnect your inner child with the parental love that wasn't there and isn't here now.
- You are letting your inner pain take over your thoughts and feelings.
- To wipe away your suffering with pleasure is to add more clutter and burden to the experience each and every time.

Craving: Sex

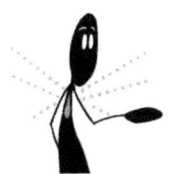

Healing Mindset

It is time to find joy and bliss in a new way. Using sex for stress release is creating a strain on your "pleasure part of self." Separate the two parts of yourself - the pleasure self from the stressful self. Because if you don't, the two intermingle into a painful self - that is tainted with frustration or shame.

There is no real and true love in a painful, shameful, or frustrated-based sexual act. It becomes a routine and thus is not real enjoyment but an addictive pattern. It is time to change the patterns by changing the root of the experience. Start by drawing, writing, breathing, stretching out your suffering, judgments, and justifications.

Take notice when your craving is based on stress relief and when it is simply a desire to connect. It is a lie to think you have to have sex or any other craving because your craving is ruling your mind and body. Desiring sex is cleaner and rewarding. Craving it is depleting and deceiving self. Real love has nothing to do with sex. Real love has to do with deep connection with touch, respect, joy, sharing, oneness, and openness.

Craving: Sex

Affirmations:
- I am the one who is in charge.
- I enjoy pleasure that is pain-free and respectful to me and the other person.
- I let go of my justifications in favor of living an authentic experience.
- I choose joy when I experience sex.
- I am grateful for deep connective touch.

Supporting Foods:
- Fennel
- Salmon
- Black beans
- Brazil nuts
- Soaked chia seeds

Craving: Spicy Foods

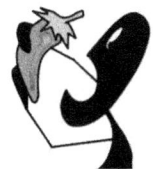

Troubled Mindset

- You are smart and brave and almost true.
- You feel the need to push the river of discovery at work, in sports, or in friendships, but you still shy away from really being honest with those hidden emotions that bother you.
- You want to deal with the bothersome hidden feelings but you can't because of all the problems that will arise if you do.
- You can't deal with a nagger, a blamer, a critic, and yet sometimes you are the nagging one, the blaming one, and the critical pointer.
- You must go on and so you do and you use food and other things to give you that punch you need of excitement.
- The push for fun and excitement is fine as long as it doesn't sacrifice your body and heart.
- Your body will always know what you are escaping from. So if you use food to escape, every time you have conflict, it will push you to get some spicy nourishment to keep your own personal excitement going, even though it appears that others are trying to take it away from you.

Craving: Spicy Foods

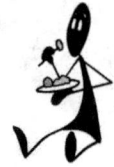

Healing Mindset

Don't be afraid. That sounds odd to you because you are pushing the excitement of life with food and other activities. However, underneath is some anger and beneath that is fear and under that is a little sadness that you are definitely are hiding from. You think that physical pain to your gut with too much spice is easier than dealing with your heart pain.

What if you stop the clock and take a moment to pause? Perhaps you can discover the excitement right there inside of you. Your escape from inner conflict is being mirrored for you in your relationships. So, take the moment and deal with it. Spice is great, but too much is a sign that you are trying to burn off something that can not be destroyed with food. Find the spice of life with discovering yourself. Discover the amazing parts of your mind, your feelings, and behaviors. You have so much to offer and so much share.

Craving: Spicy Foods

Affirmations:
- I am amazed at all the amazing creations around me.
- I find joy in the smile of a child, the laugh of a friend, the warm hug from my loved one.
- May I keep my heart open always to the gifts of the universe that are all around me.
- I am so blessed to be alive and sharing my life with all these wonderful people around me.
- I find joy in every breath.
- I find joy in the taste of all types of foods.

Supporting Foods:
- Papaya
- Pineapple
- Peaches
- Applesauce
- Carrots
- Yellow squash
- Acorn squash
- Grapefruit
- Salmon
- Free range chicken
- Turkey
- Sprouted almonds
- Cashews

Craving: Sugar

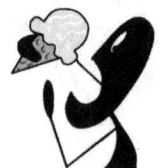

Troubled Mindset

- You are nervous about life, people, your body, and everything.
- You are anxious to get something done, but you don't think you have the time.
- The tasks at hand fill your mind with busy-ness, so filling your mouth with a quick sugar fix fools your mind and gut into thinking it settles you.
- With so much at stake, your beliefs, your pain, and your fear of the judgments of others, the sugar becomes a master and you, the slave.
- You are quickly bored, and your fantasies are too easily satisfied with sugar.
- You don't trust those who are in control of their sugar-binging.
- You don't think you can accomplish all that needs or should be done.
- You want to hide, but there is nowhere to go.
- You think and feel you deserve to have what you want when you want it.
- You think that others judge and don't care about your inner self, so you justify taking care of yourself by cheating on your body with fake sugar.
- You sense something is wrong, and you want it gone now with a quick fix... but that will make it come back larger next time.

Craving: Sugar

Troubled Mindset
(continued)

- Something sweet makes you forget for just a moment what is bothering you.
- Sugar compensates for a lack of sweetness in your life and relationships.

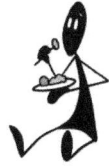

Healing Mindset

Your hidden resentments are taking a toll on your health and your mind. The sugar coating will only last for a short time. It is time to pause and notice what is genuine, authentic, valid, and supportive. Start to acknowledge what truly encourages your heart to have the passion to nourish your body with cheerful, natural sweetness. Encourage your mind to use loving and kind words for yourself with the strength of will you will take each day, one step at a time.

Craving: Sugar

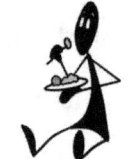

Healing Mindset
(continued)

The fake love of sugar is making your heart yearn without any genuine satisfaction in sight. So today, take the time to put a piece of food into your mouth that is fresh, natural, and not fabricated. Take the time to honor yourself with self-respecting thoughts for your mind, a caring feeling for your heart, and a sense of warmth for your body.

Difficulty with sugar cravings is a sign that your inner child needs a friend who won't judge and has the strength not to compromise. Thus, each of us needs a caring heart with a strong arm when the craving for love shows up as a mask of sugar cravings.

If you crave sugar, you might need quality fats in your diet. Thus, if you crave sugar, you might need rich emotional experiences without the anxiety from social fears. Create the path of sharing your joy with others, and you will find joy and let the sugar cravings diminish.

Craving: Sugar

Affirmations:

- I promise to love myself with a walk, positive thoughts, and a giggle.
- I am grateful for my challenge because I am learning to pause, observe, and choose.
- I put the object of my craving on the counter and pause with a nice walk.
- I want to know what it feels like to be grown up for a day.
- I enjoy finding fun in life without the need for excess eating treats.
- I face my fantasy by creating fun and nourishing experiences.
- I creatively express my food experience daily.

 ## Supporting Foods:

- Apple (Fuji, Granny Smith, Jonathan)
- Avocado
- Acorn squash
- Artichokes
- Banana Squash
- Beets (red, yellow)
- Blueberries
- Carrots
- Crenshaw melon
- Garbanzo Beans
- Cucumbers
- Celery
- Hummus
- Kimchi
- Korean melon
- Lentils
- Millet
- Quinoa
- Pumpkin
- Radishes
- Raspberries
- Salmon
- Sauerkraut
- Stevia
- Tilapia
- **Tuna**
- **Yellow Squash**
- **Watermelon**
- Wild Rice
- Healthy creative preparations of foods.

Cysts

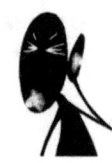

Troubled Mindset

- You are feeling guilty that you have love for the person whom you feel has betrayed you.
- You want to fight and resist, but then you wish it would all go away, and you may want to pretend it didn't happen, but negative movie reels keep rolling in your head, feeding pains from the past and reinforcing them with examples from today, generating an abnormal growth.
- Feeling sorry for yourself and for those family or friends that have been hurt won't change your situation.
- Regrets about past failures or not fulfilling certain dreams are stopping you from moving forward in your life. It is time to be clear about your role, your attitudes and your judgments.

Healing Mindset

It is time to change your heart to be clear about taking care of yourself with love, good nutrition, sleep, and exercise. Anytime you have negative thoughts towards certain people, think anew, let it go, they are on their journey. Let go of false fears and begin to trust in the promise of something good. Don't let your body become polluted with the negativity that bounces back to you. Be joyful about your creation of life - each and every day.

Cysts

Affirmations:
- I enjoy my creation of life - each and every day.
- I am clear to go and be myself, independent of the judgments and harm that have been sent my way.
- I want to be me and express my heart each day without the worries.
- I express myself, share my heart, and offer my care in a way that is not secretive, shameful, nor burdensome.
- I create with ease.
- I release the hidden resentments, live lightly, and with deep care for life and relationships.
- I love being female, and I honor and respect my body, my mind, and my heart in all situations and at all times.
- I am free to release any judgment at any time.
- I feel good about being me.

Supporting Foods:
- Meats (not fried)
- Parsley
- Safflower
- Alfalfa
- Avocados
- Fish

Dandruff

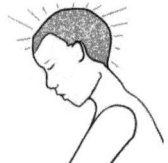

Troubled Mindset

- You are jealous, but you ignore or deny it.
- You wish things were different, but are you willing to be responsible and take your own positive action?
- You may be conflicted about what to do because your mind and heart don't agree, inducing self-doubt and blocking self-acceptance.
- You may please others to get what you want.
- You are using up your energy and drive to stay creative because you are continually placating others.
- Unable to keep it all moving, you go into overdrive.
- You may find your creativity drying up.

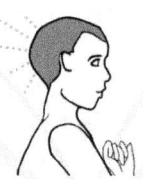

Healing Mindset

Stop. Be real with your capacities. Be true to what you want and then honor the ability and desires of others. Use your energy to be you, then watch creativity rise, and your social interactions change positively.

Dandruff

Affirmations:
- I am awake and aware of those around me and with my daily experience.
- I am safe while expressing myself and trying out social situations.
- I want to be free and be me.
- I purely live without extra worry.
- I can now relax.

Supporting Foods:

- Soured foods such as
    - Plain yogurt
    - Kimchi
    - Sauerkraut
- Raw foods
- Carrots

Dehydration

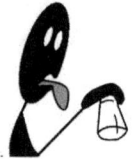

Troubled Mindset

- In my efforts to deal with life in all of its complications and demands, I come up short with being able to deal with what is happening.
- I am trying so hard, but nothing seems to be working.
- At first, I felt some discomfort with my situation, but now I feel agitated, unsettled, and hypersensitive.
- I seem to be on low-grade alert.
- I am resisting what is happening, but I can't see what to do about it.
- I feel the heat of the day, the moment, and the excess concerns that cause my body to use up vital resources in the act of dealing with the past while being afraid of what might happen in the future.
- Dehydration indicates that the use of electrolytes and minerals are off.
- You are trying too hard to manage all the details without success.
- The answers you need are right where you are. You can't see them because you are not here and now. Pause.

Dehydration

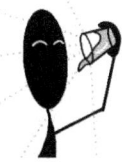

Healing Mindset

Take a moment to sip a little bit of water and let it sit quietly in your mouth. Take those thoughts of needing to act, do, run around, worry and put them aside. Let yourself enjoy the refreshment that nature abundantly provides our bodies. But if you rush around not appreciating the gift of life, it will wash over you without making a difference to your inner world.

It is time to deal with your avoidance patterns of truly being nourished and fully being cared for by nature. Each sip of water is life-giving, life-sustaining, and life-renewing. It is time to concentrate on what is real and not what is regretful or wishful thinking. Instead of jumping to food or sodas when you are anxious, pause with a sip of fresh water. Instead of thinking all is lost, pause with sensing all that you have and every moment is a gift. Be real with your feelings, your body, and your inner natural self. You can change what is happening around you once you embrace what is happening within you.

Dehydration

Affirmations:

- I choose to be in the moment and deal with what I can.
- I choose to accept what is happening, while having the courage to go forward.
- I am grateful for what I have, who I am, and the opportunity for change.
- I don't sweat the small stuff; I calmly and clearly organize it.
- I allow life to reveal its secrets with curiosity and awe.
- I succeed by accepting what is real, and acting on what I can.
- I see what is happening around me and embrace what is happening within me.
- I am feeling nourished by real food, real water, and real love.

Supporting Foods:

- Cucumbers
- Celery
- Carrots
- Watermelon
- Melons
- Blackberries
- Blueberries
- Apples
- Peaches
- Apricots
- Broccoli
- Cauliflower
- Soups
- Broths
- Some herbal teas
- Radishes
- Grapefruit
- Oranges
- Dragonfruit

Depression

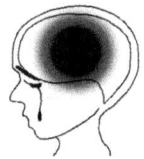

Troubled Mindset

- You feel sad and down, but underneath you are suppressing frustration and/or fear.
- You are hiding in a cave to avoid dealing with feelings, failures, upsets, and regrets.
- You lack the control to change others and your circumstances.
- You want to change your world, but your inner-world becomes too heavy and burdensome to try anymore.
- You fear being anxious more than being sad, depressed, and shut down.
- It is easier to do nothing than to do something & fail.
- You want to be right, and you think you are, but no one listens to you anyway.
- You blame others for the betrayal of your feelings, but it is an excuse so you don't have to deal with it anymore.
- You are suppressing feelings of anger and sadness because you don't think that you "should" feel that way.
- You may have a need to be right about an event, person, or situation, and can't seem to let go of it.
- Your hopes or expectations are unfulfilled.
- You may have realized that things are not the way you thought they were.

Depression

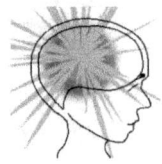

Healing Mindset

Holding on to the old is keeping you down. Emotions aren't meant to be "right" or "wrong," they just are. Feel them, free them, allow them to flow through you, and then release them. Seek understanding or acceptance of the higher purpose for what has happened. Nourish yourself with vibrant and healthy food and find joy and hope in what life teaches you.

Take 10 minutes a day to take care of you. If you are willing to move, then do stretches and exercises that get the blood flowing from head to toe. If you don't want to move, then draw or doodle while doing a breathing interval of breathing out, pausing, and then breathing in and pausing. Draw with your non-dominant hand first, and then the dominant hand. Journal your feelings with the idea of a river running through you washing away "gunk" and "clutter."

Depression is sometimes suppression of feelings and energies that need somewhere to go. Give it a path by firmly touching your body, stretching, and moving your body, singing and connecting to someone that is safe. Your brain and heart are trying desperately to work it

Depression

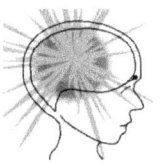

Healing Mindset
(Continued)

out, so slow down the process and find hope in the gradual process of self-help rather than getting hopeless about not being able to change the outside world.

Connect to a divine sense that is always there but when the clouds over your head are dark it is difficult to feel them. The light is always there, just let the clouds part just enough to let some of it in.

Depression

Affirmations:

- I hold onto joy, love, and expressions of laughter and sharing.
- I let go of grief, "if only," "it shouldn't have been," and "it is hopeless."
- I am hopeful.
- Life is a great teacher and opportunity.
- I remove the need to hold onto stuck thoughts and heavy feelings.
- I can gradually do life.
- I am safe to just be.
- I take a chance at feeling moments of joy, love, expressions of laughter, and sharing my inner ideas.
- I take a moment to let someone share their care.
- I part the clouds of despair to let the warmth of life and light come in.
- Underneath it all, I feel there is hope in finding my true core self.
- Every day, I take time for my inner self to have some play and fun.
- My suffering is not as big as it seems, my healing is easier than I thought.

Supporting Foods:

- Water/Get hydrated
- Raw fruits & vegetables
- Apple cider vinegar
- Soybeans
- Soy products
- Brown rice
- Millet
- Legumes
- Salmon
- White fish
- Turkey
- Cucumbers
- Watermelon
- Apples
- Cabbage
- Micro-algae

Diabetes

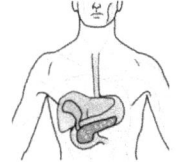

Troubled Mindset

- You are angry, frustrated, upset, and lonely.
- You experience loneliness at the gut or soul level.
- You have experienced a large emotional shock or repeated emotional shocks (perhaps both) that have gotten stuck in your mind, heart, and/or body.
- You expected life to be different, and you gave your best, but it didn't turn the way you wanted.
- You wish you could escape the reality of pain, suffering, and blame.
- You have suppressed your anger and resentment for too long.
- Your need to be right gets challenged by the discomfort that you have to get along with your relationships.
- You might even think of some as inferior and that they don't get it.
- You wish others would just change to make your life easier.
- You often feel that you are missing the love, the affection, and the approval that you deserve.
- Your craving for the sweetness in life is temporarily satisfied with food, but not for long.

Diabetes

Healing Mindset

D When you feel the desire to control others or your experience in order to get what you want: stop first and consider the consequences. You lose more in your relationships and wellbeing when you are controlling than what you gain in being right or resisting the way things are.

The same applies to eating. If you try to suppress your cravings for love, attention, and control, with eating excess foods, processed foods, or overly sweetened foods, then you will suffer a consequence of your body suffering. You use foods to suppress the emotions because you feel a need to escape reality. You acknowledge that you have made excuses, but your attitude is just pushing the emotions away and 'go on with life.' Feeling any shame, guilt, or sadness is much too painful. Instead, you resolve to find happy communication, interesting conversation, trying to control situations, or having angry forceful moments.

Look at your need to win as a positive push to find answers for your problems, but not to control. Look at the need for sweets as a positive push to create valid and authentic relationships that include respect, honor, and gratitude. See that your craving for sweets is an indication of the lack of mature patience to walk yourself through discomfort to strength in your character.

It is time to let go of the fear of discomfort, fear of failure, resentments to others and situations, the false sweetness, fear of judgments, and attacking words to others. It is time to embrace authentic expression and valid trust in yourself and others.

Diabetes

Affirmations:

- I flow with life.
- I enjoy the sweetness of each day and each person.
- I learn from everyone.
- I let go of every resentment to every person and event.
- I enjoy being real with what is sweet in life.
- I enjoy each person.
- I learn from everyone.
- I turn past resentments into opportunities for growth and learning.
- I am blessed.
- I am discovering the satisfaction of authentic sweetness in life.

Supporting Foods:

- Egg yolks
- Fish
- Garlic
- Kelp
- Legumes
- Root vegetables
- Kale
- Kohlrabi
- Whole grains
- Berries
- Brewer's yeast
- Dairy products
- Cheese
- Sauerkraut
- Soybeans
- Agar Agar
- Walnuts
- Soaked flaxseed
- Soaked chia seeds
- Garbanzo beans
- Papaya
- Pineapple
- Black beans
- Vegetable juices
- Foods high in complex carbohydrates
- High fiber plenty of raw fruits and vegetables

Diarrhea

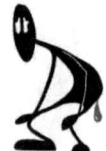

Troubled Mindset

- You have decided to let go of your goals and aspirations because you believe you cannot achieve them.
- You feel lost and helpless and don't know where to go from here.
- You may be resisting assimilating all the understanding you need to progress.
- You'd rather rush through and get it over with or just run away.
- You're carrying a fair amount of anxiety around your capability to have success.

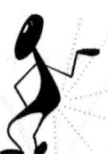

Healing Mindset

Cool your jets. Pause your steps and your mind. Decide what is important and organize yourself on a positive path to get there. Trust in the slow and steady progression. Each time your mind or body runs too fast, breathe, recenter, and trust in your forward path.

Diarrhea

Affirmations:

- I can do this.
- I have the tools and the ability to deal with my life, responsibilities, and goals.
- I let go of my blame, regret, and frustration and turn my life into a positive, enjoyable experience.
- There is nothing wrong with learning as I go and enjoying the fruits of my labors.

Supporting Foods:

- Water/Get hydrated
- Apples
- Asparagus
- Bananas
- Barley
- Beans
- Beets
- Cabbage
- Carrots
- Citrus fruits
- Fibrous foods
- Meats (moderate amounts and not fried)
- Fish
- Green peppers
- Kale
- Kelp
- Garlic
- Millet
- Okra
- Rice
- Romaine lettuce
- Watermelon

Dizziness (Vertigo)

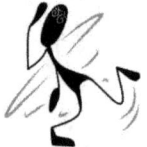

Troubled Mindset

- You might not be taking enough time for yourself, and you are overloaded to the point that you feel you can't cope anymore. This is causing you to feel unstable and off-balance.
- You find it challenging to accept things as they are and often feel that they don't turn out as you expected.
- You may be trying to control your external world, now you are beginning to realize you can't.

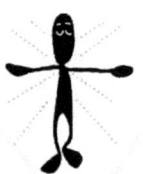

Healing Mindset

Getting real and facing problems head-on feels scarier than spinning in circles around the issues. Pause your life. Breathe and ground yourself. Running away and chasing everything at once is over the top. Go simple, think simple, then find direction and patiently follow it.

Dizziness (Vertigo)

Affirmations:
- I pause, breathe, and ground myself easily and regularly.
- I choose to focus on the simple, then act.
- I patiently follow my direction.
- I calm the overwhelm with waves of trust and comfort.
- I believe I did enough in the past, and the future holds bright for those who see the magic of enjoying the life that we have been given.

Supporting Foods:

- Bell peppers
- Broccoli (steamed)
- Citrus fruits
- Chia seeds (soaked)
- Celery juice
- Fermented foods
- Red beets
- Asparagus

Drug Addiction

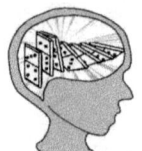

Troubled Mindset

- You are masking feelings of emotional pain that you do not want to feel.
- You've turned towards substance abuse for a short term reward, but are causing long term damage.
- You've had a lot done for you rather than learning from taking care of yourself.
- Now, you have displaced responsibility for your actions and placed it into other people's hands.
- Instead of filling your own needs appropriately, you do wrong to yourself then accuse others because you feel they don't fill your actual needs; needs that can only be filled by you, and you alone.
- When you realize why you have an addiction, you can confront the source of the problem head-on.

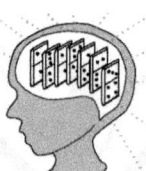

Healing Mindset

Addiction is a mask for a deeper need or pain. Heal that rift of pain that causes you to suffer, and you will find an inner strength to deal with those overwhelming behaviors. Choose today, right now, to step slowly and consistently towards the courage and action that will reroute your brain and habits into a better life.

Drug Addiction

Affirmations:

- I can choose to enjoy life.
- I choose to feel connected to others by sharing a piece of my heart; this will uplift both me and them.
- I no longer push myself.
- I am done with the silly and crazy ways.
- I see the tear of a child, feel the rose petal, and embrace the sun's ray; these are what truly matter.
- I connect to what is real and precious, letting go of anything fake.
- I choose to be authentic in heart and enjoy life through genuine care and sharing.
- I have the courage to be upset with myself and be okay with it.
- I can deal with life without resorting to excuses.
- I am good to go and fully embrace myself in any challenge that arises.

Supporting Foods:

- Sprouts
- Leafy greens
- Wild blue/green algae
- Cereal grasses
- Vegetables
- Flax seeds/oil
- Salmon
- Bananas
- Cod
- Trout
- Goat's milk
- Seaweeds
- Eat a well-balanced, nutrient-dense diet with many fresh, raw foods

Dry Lips

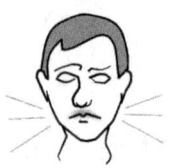

Troubled Mindset

- You may be wishing to speak but holding back until you can privately tell 'that certain someone' who you think should be different.
- The bout of thoughts that could pound in your head is relieved because you choose to be pleasant in the presence of others. However, that doesn't change the subtle thoughts that you wish you could change your life situation.
- Emotions can dry your heart if you let them, so you have kept the effort going of being the better self most of the time with most people.
- Licking your lips will only dry them more because the moisture needs to come from within.

Dry Lips

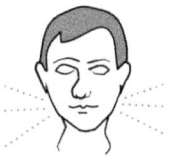

Healing Mindset

Just like the moisture needs to come from within, so does peace and acceptance in life. Emotional balance comes from your personal integrity from within.

You are honest with your abstentions from lying or deceiving but not honest with your deeper feelings. Of course, you can make a huge change for the dryness by finding one positive experience or positive trait of the one person you secretly judge. Behind all this, it is time to love yourself. Being a little bit of a perfectionist doesn't help your heart feel the depth of warmth from your relationships.

Dry Lips

Affirmations:
- I enrich each moment by being true to sensing feelings of appreciation, enquiry, and enriching the lives of others.
- For every negative feeling, I offer my heart two positive experiences.
- I am beginning the simple task of forgiving myself for my self-judgments and I see I am worthy of positive, warm love.
- I observe my deeper feelings honestly.

Supporting Foods:

- Bell pepper
- Berries
- Cantaloupe
- Cauliflower
- Celery
- Coconut
- Crenshaw melon
- Cucumbers
- Grapefruit
- Honeydew
- Lettuce
- Okra
- Oranges
- Peaches
- Peas
- Tomato
- Watermelon
- Yam
- Zucchini

Duodenum Problems

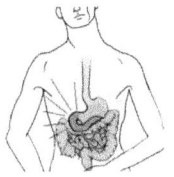

Troubled Mindset

- You carry a deep dependency rooting from a maternal need that you felt was unmet. Your life and actions have often been oriented around this chasm.
- You've lived with a hyper-ambitious drive or industrious obsession to become independent that arises from a deep dependency for approval, rather than from curiosity or joy.
- You have reached the peak of this conflict between being dependent on approval and becoming independent.
- The conflicts within yourself are carried into family life and reinforced.
- You've been angered by things others have said or done and struggle to know how to handle or process it.
- The stress with your duodenum is indicating that resolution is needed now.

Duodenum Problems

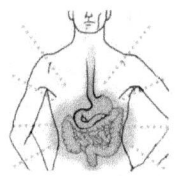

Healing Mindset

Take a step back; the hurt has felt too personal. Look at it as though it is on a stage, and you are the observer or director. Notice how the power to heal is not found with others but with your own inner child.

Connect your current capacity with that power and self-soothe through the needs of the past. Allow your ambitions to reroot and ground in true curiosity, interest, and desire to make a difference in the world. Seek clarity on the big picture and relax your overemphasis on little details.

Duodenum Problems

Affirmations:

- I am safe and filled with the love of the universe and nature.
- I am really good at separating and sorting life.
- I enjoy the challenge of daily dealings because it is an opportunity to see what is of value, what I can do with it, how to process through it, and then enjoy the fruits of my actions.
- I let the worries and doubts be signals to pay attention to.
- I embrace courage as my friend, loyalty as my motto, truth as my course, faith as my banner.
- I love myself.
- I nourish myself.
- I am awesome.

 ## Supporting Foods:

- Water/stay hydrated
- Whole grains
- Legumes
- Raw nuts and seeds
- Alfalfa sprouts
- Mung bean sprouts
- Green leafy vegetables
- Eat plenty of raw foods and vegetables
- Banana
- Broccoli
- Brussel sprouts
- Celery
- Cucumber
- Garlic
- Kelp
- Mango
- Papaya
- Pineapple
- Sauerkraut
- Brown rice
- Turkey

Dyslexia

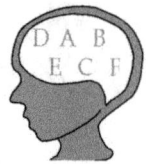

Troubled Mindset

- Life is backward sometimes.
- What you expected didn't happen, but what you feared still lingers because it troubles you that you can't get a handle on your experience.
- You've pushed yourself with too much, too soon.
- You wanted to perform at a level beyond your current capabilities.
- Your mind and heart come up with results that confuse your senses.
- Pushing yourself too hard is creating too much pressure, causing you to slip up and make simple mistakes.
- You were intent on surviving through practical issues when you began venturing to symbolic and abstract things, like letters. The mind is powerful enough to fill in the gaps of understanding, but most often, the guessing is not working well enough to keep you safe.
- It has been embarrassing to feel handicapped when missing pieces of vital information.
- You might get angry, or you might be afraid. These emotions add to the distractibility of your attention because not staying present feels safer than facing personal blame or the constructive criticism of those around you.

Dyslexia

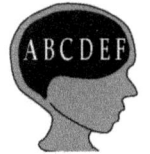

Healing Mindset

Right Hemisphere: You are focused on emotionally handling the challenge. The extra emotional exertion makes you slow but accurate.

Left Hemisphere: You're making it happen with a 'fake it to make it' type attitude. You are quick but make many mistakes.

Embrace your strengths to support you in getting a grip. It is true that you don't have all the information you need in so many situations. But that is the fun challenge of life. While others have it easy, you have it unique. What you see, feel, think, and sense causes you to paint a world that most don't get to experience! Cherish those gifts and learn to bridge the experience you have in your internal world with that of others. You will find a fascinating adventure of insight and understanding. Your gifts will blossom, your confidence will rise, and your life will be enriched. It is good to verify your ideas and your understandings, but don't negate your view. Blend your perspective and work with both worlds.

Dyslexia

Affirmations:
- I am alive with ideas and perceptions.
- I am excited to experience the many views of my mind and the minds of others.
- While I see and hear differently, I enjoy bridging the creative and logical world to my benefit.
- I am creative, expressive, and motivated.
- I am blessed with a very unique life, and I am grateful for the opportunity to share my view.
- I integrate all parts of myself while respecting myself fully.
- I am seeing my mind and heart heal gradually.
- I become safe to experience my unique perceptions while also integrating what is real.
- I feel fortunate to be me in my daily development.

Dyslexia

Supporting Foods:

- Alfalfa sprouts
- Sprouted almonds
- Avocado
- Blackberry
- Blueberry
- Broccoli
- Cauliflower
- Chives
- Dill
- Lentils
- Millet
- Onion
- Papaya
- Potato, red
- Proteins
- Quinoa
- Raspberry
- Rice
- Romain lettuce
- Spinach
- Warm foods
- Yam
- Carrots & celery (with onion, chives, or dill. Raw or steamed.)
- Barley (if not gluten-sensitive)
- Organic strawberries
- Sunflower seeds
- Sprouted sunflower seeds
- Lightly cooked vegetables

Ear

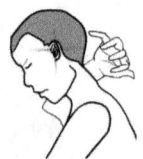

Troubled Mindset

- What you hear and what you perceive is not working out.
- You are reluctant to really catch what is going on around you, or you feel no one is listening to you.
- You have resistance to hearing or understanding a new perspective, including, perhaps especially, from your inner wisdom.
- Many of the words and sounds make you feel uncomfortable and cause conflict in your mind or heart.
- You resist the sounds because the experience is painful.
- Your blame or guilt makes new ideas throw off your balance, creating a struggle to grasp the true nature of the issue.
- You're highly sensitive and upset by critical or constructive feedback, in part because you already carry a false belief that you deserve rejection.
- Your sensitive self needs a safe place, but you still haven't found it. Instead, you punish yourself for your decisions.
- You are dismissing your inner voice and keep listening to the criticism of others as though they are more important and knowledgeable about you than you are about yourself.

Ear

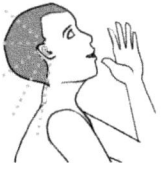

Healing Mindset

You need to listen to your true self and love yourself. If your inner voice is critical, blaming, harmful, fearful, or worrisome, then that voice is not your true voice.

Find your true voice, the voice that is encouraging and forgiving. Relax the resistance to love, peace, and joy. Open once again to the wisdom and guidance within you so you can become a part of life's blessing. Calm the sounds that cause conflict and begin the process of finding true self-acceptance and self-compassion. You are a person of worth. Find real safety that is based on facing your feelings, not hiding or running from them. Be not afraid.

Ear

Affirmations:

- I hear the quiet.
- I listen for the soft sounds of warmth of love.
- I acknowledge the simple.
- I appreciate the pure.
- I offer my mind thoughts that are honoring and respectful to my true self.
- I follow the inner core values of faith, hope, and love.
- The noise around me is my interruption to keep me safe.
- I realize now I am safe.
- I am balanced, and then I observe, and I experience my world.
- I reward my hearing with thoughts of self-respect, my feelings with warmth, and understanding, and my body with positive physical development.

Supporting Foods:

- Carrots
- Parsley
- Citrus seed extract
- Millet
- String beans
- Mung bean sprouts
- Watermelon and other melons
- Barley
- Kidney beans
- Black beans
- Blackberry
- Blueberry
- Wheat germ
- Seaweeds
- Spirulina
- Crab
- Eggs
- Tofu

Elbows

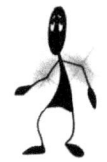

Troubled Mindset

- You are resisting the future while trying to hold up the past; this holds you back and keeps you from success or new experiences.
- You are trying to be flexible while being stubborn about things happening a certain way.
- Your insecurity is causing you to overcompensate for possible problems.
- You try to keep everyone together and everything going. But sometimes it is difficult to maintain this exertion when motivated by fear of what might happen if you don't keep juggling life and everything around you.
- You are very capable, but you've been unwise.
- You can sense some trouble, but you overreact.
- You end up not holding enough of a boundary for yourself and feel encroached on, or you are demanding your space and 'elbowing' people out of the way.
- Working with others feels difficult when you don't really understand your own circumstances and needs or theirs.

Elbows

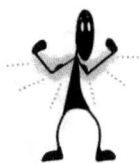

Healing Mindset

Right Elbow: You feel others are overstepping into your territory. You are not taking care of your needs so you can enjoy a fulfilled life. "How can I manifest my passion?"

Left Elbow: You are leaning too much on others. You end up indecisive, overemotional, or suppressing your feelings. Your values and your aspirations feel conflicted. You are not sure that your desire matches your soul's plan.

Care for your needs and values while respecting the needs and values of others. Recognizing your equality with others will help your sense of personal need not become inflated or diminished. Take feelings of resistance and use them as a guide that you are overcompensating with fear and control. Take your overachieving to do it all, and slow the pace. Be observant. Be honest with your real values, and then be diligent and productive with clarity and focus. Your ambition is good, but not with too much overwork or force. Be one with your life, and life will be one with you.

Elbows

Affirmations:
- I am flexible and strong.
- I am at my best when I enjoy acting on what I clearly choose to be and do.
- I enjoy watching my true self grow in strength and courage as I face the struggles of the day.
- I am capable and wise in my use of strength in action.
- I take care of my needs, then act.
- I root into my true self, and release the need for approval from others.
- I connect with my path as I embrace and act according to my core values.

Supporting Foods:
- Barley
- Wheatgrass
- Alfalfa
- Sprouts
- Celery
- Black sesame seeds
- Mulberry
- Green leafy vegetables
- Almonds
- Goat's milk
- Herbal teas
- Broths
- Eggs
- Asparagus
- Garlic
- Onions
- Brown rice
- Rye
- Whole wheat
- Fish
- Fresh pineapple
- Flaxseeds
- Oat bran
- Rice bran

Emotion: Anger

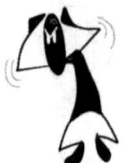

Troubled Mindset

- You have suppressed your fear.
- You are afraid of losing control of a person, thing, or situation.
- You are not holding your boundaries well and you need the capacity to hold quality personal space.
- You feel like you have lost others' respect and feel infuriated about it to mask the hurt.
- The anger you feel as a result of your need to control can destroy relationships with both people and your own body.
- Anger is helpful if channelled correctly but highly destructive if used by your pride and ego.
- When the liver struggles with immune issues, blood sugar problems, and toxins in the environment, you will be more irritable and angry. Your liver needs lots of support.
- You may be choosing to be careless and irresponsible with heated control, rather than respecting yourself, others, and life.

Emotion: Anger

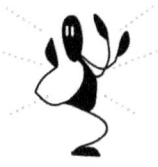

Healing Mindset

Anger becomes explosive only after we have repressed or suppressed it for so long that we have lost connection with our love. When you feel the frustration of unmet expectations but are able to maintain your love, you can express your needs in a balanced and honest way. Allow yourself to feel the real emotions behind the anger. That is the pathway back to the love that is hidden within you.

Use your anger as a motivation to move and make change. Your body feels stuck and trapped so get moving and change the state of your mind and your body. Create times of discovery and challenge your life adventure to use the intensity of anger in your favor.

If you are frustrated with someone, remember that it is a reflection of your own inner self-struggle. Be respectful to the person that delivers you a message from your inner self. They are doing you a favor that you need to deal with your ego, your pride, and things that you have pushed away for too long.

Emotion: Anger

Affirmations:

- I love life.
- I maintain positive control with trust of a higher power.
- I trust the universe.
- I allow others to be themselves.
- My desire is fulfilled with respect and cooperation.
- Everyone is my teacher.
- I appreciate the signals I receive from my emotions and take positive action to move through them.
- I have the strength to pause and move forward with courage.
- I release the excess frustrations and maintain my love.
- I observe neutrally and respectfully, then make positive movement and change.

Supporting Foods:

- Green salads with chicken
- Fish with carrots and feta
- Boiled egg over brown rice
- Soaked chia seeds
- Sauerkraut
- Red beets
- Beet greens
- **Lemon & lime**
- Bananas
- Apple
- Sprouts
- Soaked almonds
- Quinoa
- Salmon
- Papaya

Emotion: Bitter

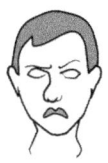

Troubled Mindset

- Just as bitter herbs are cleansers to the body, difficult experiences are to teach you and help you become more emotionally mature.
- When you hold on to excessive bitterness, it doesn't allow the experiences of life to mold you and cleanse you of emotional baggage.
- Holding onto a regret and judgment that life should have been different and adding resentment to that belief, will canker you.
- To heal and change your personal poison takes courage to stand up to your own personal struggles.
- Hating another will not make you a better person.
- Resenting self, others, and events is not allowing understanding and healing.
- Bitterness is a sign that your physical body and emotional self need some cleaning up.

Emotion: Bitter

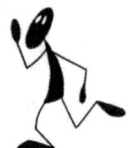

Healing Mindset

You don't have to do anything or be anything that you don't want to do or be. However, if you need to hold onto a bitter attitude about life and its problems, then you are still a slave to your situation. Part of you is bitter towards another part of you that is only hiding behind a smokescreen made of regrets, lost hopes, betrayals, and judgments.

Rebellion with a bitter attitude is enslaving your heart, liver, and eventually your soul into a deeper problem. Look at your fear of taking the chance to live the better part of yourself; the person who cares and has the strength to be respectful to those who are clueless.

It is time to grow up and live your deeper core values that brings a type of healing and strength that gives you an inner freedom that can not be purchased. Give yourself a new lightness and let the bitterness dissolve today.

Emotion: Bitter

Affirmations:

- I learn from all my experiences.
- I let life's painful events mold, shape, and refine me into a better human being.
- I enjoy all the aspects of life including the bitter/sweet.
- I amaze myself with finding moments of gratitude.
- I am grateful for the learning that people and life have offered to me.
- I breathe in curiosity and new awareness.
- I feel clean, alive, and well.

Supporting Foods:

- Fermented foods
- Jicama
- Asparagus
- Radishes
- Carrots
- Celery
- Watermelon
- Artichoke
- Figs
- Cabbage
- Sauerkraut
- Papaya
- Pineapple

Emotion: Fear

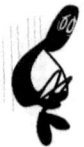

Troubled Mindset

- You have only one agenda behind the many thoughts that rush through your mind; how to be safe.
- Your need to be safe is more important than logic, and more important than truth and peace.
- If peace were your main purpose, then you would find a way to work through and face your fear.
- Courage is far away because you don't trust others, the situations, God, nor yourself.
- Fear comes as a natural survival instinct, but if used excessively, the mind becomes too narrow in its thinking, and the heart tightens in turmoil.
- The stress on the body makes you pay a painful toll that ages and sickens you.
- While you are wishing, your body is overreacting, but you are not taking action.
- You have become more irresponsible with your thoughts and feelings.
- You are in a state of lacking control.
- Notice the damage you are creating by focusing your hurt and pain from the past and forecasting it onto a possible future.
- Most likely, most of the futures you are imagining will not materialize no matter how many times the fear of it all cycles in your head.

Emotion: Fear

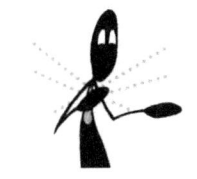

Healing Mindset

Every day, you have the opportunity and the obligation to notice your thoughts and feelings. Fear is not the enemy unless you make it your leader. Fear is meant to keep you alive in dangerous situations. And so far, you are surviving, but living in survival is not thriving. Fear is a signpost, but you have made it a roadblock.

Fear is a gift if it keeps you from falling off the cliff, but a curse if you never venture on any new path. Notice how fear effects your life. Notice where it comes from. Be wise not to blame your life on why you have fear. Fear is fear, your reaction to fear is what is spinning you in circles.

Take the time each day to embrace the possibilities of learning and growing from listening to your inner self. Take heart by allowing a gradual courage in facing life as a challenge, not an obstacle. If you want to find the real excitement of life, turn the fear inside out and let it be a part of your daily adventure of mindful discovery.

Emotion: Fear

Affirmations:
- I appreciate each moment as a gift.
- I feel amazing as I take notice of the good and positive things in my life.
- I am learning from my fears as I transition them into courage and action.
- I turn the daily obstacles into life's stepping stones.
- I enjoy creating and progressing at a pace that is safe and beneficial.
- I am the best that I can be today.
- I smile as I take the chance to be Me all day long.
- What an amazing day it is today.
- I am breathing in every moment with gratitude.
- I easily sort through the mists of confusion and find clarity and hope right at my feet.

Emotion: Fear

Supporting Foods:

- Carrots (raw or steamed)
- Parsnips
- Sweet potato
- Red potato
- Red beet
- Millet
- Barley
- Dark brown rice
- Quinoa
- Amaranth
- Seaweed
- Parsley
- Tofu
- Black beans
- Kidney beans
- Mung beans
- String beans
- Blackberry
- Banana
- Watermelon
- Raspberry
- Blueberry
- Warm soup
- Applesauce
- Cooked garlic/onion
- Romaine lettuce
- Chard
- Sprouts
- Umeboshi
- Kuzu
- Boiled egg over brown rice
- Salmon
- Lightly steamed vegetables
- Feta or high quality cheese
- Jicama
- Papaya
- Micro-greens

Emotion: Greed

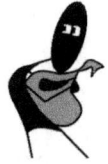

Troubled Mindset

- Behind any project or task that focuses on material gain, or power over others, is an essence of greed flowing through its veins.
- The vanity is falsely justified to continue the process of using others, or one's own body, to get whatever lie is being spoken to the unsuspecting heart.
- What is behind the need to greed? Is it some painful experience from the past that pushes you to sacrifice that which is truly valuable for the glitter that passes so quickly?
- Is it the competitive nature that won't allow you to lose at any cost even if it leaves an unresolved emptiness?

Emotion: Greed

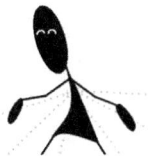

Healing Mindset

Leave it alone if your need for greed is more important than your health, your relationships, your financial core safety. Especially consider surrendering your addictive needs if you have to lie, cheat, steal, belittle, harm others or self, because greed is never satisfied. It will consume your heart and mind until your body is a slave to its demands.

Let greed be a signal that you have needs for adventure and discovery. Greed is meant to be a sign that you have deviated into the path of shadows. Get back to seeking wealth, intellect, and positive creation while staying true to core values that support your relationships to others, the divine, and your personal health of heart, mind, and body.

Emotion: Greed

Affirmations:

- I love the bliss of accomplishing projects that are made from personal integrity and true grit.
- The excitement of gain is now tempered by how to create wealth of experience for the many.
- I take time to keep my head on straight and my heart at peace.

Supporting Foods:

- Almonds, soaked
- Asparagus
- Beets
- Bell pepper
- Broccoli
- Brussel sprouts
- Butter
- Cauliflower
- Chia seeds
- Cucumbers
- Delicata squash
- Flax seeds
- Hubbard squash
- Leafy green lettuce
- Leafy red lettuce
- Mahi Mahi fish
- Microgreens (including wheatgrass, etc.)
- Millet
- Steel-cut oats
- Papaya
- Pineapple
- Quinoa
- Romaine lettuce
- Salmon
- Sprouts
- Sweet potato
- Tuna fish
- Yellow crookneck squash
- Zucchini
- Reduce excess steak, beef, swordfish, or animals that are heavy in their meat or aggressive in their nature.

Emotion: Guilt

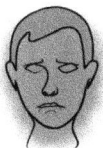

Troubled Mindset

- Feelings are not "truth", but they can speak loudly when you are running or drifting from them.
- Guilt can be a gift to society if it is used as a signal. Or, it can make people miserable if it is used to blame and overly punish others or yourself.
- For those who feel guilt; notice how you are controlling your actions and words with fear and sadness rather than reality.
- As a human, you make mistakes. Thus the guilt is a sign of conflicts from three sources; your inner values, your actions, and the judgments of others.
- With guilt, you are turning your fears and embarrassments into a set of false values. Real values and purpose are not built on guilt, shame, or fear.
- You have let your rough past consume your future.
- It is good to have a conscious, but let it bring awareness not punishment.
- It is possible that your self-judgment is greater than your crime. Notice how it affects your thoughts, your relationships, and your ability to sleep.
- If it causes you to over-eat, that feeds the problem.
- Guilt is a tool, not a weapon.

Emotion: Guilt

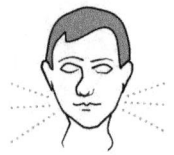

Healing Mindset

It is time to separate the burdens from the realities of your situations. You have let your guilt go too far. It was only supposed to wake you up so that you wouldn't trip again, but now it is a boulder blocking your progress on your path. Appreciate the signals from guilt, and then throw them to the wind.

Learn from the missteps so you can take many positive steps in the future. Be wise to watch when guilt leads you to shame.

Be grateful that you can still sense "a poke" from your inner self when it is appropriate to make a change. It will keep your ego in check. But a false humility dressed in guilt is still ego turned inside out. Be good to yourself and start respecting your heart, your body, and your mind without the driving chains of guilt.

Emotion: Guilt

Affirmations:
- I use my emotions for my greater good.
- I am grateful for the awareness my inner self gives me.
- I take time for me, when my heart feels down.
- I am an amazing soul with so much to offer.
- I experience each day with a passion for life.
- I feel the sun shine through my soul, delivering warmth and goodness to my heart.
- I offer quiet relief for my busy mind.
- I give my heart and my body a moment to breathe and enjoy.

Supporting Foods:
- Kidney beans
- Black beans
- Brown rice with spices
- Celery
- Warm squashes
- Soothing healthy vegetable drinks
- Pumpkin
- Papaya
- Cauliflower
- Thyme
- Basil
- Cucumber
- Coleslaw of cabbage and carrots
- Jicama
- Red beets
- Watermelon
- Blueberries

Emotion: Hatred

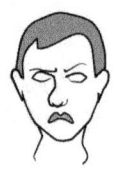

Troubled Mindset

The words and phrases that your mind repeats over and over sound a lot like this: "I have yet to find the opportunity to forgive that person. They do not deserve it. You have caused too many problems for me to forgive and let go. Besides, how can I trust you?" The only reason for forgiveness is to let go of the dark pounding of the cycle of thoughts that haunt your mind daily.

Those thoughts that cause you to hate others, hate yourself, or hate your situation in life, will only bring more problems and a skewed reality. Think of the problems that result from digging a deep trench in the pathways of your mental processes which lead to the biology of your brain and body supporting the negative thought patterns. The end is a miserable soul and the time wasted on focusing on internal dialogue that is not worth saving or sharing.

Hatred is not a core emotion; it is the mind's way of compelling you to push forward when you've experienced significant pain and suffering caused by others or yourself. It comes after a deep decision, typically following a broken trust, rejection, or betrayal.

Emotion: Hatred

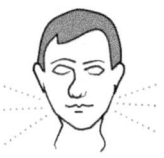

Healing Mindset

It is time for the wisdom to uncover some message that your inner self is trying to get through to you. You are fighting the inner truth that would have you let go and be free of this daily troubling torment you give yourself.

Ask yourself, "Why would you want to be subjected to negative thoughts and feelings that only hurt your mind, your body, your heart, and hurt others around you?" Your bitter attitude makes you "bark" at others around you, even if they didn't cause the problem.

Take some personal inventory. Wake up your inner parts inside that want to be free and no longer chained to this misery. If you could only see your real self: the person who cares and who is capable of handling the dark storms of life. See the person inside who can handle the negativity of others without becoming the negative energy of another. You can do this. Learn and grow. Learn how to be mature even while others are immature.

Emotion: Hatred

Affirmations:

- I choose this day to be my positive, productive self.
- I am capable, flexible, and strong.
- I am curious, what will happen when I let go of negative thoughts and feelings?
- I am mature and able to positively respond to the words and actions of others.
- I productively learn from the expressions of others.
- I am highly effective in expressing my feelings in my relationships.
- I am cool, calm, and collected in any storm.
- I am strong and kind.
- I am free to forgive and let go of all burdens.
- I let God forgive those in trouble or who have troubled me.
- I feel inner peace as shadowy clouds drift away.

Supporting Foods:

- Blueberries
- Papaya
- Watermelon
- Celery
- Apples
- Garlic
- Onions
- Green beans
- Peas
- Grapefruit
- Lemons

Emotion: Irritation

Troubled Mindset

- Just as the name implies, it is the body's attempt to send a message that things are not right and there is no immediate solution in sight.
- What the mind wants does not match what is possible, nor can it happen.
- If you force it, the temporary relief does not solve the bigger problem nor the cause of it all. This is true whether it is body discomfort, or an upset with someone's actions or sounds that they create with their mouth.
- If this feeling and thought is left unchecked it leads to hatred, animosity, and intentional mischief.

Emotion: Irritation

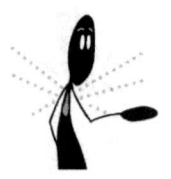

Healing Mindset

How can you calm the flames that have no fire? How can you be free of major internal discomfort without resulting in harmful responses to others or yourself?

Start with yourself and your body. If your body is too hot, sweaty, cold, or in pain, allow the mind and the option to change your focus of thought and purpose. Allow your heart to recall what your real treasure is instead of the momentary satisfaction.

Similar to a child experiencing a shutdown moment, the ego body is in survival mode and needs both a plan and an understanding heart. If there's irritation directed towards another, the mind needs the heart to assist the inner teenager in recognizing what is more important than selfish needs—an opportunity to learn how to navigate the mountain of personal growth, finding peace in the storm and boldness in the shadows.

Emotion: Irritation

Affirmations:

- I see the rays of a brighter day beyond this temporary moment of discomfort.
- My disappointment is a door to seek the positive path of personal growth.
- I go into the moment, finding the release on the other side of pain where I find spring beginning to rise.
- I find joy in the simple.
- I find truth hiding behind the willingness to look past the shadows.

Supporting Foods:

- Apple
- Asparagus
- Avocado
- Barley (sprouted)
- Beet
- Black cherry
- Brussels sprouts
- Wheat grass
- Carrot
- Celery
- Chia seed
- Fennel
- Garlic
- Globe artichoke
- Grape
- Greens
- Flax seed
- Lemon
- Lime
- Mulberry
- Mung bean
- Pear
- Plum
- Raspberry
- Rye
- Seaweed
- Tomato
- Walnuts

Emotion: Shame

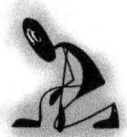

Troubled Mindset

- Your mind is trapped in a constant cycle of inner turmoil.
- Your thoughts betray you.
- The monkey mind has become a badger, gnawing at you to change something that you cannot.
- Shame is not the truth, but it is a taskmaster.
- It makes you think that if you were different or if you had not done something, then everything would have been fine.
- Watch the "if only's," as they only make you miserable.
- If the shame is coming from yourself or others, it is time to find a way out because the inner contempt is slowly destroying you.

Emotion: Shame

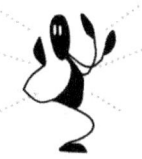

Healing Mindset

Blame and shame are a game with a miserable name. You can't win, nor can anyone, because the object of this game is to shut down progress, creativity, and joy. However, if you take the shame and look at its original purpose you will find an opportunity for positive change.

Shame wants you to never make a mistake so you won't be hurt, embarrassed, or betrayed ever again. Most of that is false, except for the learning from the mistake. You can't guarantee success, but you can guarantee learning and growth. Focus on the positive growth, even if others want to harm you with shame. You determine your inner climate by focusing on your truth, your values, and your capacity for growth and learning.

Emotion: Shame

Affirmations:

- I choose this day to feel the joy of the simple.
- I choose to reflect the light of the day rather than the shadow of their night.
- I breathe new life into my body and new ideas into my mind.
- I expand my thoughts and awareness to new possibilities.
- I am a soul with purpose and love.
- I accept the love from those who safely care for my well being.
- I renew my sense of goodness and start a new life today.
- I take the past and make it fertilizer for my future.

Supporting Foods:

- Warming soups
- Okra
- Cauliflower
- Asparagus
- Broccoli
- Romaine lettuce
- Jicama
- Radishes
- Spinach
- Almonds
- Almond milk
- Oranges
- Lemons
- Grapefruit
- Raspberries
- Blueberries
- Watermelon
- Celery

Emotion: Worry

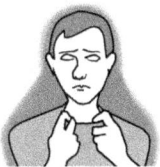

Troubled Mindset

- Spinning your wheels with the break on is causing your mind and body to work too hard, too much, and too often. You ask yourself, "But what am I supposed to do? I have to worry all the time." Thus, your worry is your boss. You are a slave to the constant concern that reaps no benefit nor positive consequence.
- Worry doesn't solve problems; it just makes sure you remember that you have problems. Maybe you should hire someone to call you every hour with a worry so that the rest of the hour you go about your daily living. ;)
- Worry is a consequence of not trusting life.
- You are letting your mindset focus on your worrying thoughts, believing that thinking them will prevent your scary situation. However, it only magnifies it.
- Worry is addictive, and the mind responds to the adrenaline produced by worry with spinning more biochemicals in the brain to keep the worry going.
- Blood sugar is up and down, which leads to food issues and fatigue or hyperactivity in the body or mind.
- Worry is a false path because it does not have an outlet or completion.

Emotion: Worry

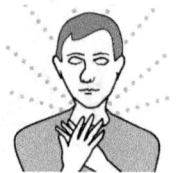

Healing Mindset

Use your worry as a signal that you feel out of control. Once you recognize that your heart and body are scared, return to the energy of the earth. That means to breathe with interval breathing, walk to connect with your natural surroundings. Find a moment that your thoughts are simply of nature or other simple things.

Since worry goes in the opposite direction of a solution, you will know what direction NOT to go to. The path to finding the common ground of the 'simple' first, allows the mind to rest and the heart and body to catch up. Being out of control and lost in the fog of confusion is not the worst thing, but always staying in the worry could lead you to the worse things.

The challenge of finding clarity is quite rewarding if you embrace the worry like you would a small child. Lead the child self with respect and understanding down a gradual path of finding what is real and what isn't. Acknowledging what you can do about a situation and what you can't.

Emotion: Worry

Affirmations:

- I worry less and courage more.
- Don't worry, just be.
- I taste the amazing goodness of life.
- I focus on what is real, what is positive, what I can do.
- I enjoy the time of daily reflection and planning.
- I am grateful for each challenge in my life.
- I notice the moment; it is so cool to pause.
- I appreciate my desire to take care of everything and pause to take care of me.
- My mind means well, my heart wants good, and my body wants safety.
- I am calm in the storm and energized in the sun.
- I take clear action.

Supporting Foods:

- Jicama
- Parsnips
- Yams
- Sweet potato
- Carrots
- Salmon
- Cod fish
- Grass-fed beef
- Soaked chia seed
- Quinoa
- Millet
- Amaranth
- Papaya
- Celery
- Red beets
- Radishes
- Dark green vegetables
- Orange & yellow vegetables
- Parsley
- Green beans
- Lettuce

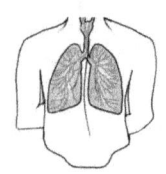

Emphysema

Troubled Mindset

- Experiencing life has become too dreadful or painful, so the body is closing off part of the physical and emotional experience.
- The problem is, you are shutting off parts of life that are necessary to stay alive.
- That also includes warmth, sincere love, authentic connection.
- Living in a pipe dream is neither healthy or helpful.
- Fear of feeling lonely, sad, accused, or blame is sending the wrong message to your body.
- When you are rejected, the other individual is rejecting the parts of themselves they cannot deal with.

Healing Mindset

It is time to pause the moment and breathe slowly with calmness, peace, and simple purpose. Nothing matters but this moment. Other problems are just little storms that will come and go, but your inner core needs you to love and accept yourself fully today.

Think of the upsetting nature of others as immature bouts of little children stuck in adult bodies. Think of your reaction to their overreaction as a minor bump and start breathing again. Allow more of life to be experienced, and your body will create more room to receive the oxygen and the positive things of life.

Emphysema

Affirmations:

- I have plenty of room for air and oxygen.
- Now, I open my inner windows and doors to receive the life-giving force, love, and vitality.
- I am starting to have faith to live another moment and another day.
- I am grateful that I can breathe in what I can.
- My capacity to receive love and nourishment is increasing daily.
- I am safe.

Supporting Foods:

- Apple
- Carrots
- Cauliflower
- Celery
- Chard
- Chickweed (for some)
- Cantaloupe (for some - if candida or fungus, do not use)
- Citrus
- Fennel
- Fenugreek seeds
- Fish
- Garlic
- Greens
- Kelp
- Onions
- Papaya
- Peach
- Pear
- Persimmon
- Pumpkin
- Radish
- Seaweed
- Tomato
- Turkey (for some)
- Yam
- Use garlic & onion to sniff when there is lung congestion.
- Possibly brown rice

Endometriosis

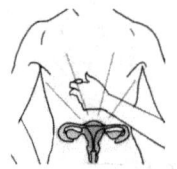

Troubled Mindset

- Being a woman is scary, and you are angry about it.
- You blame and reject your femininity, feeling it to be the source of your inner conflicts.
- Being stuck with your problems is not fair, and you wish it would change, but you are afraid of what will happen when it comes around.
- You want to create a new life, a child, but what if you can't deal with the challenges of the future?
- You've allowed self-degrading beliefs to come into your mind. For example, you might believe that you are not as capable as others in action, knowledge, and learning.
- You may take on the blame or shame too easily.
- You may feel unacceptable, depleted, and unsupported.
- You wish that you were stronger so that you could be safe, defend yourself against certain men, and have your future children be safe.

Endometriosis

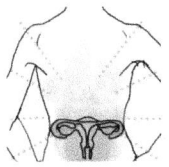

Healing Mindset

The gift of creation is unique to women and is prized by the Gods above and the Earth below. Your troubled past can be cleansed easily if you accept that life is full of stress and turmoil that is meant to be processed.

A female and mother role is to cleanse monthly, nourish daily, care for self and others in the moment. Embrace the goodness of joy in those around you. Being female is stronger than males because you hold the gift of creation and tender love. Males are to offer support and strength, but not use it against you nor drive you to it. Accepting the male energy that is strong and supportive is to accept your own female and male energies as a balanced set of love and strength.

Endometriosis

Affirmations:

- I embrace my gifts as they are and enjoy growing my positive character traits daily.
- I am safe being a woman.
- I enjoy both my feminine and masculine sides.
- I am tender and firm, caring and directed, understanding and insightful.
- I let the fears and upsets that fester my insides heal and become wisdom, warmth, and renewal.
- Once I was troubled, but now I am reborn.
- I am free to be me every day while I create a positive life for myself and my family.
- I easily heal and enjoy a positive cycle of body function.

Supporting Foods:

- Alfalfa
- Avocados
- Fish
- Meats (not fried)
- Parsley
- Safflower
- Raw vegetables and fruits
- Whole grains
- Raw nuts and seeds
- Green drinks
- Kelp
- Dark green leafy vegetables

Epilepsy

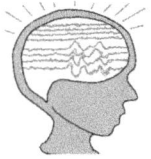

Troubled Mindset

- You are not satisfied with yourself and have consigned to deal with yourself through self-abuse.
- Harsh self-judgments, such as believing there is something wrong with you, root from asserted feelings of being overlooked, rejected, wronged, or defiled from people who you expected to know better.
- You're putting too much emphasis or attention to these negative feelings, making them intensified and your feelings of inadequacy worse.
- Feeling surpassed by the world reinforces your anxiety and resentment around your competence and ability to cope with life.
- You wonder if you will ever be 'good enough,' arising from feeling that too much was expected too soon and believing love is conditional on behavior.
- If epilepsy is in childhood, it comes from a fear or sense of being mentally defective.

Epilepsy

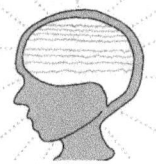

Healing Mindset

Start with kindness towards yourself. It may seem 'out there' when you start, but consider it's deep importance. Dedicate yourself to be kind and forgiving toward yourself, especially when you make mistakes. You may really enjoy experiencing love with no conditions.

There is no competition worth any level of self-brutality. Compassion for yourself in the darkest moments will have the greatest impact. Connect with the truth that love is like the sunshine; it is available to all, including you, no matter their performance.

Epilepsy

Affirmations:
- I am bridging the gaps in my life that have been filled with stress and activity.
- I calmly approach each day with opportunity and balanced adventure.
- Although my body and brain are still sorting things out, I can settle my energy to the earth and natural things.
- I am not pushed nor pulled.
- I am connected to all parts of my personal self with gratitude for life and adventure.
- I calmly change the vibration of worry to insights of learning and connection.
- I am perfectly human and humanly qualified to breathe, smile, and share my heart with whoever is ready to receive my personal joy.

Supporting Foods:
- Chia seeds, soaked
- Flax seeds, soaked
- Salmon
- Avocados
- Sour milk products like plain yogurt and kefir
- Beet greens
- Chard
- Eggs
- Green leafy vegetables
- Raw cheese
- Raw milk
- Raw nuts
- Seeds
- Soybeans
- Seaweed
- Red grapes
- Peas
- Carrots
- Green beans
- Fresh vegetable juice

Eyes

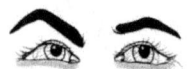

Troubled Mindset

- You may be trying not to 'see' the truth, but stay in denial about something you wish were not true.
- You'd rather deny it than risk feeling the hopelessness of trying to fix it and failing.
- You may use denial as a protection from allowing others to see into your soul. The side effect is that it makes it hard to see yourself with clarity too.
- When you choose not to see the truth and stay in denial, you end up imbalanced and becoming inflated or deflated about who you are.
- You have tended to pay more attention to the negative side of things.
- Your suspicions of individuals, constraints/barriers in life, or fearing what 'might' happen, make the issue worse.
- Your right eye is more about what is going on externally.
- Your left eye is about what is going on internally.

Eyes

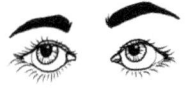

Healing Mindset

Begin the process of change by dropping the tug-a-war with truth. Recognize it each moment, then breathe through and release the tension. Life is a journey through experiences that teach us.

When we see things as they are, we advance our understanding. Consider nourishing the joy of what is. Let go of your doubts and forced expectations and embrace growth from life. Be the positive force for good that brings more light into the eyes of others.

Eyes

Affirmations:
- I realize my vision is an amazing view into the many parts of my soul and the souls of others.
- I want to see what is and stay open to what can be.
- I am growing and learning from life.
- Although I don't see all, I believe in the possibilities of life.
- I will color my experience with fun, curiosity, insight, and love.
- I thank the divine for giving me sight, insight, and foresight.
- I desire and hope with positive expectancy.
- Eyes on the back of your head is better than 20/20 "hindsight."

Supporting Foods:
- Water/Get hydrated
- Carrots
- Cantaloupe
- Green leafy vegetables
- Black-eyed peas
- Organic sweet potato
- Green beans
- Yellow vegetables
- Nuts and seeds
- Wild-caught seafood such as
  - Salmon
  - Mackerel
  - Sardines
  - Halibut
  - Tuna
- Red bell peppers
- Corn
- Peas
- Mango
- Kiwi
- Papaya
- Blueberries
- Blackberries
- Cherries
- Eggs

Eyes: Red / Blood Shot

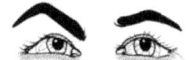

Troubled Mindset

- You feel like you have been hit by too much in life and you need a break.
- You are tired, overwhelmed, and frustrated with what is happening to you.
- You are sad about events and about people.
- You quietly suffer but now openly can't stop showing your suffering eyes.
- Your body needs support but there is not enough time, energy, and people there for you.
- You don't want to see nor experience what is going on around you.
- You are suffering with deep pressure, grief, and pain.
- You could have hidden resentments but who can you tell them to.
- You wish it would be different but every thought of your wish of regret, sadness or resentment pushes the inflammation into more irritating redness.

Eyes: Red / Blood Shot

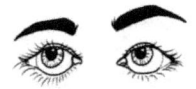

Healing Mindset

Your body needs extra support to keep going, so be sure to allocate time for yourself without the self-imposing restrictions. While you might feel pressed for time, consider allowing time to serve you rather than being confined by its demands.

How do you achieve this? Rather than trying to find available time, intentionally plan and create brief moments (3 to 5 minutes, 3 times a day) dedicated to sitting, breathing, listening, calming, appreciating, and quieting your busy mind and body. Establish daily moments that are already scheduled, and as you consistently adhere to this rhythm of creating personal self-time, it will reciprocate by honoring and respecting you.

Instead of allowing stress reactions from conflicts and overwhelm to control you, empower your inner self to rediscover your true essence every day. In doing so, you'll find that answers begin to emerge to guide you through life's journey.

Eyes: Red / Blood Shot

Affirmations:

- I am learning to be calm when others are not.
- I offer my body time, my mind peace, my heart healing, and my body nourishment.
- I will go forward after I step back to give myself a moment.
- I recharge and rejuvenate first and then move forward.
- I pause to breathe, ahhh.
- I think I just caught my breath and my life.

Supporting Foods:

- Water/Get hydrated
- Carrots
- Cantaloupe
- Green leafy vegetables
- Black-eyed peas
- Organic sweet potato
- Green beans
- Eggs
- Nuts and seeds
- Wild-caught seafood such as
  - Salmon
  - Mackerel
  - Sardines
  - Halibut
  - Tuna
- Red bell peppers
- Corn
- Peas
- Mango
- Kiwi
- Papaya
- Blueberries
- Blackberries
- Cherries
- Eggs

Eyes: Stye / Suffering

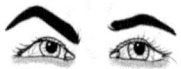

Troubled Mindset

- Your world is changing around you without your permission or control.
- You don't want to see nor experience what is going on around you.
- Anger is being suppressed so well that you think it's just a physical problem. But look around and you will notice that somewhere, and to someone, you are irritated and upset with them.
- You wish it would be different, but every thought of your resentment pushes the inflammation deeper into your eye area and causes more irritation.
- You are overwhelmed with the thought that something will happen beyond your control and you won't be able to recover.
- You want to stop the slide of suffering and feelings of being out of control.
- You are either so mad with frustration or trying to stay calm by suppressing the chaos.

Eyes: Stye / Suffering

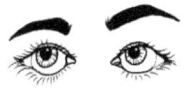

Healing Mindset

It is time to stop thinking that "your way" is the only way. It is getting you into trouble inside. It is time to take your feelings of survival and transform them into a path of discovery of how to live with hope, gratitude, adventure, and wisdom.

Just because others are wise, doesn't preclude you from using your precious energy fuming about it. Use your life to make a difference for yourself, with daily moments of change of heart. Change your mind, heal your heart, and move your body to create productive thoughts, beneficial feelings, and movements full of vitality. Spend little time in your troubles and more time in your creations. See where you are learning and give space for the other person to learn as well. Remember to be firm with a gentle heart.

Eyes: Stye / Suffering

Affirmations:
- I see clearly now.
- The hope of tomorrow starts with the clarity of today.
- I turn wishes into productive creations.
- I choose my positive perspective.
- I am grateful that I am pushed to find the real me.
- Behind the clouds, I will find hidden truths of clarity and insight.
- I take part in being responsible for what I can and let others do the same.

Supporting Foods:

- Asparagus
- Beets
- Blueberries
- Blue corn
- Broccoli (steamed, organic)
- Carrots
- Cauliflower
- Celery
- Cucumber
- Kidney beans
- Lemon
- Lime
- Lentils
- Millet
- Papaya
- Pineapple
- Turmeric
- Yam
- Zucchini

Face

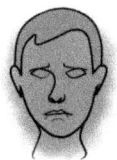

Troubled Mindset

- "Losing face" or "Can't face up to them/it."
- In a world of show and constant judgments, the face has to hide some feelings and emotions but often displays the frustrations of the internal conflicts.
- You don't have a clear sense of the defining features of your true identity, making it hard to present yourself to others.
- The idea of hiding self-doubts, self-blame, and beliefs of personal inadequacies comes to a head when the forces of nature can't keep up with the desire to still experience life and push forward.
- Part of you may be avoiding facing yourself because you have bought into the idea that you have to 'fake it to make it,' yet you resent that.
- To face life is to face your fears, your self-hate, your worries, and your overwhelm in social situations.
- Slow the negative thought flow and encourage yourself.
- Your right side has to do with figuring out how to share who you are with the world.
- The left side of your face has to do with believing that you are somehow inherently bad, and therefore unacceptable.
- Your forehead has to do with current negative thinking.

Face

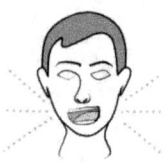

Healing Mindset

You are not bad. You are not the problem. Reconnect to your heart and appreciate the innate divinity of your soul.

You may experience problems, but that is normal. Don't let the judgments of others or your self-criticism be your boss. Release your judgments toward yourself and self-limiting beliefs to help as you rise above the anxiety and fear of rejection.

Find your inner truth, your inner beauty, and your inner connection. Your face reflects conflict, not truth. Resentment to others or to yourself is only an experience. So it is time to stop the manufacturing of inner suffering and start the creation of healing, love, and self-appreciation. The glorious experience of finding beauty in all things will reflect on your face. Be the beauty that you want displayed to the world.

Face

Affirmations:

- I can do this.
- I can face my life and my feelings.
- I appreciate that my feelings and inner conflicts can't hide anymore because I am ready to look, deal with, release, and heal my emotions and thoughts.
- I love and respect my inner beauty and take care of myself.
- I let the beast out and send it on its way.
- I let the light shine on my face and skin today.
- I am soft and firm with my heart and the understandings that come to me.
- Let's face it, a smiley face is better than a frowny one.

Supporting Foods:

- Drink at least 2 quarts of water every day.
- Eat a balanced diet, including raw vegetables
- Fruits
- Millet
- Brown rice
- Seeds and nuts
- Garlic
- Onions
- Eggs
- Asparagus
- Bell peppers
- Yellow and orange vegetables like carrots and yellow squash
- Apples
- Citrus fruits
- Tomatoes
- Grapes
- Blackberries

Fainting

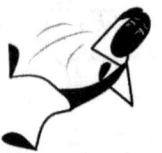

Troubled Mindset

- "Checking out" because you are not up for figuring this out.
- You carry a limiting belief that you don't have the capacity, strength, or support to fix it anyway.
- Your plans are not leading you to the expected outcomes, and you feel overwhelmed under the weight of too much pressure, believing a catastrophic ending. Alternatively, you might not have plans because you believe you can't make any at your age, also anticipating a catastrophic ending.
- You may be resisting facing life's challenges and learning new things.

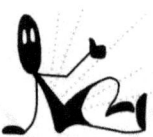

Healing Mindset

Every moment is a gift. Each breath is a new opportunity for adventure and insight. Live in this moment, and don't over-concern yourself with future outcomes. You carry a purpose and the capacity to fulfill that purpose. Release the fear, tap into your strengths and resources, and follow through with your initiative.

Fainting

Affirmations:
- I embrace each moment as a gift.
- I breathe with appreciation for a new opportunity for adventure and insight.
- I trust the future to work out for the best.
- I support myself.
- I allow myself to be supported.
- I breathe in new opportunities and breathe out false expectations.
- I value my capacity and trust in the moment.

Supporting Foods:
- Asparagus
- Avocado
- Bamboo
- Beets
- Broccoli, organic
- Carrots with celery
- Cauliflower, organic
- Celery juice
- Dulce
- Green leafy vegetables
- Halibut
- Kelp
- Moringa
- Nutritional yeast
- Phytoplankton
- Seaweed
- Salmon
- Spinach
- Trout
- Yam

Fatigue

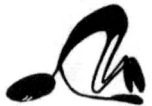

Troubled Mindset

- Your mind is living in denial; your heart is living in pleasing others; your body is living in overwhelm.
- You'd often prefer to stay in denial about real issues, or proper limits, because of the emotional weight of fear, anger, sadness, or frustration.
- No matter how hard you try, it is never enough.
- Your perfectionistic and pleasing tendencies are wearing you down.
- As you overdo it, you stop enjoying it.
- You give your energy in the form of wisdom or insight without replenishing yourself with new learning and growth, or you give by physically doing for others without renewing your body.
- You plan, but struggle to keep up with the deadlines.
- Even when you 'relax' you are internally running around to mentally 'keep up,' which wears you down and keeps you tired.
- You care to share, but your efforts don't reap the love and results that you were wishing for.
- Your body is trying to carry your emotional agenda to the brink of physical destruction.

Fatigue

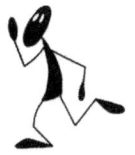

Healing Mindset

Be careful to watch what is happening. If you are going to do everything, then don't. You don't have to save the world so that you can be happy and safe. Find resolution for the past and hope for the future without focusing on pleasing everyone.

Look inside; there is a beautiful soul that needs your time, attention, care, and understanding. Every day, take care of you. Set and follow simple rituals of self-care that always happen and happen without worry or regret. Justification for stopping self-care is a lie you have told yourself that leads to more problems than anyone should deal with. Bring joy back into what you do by honoring your true limits.

Fatigue

Affirmations:

- I can be happy without pleasing everyone.
- I do not have to be saved to get well.
- I do not have to save to be happy.
- God is my support.
- I am willing to see what is real.
- I am grateful and happy.
- I look at my inner struggles as messages from my body to stop and listen.
- I listen to my inner heart messages understanding that love is needed but not in pleasing.
- The fretting of the past is now the simple function of happily focusing on living simple rituals of self-care and functioning in the moment.

Supporting Foods:

- Drink plenty of water
- Fresh fruits and vegetables
- Whole grains
- Seeds and nuts
- White fish
- Spirulina
- Chlorella
- Alfalfa
- Wheatgrass
- Brewer's yeast
- Citrus fruit
- Bell peppers
- Broccoli
- Legumes

Feet

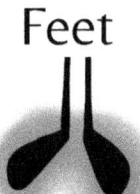

Troubled Mindset

- It's all about your direction and foundation.
- The future seems scary as you resist, in one way or another, to move forward, yet you insist you must keep moving.
- You fear making mistakes with no place to land or call home when the winds of life threaten to blow you down.
- You lack the confidence to 'stand on your own two feet' when you face life's challenges.
- Your feet are trying to get your attention to resolve the issue with your conflicted path.
- Cold feet? You are fearing and not fully embracing your path. You're holding on to reservations that need to be resolved to move forward with confidence.
- Sweaty feet: The details are creating an emotional load that prevents you from seeing the big picture.
- Pigeon-toed: You may find that your direction is hindered by indecisiveness. You are doing what you are told rather than heeding your true feelings or soul's plan.
- Feet pointed outward: You are split in the direction you are taking. You are not sure of yourself. The left is your spiritual direction, the right is your physical direction.
- Smelly feet: You are disgusted by the way you think you should go.

Feet

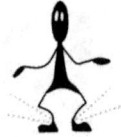

Healing Mindset

Understand your conflict. See it clearly; perhaps, journal it out. Honestly reflect on your resistance, frustration, heartache, or fears about your direction. You won't move forward easily when you're in conflict in one way or another. Once you resolve, breathe as you ground your energy. Imagine yourself 'rooting' in like a tree to get your bearings and feel safe. Stand in the state of safety and security, feel and embrace the experience of being fully present in the moment then move forward.

Left foot: Start by focusing on yourself. You put others before yourself and neglect your needs, including emotional needs. Release the pain of past relationships so you can move forward in a positive direction.

Right foot: You are feeling overwhelmed with too much responsibility. Flow with life rather than forcing things to happen. Force will backfire, and you'll just 'shoot yourself in the foot.' Trust that there is a map and that all you need to do is follow it.

Feet

Affirmations:
- I walk with confidence.
- I stand in strength.
- I move with balance.
- I thrive in connections to my core self.
- I go forward with a clear direction.
- I am hopeful, helpful, and energized with life force.

Supporting Foods:
- Drink steam-distilled water
- Eat a well-balanced diet of raw fruits and vegetables
- Whole grains
- Fish
- Chicken
- Yogurt
- Kefir

Fever

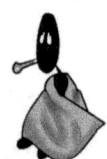

Troubled Mindset

- The world is a scary place out there, and your body is trying to protect you because you haven't taken care of yourself physically and/or socially.
- All the while, you are upset about some situation.
- You're 'burning up inside' with unexpressed anger.
- The chaos may be getting to you.
- You are resisting authority figures, not wanting to be given commands when you feel you or your contribution is undervalued.
- You are angry and feel as if life is not fair.
- You are extra concerned about possible negative outcomes.

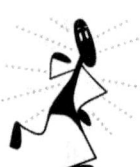

Healing Mindset

Take a step back. Breathe and reconnect to your body as you relax the need to control the situation. Trust that things can still work out for the highest and best, no matter the outcome. Do what you believe is right without losing your grounding and balance. Remember that your innate value does not change no matter how others treat you. Stay true to who you are. In your weakness, the body is trying to protect you. Learn that courage is better than inner turmoil.

Fever

Affirmations:

- I appreciate my body wanting to take care of me.
- I will listen and pause life so that my inner turmoil won't burn me up.
- It is time for me to be true to me.
- I honor and respect my body.
- It is time for me to be courageous in life's situations.
- I am changing for the better.
- I turn fear into trust and courage.
- I turn anger into positive action.
- I turn feelings of personal attack into wisdom and productive action.
- I wisely pace my mind, my heart, and my body.

Supporting Foods:

- Drink plenty of water
- Juices
- Teas
- Broths

Fibromyalgia

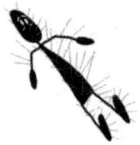

Troubled Mindset

- You are resisting the deep feelings of regret, sadness, guilt, and resentment.
- You suppress your envy and judgment of others while openly resent yourself and your situation.
- You feel unwanted, overwhelmed, worried, and weak.
- Resisting life, especially in the aftermath of challenges that have knocked you down, leads you to wonder if there is sufficient energy available and brings a sense of hopelessness regarding potential solutions to your situation.
- You hide behind your problems and use pain to avoid the overwhelm of dealing with emotional conflict.
- You may have forgiven externally, but inside you're still holding on to it.
- You haven't been paying enough attention to what your body or your intuition is telling you.
- You are becoming stubborn, listening less to your body, and living in a shadow of struggle and survival.

Fibromyalgia

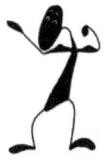

Healing Mindset

Listen to the inner voice that supports your core truth. Self-blame, regret, gloom, and suffering are signals that you are avoiding the courage to face your emotional pain.

Listen to your body's intuition. The struggle has a clear message if you will calm down the foggy mind. Random pain is not random; each one is a signal. Stop fearing the pain, and stop fearing the healing of it. Breathe slowly and learn how to gradually help your body, your heart, and your mind. Feelings are not truth. Feelings are messengers of lost and confused parts of self that need love, direction, and integration.

Fibromyalgia

Affirmations:

- I choose to take care of me.
- I choose to listen to my inner guides and divine influence.
- I choose to be truthful and to let go of any resentment.
- If I can create pain, I can heal it.
- My pain is only a signal that I got stuck on the way to finding myself.
- So, I choose this day to take care of me, my mind, my heart, and my body.
- I choose to be honest with myself.
- I choose to let go of any resentment toward myself or others because I know that darkness feeds struggle.
- I feed my inner light with self-care, self-love, and self-appreciation.
- I cleanse my body and my mind.

Fibromyalgia

Supporting Foods:

- Raw fruits and vegetables
- Fresh vegetable juices
- Raw nuts and seeds
- Plenty of water
- Herbal teas
- Millet
- Brown rice
- Turkey
- Chicken
- Deep-water fish

Flu (Influenza)

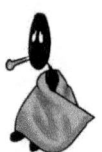

Troubled Mindset

- Resistance to change.
- You feel guilty for not doing what someone else has wanted you to do.
- You fear something awful may happen.
- You feel vulnerable and victimized by the change and negativity that surrounds you.
- You feel like a lot is expected of you but are not offered support or protection through your responsibilities.
- You feel weakened by your fearful beliefs and perspectives and are having a hard time carrying your burdens.

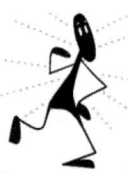

Healing Mindset

Relax the resistance and open your mind to a higher perspective to help you pull out of the 'group think' that constrains you. Free from fear and full of trust, move with the shifts in the weather, circumstance, or even internal adjustments as you release the old and embrace the new. Support yourself with quality nutrition, plenty of water, and calming sounds and surroundings to bring healing to your body and mind.

Flu (Influenza)

Affirmations:
- I use this time to release old and unwanted clutter from my mind, toxins from my body, and negative emotions from my heart.
- I appreciate my immune system.
- I am supporting my internal defense systems to learn, mature, and become strong for healthier living.

Supporting Foods:

- Water/Get hydrated
- Turkey soup with healing spices
- Jicama
- Celery juice
- Carrot juice
- Congee (extra slow cooked rice)
- Cinnamon spice
- Clove spice
- Ginger spice
- Thyme spice
- Micro-greens
- Fermented foods
- Squash
- Warm broth soups
- Watermelon
- Asparagus
- Steamed broccoli
- Steamed cauliflower
- Chicken soup
- Garlic
- Steamed red beets
- Green onions
- Parsley

Fungus

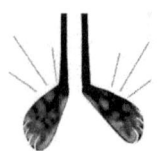

Troubled Mindset

- You have a lost sense of self.
- You hold onto too many ideas, beliefs, feelings, and/or secrets.
- Once you decide to take action, you confuse your scattered action with what is purposeful and beneficial.
- You have old patterns that keep you stuck, and it is time for a new way of thinking.
- There may have been a purpose for the former way of thinking or doing things, given the circumstance of your family or ancestry, but those ways no longer serve you.
- These habitual patterns have gone stale and swampy.
- It's time to live in a way that serves your life for the highest and best good, today.

Healing Mindset

Flow with life instead of trying to fight change. Embrace the idea that you were meant to have joy in areas that have up to this point just been in 'survival' mode. Heal from the inside out and rise into your best self. Find who you really are, what you truly want, and be honest in all your communications. Be honest with your thoughts. Don't give into blame or shame. Be open to strengthening yourself and others with positive values. Check the body area for more details.

Fungus

Affirmations:
- I celebrate the day.
- I encourage myself and others.
- I am firm in my beliefs and caring in my approach.
- I let those crazy thoughts scatter away and I clearly think and feel what is coming from my core self.
- I empower the best in myself and others.
- I eat, sleep, stretch, and breathe to strengthen and empower my mind, heart, and body.

Supporting Foods:
- Eat plenty of raw vegetables
- Broccoli
- Asparagus
- Avocados
- Onions
- Peas
- Brussel sprout
- Carrots
- Bell peppers
- Chlorella
- Garlic
- Kelp
- Kombu
- Dark green leafy vegetables
- Watercress
- Fish
- Chicken

Gallbladder

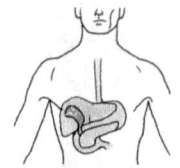

Troubled Mindset

- You have been upset and stubborn.
- You may feel resentful and often hateful.
- You act impatient and indecisive.
- You want to "huff and puff" and "blow the house down," but then again, you don't want to "burn your bridges," so you hold back and speak sideways with "stabbing" comments to those that bother you.
- Stubbornness is holding you back from a willingness to move forward and live/just be.
- Something in your past is contributing to resentment, anger, or bitterness in your present.
- You may feel like a victim and feel a need to force things to go your way to make things work out.

Gallbladder

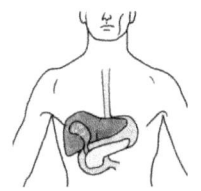

Healing Mindset

Your focus has been about detecting the wrongs of the world rather than enjoying its beauties and growth. There will always be problems, misdeeds, or limitations. It's not so much about the final result or "fixing it" as it is about the 'way' of getting there.

Use compassion, kindness, and be flexible. Value people, be gentle with them and with yourself through the weak times. Look deep inside yourself and believe in your capacity to let go and forgive. It is within you.

There is purpose in your experience that is meant to help you grow and use your strengths to benefit all. Transform the hurts of life into nourishing soil that provides a foundation of positive growth.

Gallbladder

Affirmations:

- I love myself.
- I forgive others.
- I clear the clutter and choose with awareness.
- I act and experience life.
- I transform any resentment into self-responsibility.
- I am decisive.
- I am able to direct my heart for safety and good.
- I am strong.
- I play.
- I transform confusion into clarity of mind and action.
- I transform my rage and emotions into the depth of character.
- I am teachable.
- I enjoy life's pleasures that are supportive to my body and soul.
- I forgive myself and others.
- I see the value in others and creatively communicate.
- I am confident in making decisions by listening to my core values.
- I clear clutter and choose awareness.
- I transform confusion into clarity of mind and action.
- I transform my rage and emotions into an inner depth of character.

 ## Supporting Foods:

- Apple
- Asparagus
- Beets
- Barley
- Corn silk
- Globe artichoke
- Parsley
- Parsnip
- Pear
- Radish
- Applesauce
- Eggs
- Yogurt
- Broiled fish
- Turmeric
- Fresh apple juice
- Pear juice
- Beet juice

Gallstones

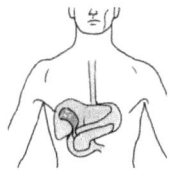

Troubled Mindset

- Your regret has turned to stone.
- You've lost the real reason for your upsetting feelings.
- You resent what they did, what should not have happened, the choices you made, the expectations unfulfilled, and everything else.
- The bitterness and resentment have settled, and you continue to withhold love from those you care about most to cope.
- Your suppressed feelings are trying to burst out, but you push them down.
- You're wishing that something else will change so you won't have to face your fears.
- It feels hard to forgive, and you seek someone to blame.
- You are angry to the point of rage or resentment.
- Your anger has a short fuse despite your best efforts.
- Your true character is hiding behind some hidden agenda.

Gallstones

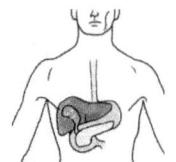

Healing Mindset

Be honest with all your agendas. Come to grip what is really true and real. If anger looms, then follow the path to release it. Look and find the expectations that turn into resentments because these are what hurt you, not the events.

Choose to choose, to take a stand without force or regret. Experience life as a learning and growing. Experience and enjoy each step. Subtle judgments don't serve you. When you notice them, acknowledge them neutrally (without additional judgment of yourself), then choose to return to love and compassion.

Clear your mind and heart and let your body live. You have it within you to be clear, decisive, experience strength and fortitude, and play. Guide your heart towards the good. Allow the intensity you've experienced to create a depth of character that brings about positive action.

Gallstones

Affirmations:

- I love myself.
- I forgive others.
- I clear the clutter and choose with awareness.
- I act and experience life.
- I transform any resentment into self-responsibility.
- I am decisive.
- I am able to direct my heart for safety and good.
- I am strong.
- I play.
- I transform confusion into clarity of mind and action.
- I transform my rage and emotions into the depth of character.
- I am teachable.
- I enjoy life's pleasures that are supportive to my body and soul.
- I forgive myself and others.
- I see the value in others and creatively communicate.
- I am confident in making decisions by listening to my core values.
- I clear clutter and choose awareness.
- I transform confusion into clarity of mind and action.
- I transform my rage and emotions into an inner depth of character.

Supporting Foods:

- Apple
- Asparagus
- Beets
- Barley
- Corn silk
- Globe artichoke
- Parsley
- Parsnip
- Pear
- Radish
- Applesauce
- Eggs
- Yogurt
- Broiled fish
- Turmeric
- Fresh apple juice
- Pear juice
- Beet juice

Gangrene

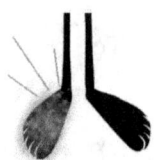

Troubled Mindset

- The feeling or belief is: "I have lost something precious, and there is no way I can replace it."
- You may be blaming yourself for your errors, or the errors of others, that you can't reason through.
- You harbor resentment towards life and yourself.
- Shame and guilt act as powerful influences, fueling negative thoughts and words that, over time, are transforming into a toxic presence within your body.

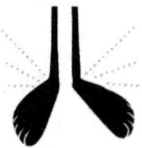

Healing Mindset

It's time to confront the immediate challenge and halt the negative thoughts of shame and gloom. Consider positive ways to learn from your situation. Engage in meditation to clear your mind and heart of thoughts and feelings that poison your life.

During meditation, visualize assisting your body in the cleansing process and empowering your immune system to work for you, not against you.

Gangrene

Affirmations:

- I am healing the emotional pain that I have caused or that others have caused me.
- I am releasing my hopelessness and grief.
- I transform negative energy by burying it deep in the earth. Then, I use this transformed energy to create and build upon things that bring joy into my life, a little more each day.
- I am grateful for the lovely moments.
- I close my eyes on the illness and open my heart to healing from all the kindness and caring that the universe and my loved ones can give me.
- I am worthy of love.

Supporting Foods:

- Garlic
- Shiitake mushrooms
- Onions
- Leafy greens
- Green drinks
- Bananas
- Citrus fruits
- Bell peppers

Gas/Flatulence

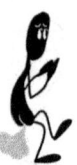

Troubled Mindset

- You are reacting to the good things of life.
- You are pushing yourself too much to do good, be good, be right, and to properly process everything around you.
- Part of you holds back due to trouble expressing how you feel.
- Your ideas are unprocessed because of the underlying fear that keeps the inner commotion and tension.

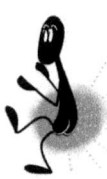

Healing Mindset

Learn to love your filters that are filled with past judgments. Gradually work through your judgments until you are clear and objective with your actions and reactions to life. Expect to be disappointed sometimes. Expect the unexpected. Enjoy the ups and the downs. Life is a lot of fun, especially when you take the bad with the good and work it through filters of enjoying all aspects of life experiences.

Gas/Flatulence

Affirmations:

- I easily assimilate food and life.
- I use any fear as a door to clarity and calm them to the earth.
- I am sense life in its parts and whole.
- I enjoy the wide variety of life's events and experiences.
- I clearly process and balance the emotions of my day.

Supporting Foods:

- Rice congee
- Cooked carrots
- Lemon
- Lime
- Alfalfa
- Watercress
- Barley broth
- Fresh pineapple
- Fresh papaya

Foods to Avoid:

- Limit
    - Peanuts
    - Lentils
    - Soybeans
- Avoid
    - Dairy
    - Processed food
    - Beans
    - Red meats
    - Fried foods
    - Sugar
    - White flour products

Hair Loss

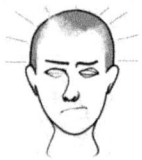

Troubled Mindset

- Your inner strength is depleting as you worry about things beyond your control.
- Alternatively, you might be upset about aspects of your life situation that you can potentially change.
- People are people, and if you continue to worry or resent about what they might do or should do, it is like pulling your hair.
- Your hair won't have the support it needs to stay strong because your energy and focus is on everything that you can't control.
- Your inner direction is too focused on wishing others would be different.

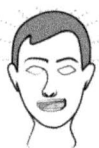

Healing Mindset

You can take a deep breath and trust that life is an experience of relating to people who might make a mistake or who might not give you what you want or who might have problems that you can't do anything about. You can take the challenge of learning to guide instead of trying to drive. You can only drive your own life story. Others will mess up and have problems, that is how they learn. Start the process of enjoying the journey of relationships.

Hair Loss

Affirmations:

- I am in control because I have surrendered my need for control.
- I am balanced and strong because I give my worries or my demands to the light and to the earth.
- I am nothing without the divine, but I am strong and blessed with it.
- When someone is in need, I trust in God first, then I help.
- When I wish or demand someone else to change, I transform that demand into a puff of air, releasing my forced will to the wind.
- I receive true balanced strength from an inner wonderful force of love and kind sharing.
- I appreciate this inner joy that comes with surrendering to the love that is only shared with honoring and respect.
- I am safe living with honor.

Supporting Foods:

- Brewers yeast
- Brown rice
- Bulgur
- Green peas
- Lentils
- Oats
- Soybeans
- Sunflower seeds
- Walnuts

Hands

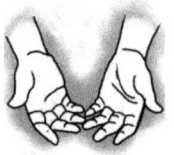

Troubled Mindset

- It's about what you're doing.
- You may be trying to hold on too tightly to something in your life, or you just can't get a grip on it.
- You may struggle with your ability to 'handle' what life throws at you.
- There may be an imbalance with giving and receiving; you don't feel it's fair, or you aren't enjoying it.
- Cold hands: Your hearts not in it. You may need a break, or you may need to change things up quite a bit.
- You don't love what you are doing, and you need to refocus your energy. Be fully present with whatever you choose to do.
- Sweaty hands: You've lost sight of the purpose. You're anxious about the details and fear you might make a mistake. Take a step back and look at the big picture.

Hands

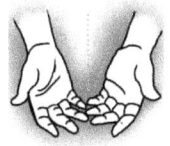

Healing Mindset

Left hand:
You feel as though there is an emptiness in your life that you don't know how to fill. You feel lonely and are unsure of what steps to take to rectify this feeling. Step up and take charge of your life. Discover what helps to fill this void and pursue it.

Right hand:
You feel as though you've lost the ability to think and act creatively. You are unsure of or frightened by the thought of how this lack of creativity will affect your work. You may feel betrayed by someone you depended on. Recenter to empower yourself with understanding and renewed strength.

Hands

Affirmations:
- I get it.
- Life is easy to manage.
- I enjoy creatively managing life.
- I love to create and complete projects.
- I love to touch and share my heart.
- I accept what is offered, and in return I share my caring heart.
- I am present in this moment as I act.
- I connect to the purpose of my doings and/or my work.

Supporting Foods:

- Alfalfa
- Cabbage
- Celery
- Flaxseed soaked
- Oats & oat bran
- Rice bran
- Fresh pineapple
- Brown rice
- Wheat
- Rye
- Asparagus
- Farm fresh eggs
- Garlic
- Onions
- Green leafy vegetables
- Oatmeal
- Fish
- Amaranth
- Salmon
- Ginger
- Parsley

Hands Chapped

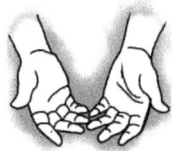

Troubled Mindset

- You are trying to stay to clean from the filth around you.
- You concern yourself too much with being "hands-off" from what you consider unclean or dirty. Yet, you want to stick your hands into helping and being apart of the mix. This dichotomy or inner conflict goes deep into your system so you are in denial that you are both nice and cold to those around you.
- You need healing to your inner pain that festers. This pain came long ago and is mostly forgotten and you deal with daily stresses with positive function but hidden suffering.
- You worry and fret, before, during, and after the use of your helping hands.
- In the cold months, it is worse because you need to take care of yourself but don't realize that it includes some embracing of inner truth and accepting of sincere love.

Hands Chapped

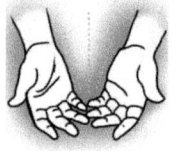

Healing Mindset

Be honest with yourself and realize that those subtle resentments do add up in your physical body. Subtle wishes mixed with too much regret and little hatreds do cause physical reactions in your gut and eventually manifesting on your hands.

Choose today to notice any judgment and send it to the earth, notice any sadness and warm it with understanding and appreciation, notice any frustrations and encourage yourself with simple positive challenges. Worry is leaving and enjoying life's trip is on my horizon.

Hands Chapped

Affirmations:

- I am ready to let the warmth of God's love in.
- By doing so, I am ready to let go of any and all resentments to anyone in my life past or present.
- I acknowledge the healing hands of the divine upon my belly and my hands.
- I realize that I need positive protection for my skin, and I stop letting go of skin oils by too much worry and judgment.
- I am encouraged with my progress of faith in dealing with others, breathing through my fears and pain.
- I turn regret into hope and strength.
- I feel my hands and my inner physical self healing the sores of my life.

Supporting Foods:

- Drink at least 2 quarts of water every day
- Raw vegetables
- Fruits
- Millet
- Brown rice
- Seeds & nuts
- Garlic
- Onions
- Eggs
- Asparagus
- Carrots
- Yellow squash
- Bell peppers
- Apples
- Citrus fruits
- Tomatoes
- Grapes
- Blackberries

Hay Fever

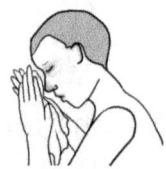

Troubled Mindset

- You're stuck in a state of chronic grief because when your feelings begin to come up, you pull them right back in.
- You're always wondering if you are okay or if they will be okay if you are not okay, or some other mixed emotional belief.
- You feel dissatisfied with yourself and uncomfortable with others.
- Your unresolved emotions are feeding your fears and reactions.
- There seems to never be enough of whatever it is you need to do what you desire.
- You think that life is dangerous, but you still want to experience it.
- The unresolved feelings of rage, fear, grief, and sadness aggravate your body system.
- You feel you deserve some punishment, but somehow know it is not true.

Hay Fever

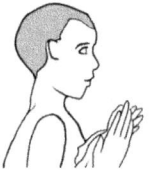

Healing Mindset

It's time to take time to heal your inner conflicts. Identify what triggers you. Most of your beliefs are not valid because they are based on emotional filters that protect a child, not an adult.

When emotions come, find a safe space to let them flow without needing them to be right or wrong, just feel. Breathe through them to release as they naturally process through your system. Find and connect to a core part of yourself. Find the values that work for you and let go of the ones that were not yours to begin with. Believe that you are meant to be a part of life's joy.

Hay Fever

Affirmations:
- I believe in me.
- I believe in God and nature.
- All things work for my good.
- I am acclimating to life gradually and slowly.
- I am safe in the sun and the rain.
- I honor and respect my body.
- I appreciate all that my body does for me.
- I calm my immune system, and I value the gradual maturation of my body's defense systems.

Supporting Foods:
- Eat a variety of fruits and vegetables
- Bananas
- Carrots
- Grains
- Raw nuts and seeds
- Plain yogurt
- Soured foods
- Kefir
- Kimchi
- Sauerkraut
- Garlic

AVOID:
- Chocolate
- Processed foods
- Dairy products (except yogurt)
- Soft drinks
- Sugar
- White flour

Head

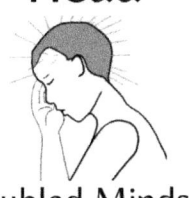

Troubled Mindset

- "Who is in charge here, anyway?"
- You'd like to be the one to call the shots.
- You are frustrated with how things are being done by the authority figures in your life.
- Your attempts have not helped the way you wished.
- Your judgment of others crossed with your self-criticisms amplify the already strong internal conflict.
- Nothing feels fair.
- Your masculine side is 'heading' things up by trying to 'fix' it, while the heart of the issue is being ignored, dismissed, or suppressed.
- You have a lot on your mind and feel the weight of responsibility.

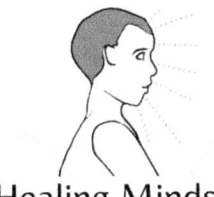

Healing Mindset

Choose to relate to the issue at hand by allowing your heart to play a role. It will help relax the pressure and conflict. Face the real heart emotions with the courage to connect. Consider coming to terms with the conflict you have carried and your higher self or divine authority figure. Experience the joy of learning, growth, and new insights as you walk through your circumstances with hope for the future.

Head

Affirmations:
- The answers I seek come easily as I connect with the source of strength and truth.
- I honor my heart, and I respect my body.
- I think, therefore I discern.
- I hope, therefore I experience.
- I pray, therefore I plan.
- I resent no more.
- I am level headed, clear-minded, and open-hearted.

Supporting Foods:

- Water/Get hydrated
- Almonds
- Almond milk
- Watercress
- Parsley
- Garlic
- Cherries
- Pineapple
- A little salt water
- Ginger tea
- Lemon
- Grapefruit
- Okra steamed
- Zucchini steamed with a little salt
- Figs

Headache

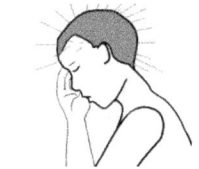

Troubled Mindset

- It feels like a tornado hit. "Just make it all stop!"
- Circumstances outside of your control are congesting your head with fear and anger.
- You don't trust the 'higher power' or divine essence to make things "right," or to make them the way you want them.
- To counterbalance the lack of assurance you feel, you begin overthinking, overanalyzing, and suppressing your emotions.
- At some level, you don't believe you are smart enough, but these compensations make things worse. You end up angry, and perhaps mad about being angry.
- The self-judgments challenge your self-worth, which is angering, then the cycle continues.
- Back of head: Suppressed anger, excessive pleasing, fear of seeing, fear of connecting, wanting to escape. You may demand more of yourself than you can or have given.
- Forehead headache: Worry, overly concerned, self-pity, self-blame, intense anger suppressed, sadness. Holding a negative perspective and struggling to see the good.
- Top of head: Suppressed emotions of all types. Anger to someone close. Fear of moving forward, trepidation. Learning feels overwhelming.

Headache

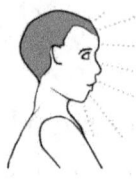

Healing Mindset

Begin by opening yourself up to feeling deeply. Your heart and mind are meant to work together. Your mind has been taking too much of the show. Your emotions can give you experience and knowledge. Choose to allow yourself to change the pattern of suppressing your emotions, then walk the path.

Be patient and have faith in yourself and others. Trust life with all its possibilities, focusing on congruency and abundance.

Headache

Affirmations:
- I will trust life with all its possibilities.
- I focus on creating congruency and abundance.
- Frontal: I love and respect myself and others.
- Life is an opportunity.
- I thank the universe for choices; they are good for the mind and enriching to the soul.
- Back: I spontaneously live in all areas of life.
- I am richly connected with the universe.
- My past is wisdom, and my future is enriched.
- Top: I am open to receive God's love and wisdom.
- I release my trapped feelings into a freedom of expression and movement.

Supporting Foods:
- Water/Get hydrated
- Almonds
- Almond milk
- Watercress
- Parsley
- Garlic
- Cherries
- Pineapple
- A little salt water
- Ginger tea
- Lemon
- Grapefruit
- Okra steamed
- Figs
- Zucchini steamed with a little salt

Heart Problems

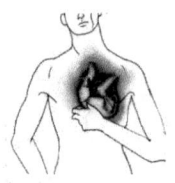

Troubled Mindset

- You have kept your heart closed to love for fear of rejection as a default response.
- The stagnant flow of emotion leaves you 'heavy-hearted,' resentful, grieving, and wounded.
- All roads lead back to the heart. It is the center of energy, life, hope, and healing.
- Love begins in the heart and concludes there. However, allowing shattered hopes and damaged dreams to transform into suffering, followed by blame and resentment, will only burden the heart further.
- All life in the body flows through the heart and back out. Any emotional upset could keep the heart hostage until you choose to deal with it properly.
- You feel it is not fair that certain people have hurt you.
- The insistence on being right that you were wronged will eventually destroy your--self.
- There are emotions of resentment, grief, woundedness, and a 'heavy-heart.'

Heart Problems

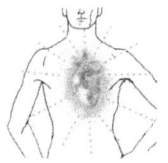

Healing Mindset

Seek peace instead of power. Your mind and body were created to enjoy experiencing love. You've been driven to maintain control and still get what you want, but it's time for that to change.

Have a heart by letting the resentment be a signal that it is time to get out of the dark clouds and share some sunshine. The caring will heal your heart and do someone else great good. Because the heart is an indicator of many emotional and physical issues, use the moments of heart symptoms to enrich your life with good communication, good food, good sleep, good meditation, and a good smile. You need a good old laugh.

Heart Problems

Affirmations:

- When I worry or fret - I laugh at my reflection and smile.
- I laugh at my face displaying danger, and take a deep breath, calm, stretch.
- I come back home to myself when I forgot to say hello to my beautiful day.
- I smile at the cute little things that a child, a dog, or my partner does or says.
- I frown on worry, over-concern, resentment, or blame.
- I hurry to praise others and myself.
- I slow down and feel my emotions of peace, warmth, and understanding.
- I ponder my life with intrigue, hope, and gratitude.
- I care for those who share and pray for those who don't.
- I serve others graciously.
- I discipline effectively.
- I am free to love others as they are.
- I give others the things that help them grow.
- I'm loved, I have joy, and I love others and myself.
- I give thanks often.
- I welcome abundance and wealth into my life.
- I give freely to others in need.
- I honor the warnings of the body, and respect the wise use of energy and thought.

Heart Problems

Supporting Foods:

- Apples
- Black beans
- Broccoli
- Brown rice
- Butter (appropriate amounts/organic)
- Cabbage
- Cauliflower
- Corn
- Garbanzo bean
- Fenugreek
- Fenugreek sprouts
- Kale
- Lentils
- Oats
- Red legumes
- Romaine lettuce
- Shiitake mushroom
- Wheat (If not gluten sensitive)

Heartburn

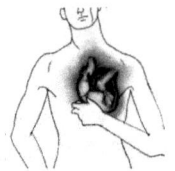

Troubled Mindset

- Are you trying to digest that which belongs to someone else?
- Are you pushing life without regard to what living is all about?
- You are pushing and pulling just to get through your day and your night. "Why can't I get it?!"
- Frustrated with yourself, you feel like you are failing to grasp something in life.
- Just like your body assimilates food, you are trying to assimilate life, but you are trying to do it in a way that does not honor or nurture you.
- You are trying to hold emotions in that could get you upset and irritable. So you think it is better to ignore and delay than to face what is right there in front of your face and your belly.
- It all makes you angry, then with heat, it 'bubbles' back up.
- Excessive responsibility and resistance to happiness reinforce a pattern of dissonance. "I'd rather burn than feel."

Heartburn

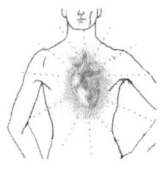

Healing Mindset

Watch yourself. Relax. Eat in quiet. Think simply. Life doesn't have to be so hard and so rough. Relax and calm the daily pressures. Weathering the storm is easy when you have clarity, patience, understanding, and focus. The key is to bring harmony to your gut by bringing awareness and balancing to your heart's feelings and mind's beliefs.

There is no magic pill for getting rid of emotional conflict. It is time to take a deep breath and embrace your challenges and heal your body and soul.

Heartburn

Affirmations:

- I am getting more accustomed to experiencing the emotions behind my pain.
- I'd rather be real and have some emotional pain than to continue this physical drama.
- My organs work together, play together, heal together.
- I am calm, cool, and collected.
- I laugh a little, play a little, and smile a lot.
- I embrace my challenges and heal.

Supporting Foods:

- Plenty of fresh fruit and raw vegetables
- Carrots
- Whole grains
- Fresh pineapple
- Papaya
- Brown rice
- Barley broth
- Eat slowly and chew food thoroughly

Hemorrhoids

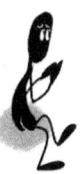

Troubled Mindset

- You try to give out your love, but it feels like "crap."
- Your insights have seldom been understood or accepted.
- You have come to believe that any intervention you take will make things worse, so you 'pull in the reigns' any time you consider opening your mouth.
- You end up resting on your resentment and anger over this unfair deal, feeling powerless to change things.
- The tug-of-war originates from the fear that if you release your anger, you will open your mouth, and if you share, you will make things worse.
- You hang on to your anger and remain tight-lipped as a protection, but it isn't working.
- While you are sitting on your emotions, your lower gut is trying to hide and suppress more than it can handle.
- You feel manipulated so you manipulate your inner feelings and communications so that you can attempt to control any possible negative attack from the villain in your life.

Hemorrhoids

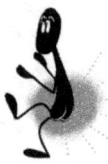

Healing Mindset

Start with balancing your internal world. Process the anger that is happening today and the hurts from years and years ago. Once you process your anger, your body will have room to heal, and your words will have a greater effect because the feeling behind them will be cleaner. You will, in effect, drop the rope of tug-a-war with yourself. Trust that you are able, and meant to be a unifying force for good as you play your part with love.

Hemorrhoids

Affirmations:
- I show self-respect when I feel down and heavy.
- Even though I feel concerned, I trust that I am safe to be me.
- I want to be strong and kind, so I respect my intentions by honoring my body first and then my heart.
- Sometimes it is fine to take a moment for me, so I relax and enjoy the moment of self-nourishment.
- I love myself with truth, understanding, and sharing what is appropriate in each relationship.
- I can do this. I find comfort in focusing on the positive intentions of others rather than their negative actions.
- I transform my will into personal power and encouraging joy. There is hope.

Supporting Foods:
- Drink plenty of water and juices
- Eat foods high in fiber
- Dark green leafy vegetables
- Wheat bran
- Oat bran
- Whole grains
- Brazil nuts
- Broccoli
- Cabbage
- Brussel sprouts
- Cereal grasses
- Green beans
- Guar gum
- Lima beans
- Pears
- Peas
- Alfalfa
- Carrots
- Molasses
- Eggplant
- Apples
- Bananas
- Beets
- Clams
- Figs

Hepatitis

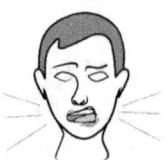

Troubled Mindset

- You make excuses for your behaviors when you know the reality is the opposite.
- The demands of your life began before you learned how to cope logically and responsibly.
- There have been heavy burdens and bitterness placed on you and by you. Thus, you cope by holding judgments and criticism to yourself, and deeply to others.
- You think you deserve more than you are getting.
- You have defensive reactions because you feel others betray you and don't care.
- Your hurt has left you defensive and resistant to growth or change.
- You are easily frustrated when you struggle to take effective action in your life.

Hepatitis

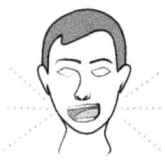

Healing Mindset

You can't have your resentment and your healing too. You will have to choose between taking care of your body or holding onto the bitterness. Your body needs you to bring in prebiotics, quality foods, and appropriate exercise. Likewise, your heart and mind need you to clean out the toxicity in your thinking.

It is time to change the patterns and find the positive, healthy balance of self-nourishment and giving time to helping others in their struggle. Allow deep nourishment to your soul by catching every negative thought and turning it into new learning. Courage starts with your honesty about what really matters. Entitlement is a destroyer, so take the opportunity to mature your responsible soul.

Hepatitis

Affirmations:
- I find opportunities everywhere to become my real self.
- I am so grateful for each day and each breath.
- My struggles have brought me the opportunity to become strong and industrious.
- I am insightful.
- I choose to praise others today.
- I choose to honor and respect my real core self with self-care, self-love, and peace.

Supporting Foods:
- Raw fruit and vegetable diet
- Artichokes
- Carrots
- Cereal grasses
- Garlic
- Red beets
- Cucumber
- Figs
- Celery
- Drinks and other vegetable juices
- Grape juice

Hernia

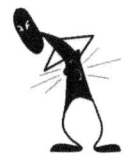

Troubled Mindset

- Your anger is pushing through despite noble efforts to dismiss or reject it.
- You are afraid to admit you might be wrong.
- You are afraid to tell them they are wrong.
- The pestering or nagging of another is centered inside, and you quietly are fighting your feelings towards them.
- You don't want to hurt people or cause contention, so you pretend there isn't a problem.
- The pretending of emotions only fuels the anger within you.
- You'd rather try to turn away from the real feeling of unresolved emotions and feelings than to confront being responsible for your part in a relationship.
- You end up feeling controlled, belittled, exploited, manipulated, and angry about it until you explode under the pressure.

Hernia

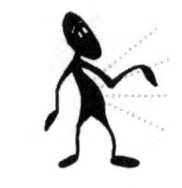

Healing Mindset

Find freedom in transformation. It is time to find somewhere you can go to release your feelings. If you do feel controlled, belittled, exploited, or manipulated, then end the madness of pushing the internal negative self-talk and resentment.

Face yourself and your internal dialogue. Find ways to move through your fears and tears. Become creative and open to new ways of expression and living. Allow life to nurture you in new ways.

Hernia

Affirmations:

- I find new ways to ground myself.
- I find safety in my creativity.
- I am aware of any secret feeling, and I release the need to hold on it anymore.
- I find ways to be nurtured that is honoring to my heart and body.
- I am true to my core values.
- My courage comes from my soul and my authentic heart.
- I am glad that I no longer carry their burden.
- I have the self-respect to care for myself and then share kindness.

Supporting Foods:

- Fennel congee
- Green beans
- Peas
- Broccoli
- Cabbage
- Carrots
- Apples
- Salmon
- Flax seed soaked
- Chia seeds soaked
- Garbanzo beans
- Hummus
- Drink lots of water
- Include extra fiber in the diet.

Hiccups

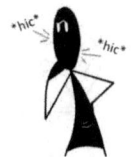

Troubled Mindset

- "Slow down! You go too fast, got to make the morning last."
- You are rushing through your eating, speech, and/or emotions.
- "Oops! Missed it!" You had a chance to be real with your feelings but passed it up.
- You gasped and gulped as you played tug-a-war between pleasing others and being true to yourself.
- This is in part because of your frequent struggle to understand and express your feelings.

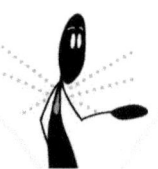

Healing Mindset

Take a moment and pause. Give yourself a chuckle because you are a little scattered. You may have two eyes, two ears, and two nostrils, but only one stomach. It needs your attention when you chew and swallow. Start with being aware. Acknowledge your feelings and choose consciously how to express or act upon them.

Hiccups

Affirmations:
- I smile at myself because I want to go and be and do things fast and now.
- I honor my creativity and my excitement.
- I enjoy taking time for me, myself, and my tummy.
- It is awesome that my body reminds me to slow down and enjoy the day.

Supporting Foods:

- Eat slowly and chew food thoroughly
- Eat a spoonful of honey or peanut butter
- Suck on a lemon
- Slowly sip icewater

Hip Problems

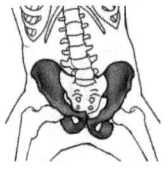

Troubled Mindset

- Instability in life shows up in the hips because of physical and spiritual imbalance.
- Decision making becomes very difficult as you reluctantly attempt to move forward.
- You may feel fear or worry as you wonder how you are going to fit in with your group or environment.
- You feel your value is in question, especially if you make the changes your hip is pleading for in order to ground with stability.
- This may include holding appropriate boundaries by not over carrying the mental/emotional burdens of others but supporting them in carrying their own.
- It's like you've got the whole world on your hips.
- You've got the burdens of others on your sides.
- You've got too much concern that you've got to hide all your worries and problems inside.
- You think that those in your life need some sort of help because they are in so much turmoil.
- You use your hips to ground and stabilize your life, but when you try to stabilize the whole world, it is too much burden.

Hip Problems

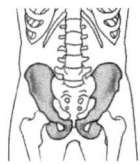

Healing Mindset

Left hip: Wake up to a new way of relating to yourself and others. Grow in your spiritual capacity as you deepen your connectedness, belonging, and close intimate relationships. Has more to do with female attributes or females in your life.

Right hip: Seek with a sense of adventure as you find your place in the world. Observe keenly your similarities and move forward with a foundation of clarity as a team player. Has more to do with male attributes or males in your life.

Suggestion: Help yourself help you by getting that energy of worry, overwhelming concern, and inner struggle out of your life. Are you really solving anything by carrying everyone's problems? It hasn't worked, it doesn't work. Your burden is mostly made up, so write, pray, move your painful emotions to the earth and sky and find freedom by supporting people through their problems instead of enabling them through their stories. Become connected with the flexibility of respecting yourself enough to stop the burdensome weight of worrying about others.

Hip Problems

Affirmations:
- I am safe & grounded.
- I don't need others to save or make me safe.
- I choose to enjoy my life with my relationships.
- I balance my finances and relationships.
- I trust that others can take care of themselves.
- If others need help, I set my boundaries to do what they ask and no more.
- I transform worry into courage for myself to be respectful of their journey.
- I encourage instead of discourage.
- I trust.
- I am flexible.
- I revitalize my life force energy every day.
- I enjoy life in every situation.

Supporting Foods:

- Purple and orange fruits and vegetables
- Bone broth

Hives

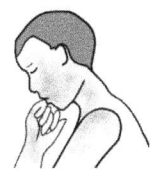

Troubled Mindset

- You are running away from a major conflict.
- You think it is unresolvable.
- You think it could be your fault, but then again, you want to blame someone else.
- At some level, you seem to believe anything that goes wrong in the world is your fault.
- Any issue, sorrow, or struggle, that others experience, especially family, is like a personal attack to your value.
- This perception is unfair, for you and others, because it triggers a big response to the perceived unfair attack.
- You are scared to face your enemy.
- You've tried to take on the load and care for others to 'correct' the injustices or sorrows as an effort to gain acceptance, but it's backfiring.
- You do not feel valued, appreciated, nor safe.
- You want to explode with frustration, but you can't, so you let it erupt inside.
- Ask yourself, "What am I really afraid of anyway?"
- Your imagination has gone too far into paranoia, and you think it is unfair and unsafe to deal with it.
- You have become too emotionally sensitive for your own good.

Hives

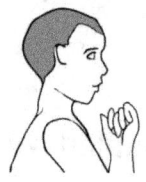

Healing Mindset

You have got this. Be real with the person in the mirror. Release the belief that it is up to you to fix the struggles others face, let them learn from their experiences as you do yours.

You have a part to play, but it is within the realm of your responsibility to yourself and your divine purpose. Take a deep breath. Now take those feelings of fear and anger and find a better use for them. For example, fear can help you be aware instead of freaking out. Anger can help you take action instead of a rash creation.

Your emotional sensitivity is a warning to stop, be real, let go, and learn to become courageous and honest with your situation. Find the humor, the joy, and the intrigue in all areas of your life.

Hives

Affirmations:

- I am keenly aware of my surroundings, and I am safe.
- I enjoy life in all its creations.
- I have moments to live and days to explore.
- The adventure of life is fun.
- I am free and expressive.
- I show respect for my body by remembering to clear my mind of chatter and to breathe fresh new life.
- I am okay.
- Things are good.

Supporting Foods:

- Turmeric
- Garlic
- Whole grains
- Brewer's yeast
- Fish
- Kelp
- Soybeans
- Dark green leafy vegetables
- Citrus fruits
- Asparagus
- Avocados
- Broccoli
- Bell peppers
- Oatmeal
- Sweet potatoes
- Legumes

Hodgkin's Disease

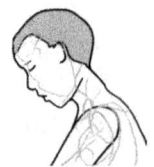

Troubled Mindset

- You have feelings of deep hopelessness.
- You never feel good enough. And trying harder to find love and appreciation has become too much.
- You have a 'do or die' attitude towards gaining acceptance from others.
- You need approval and love so much that it consumes your thoughts and mind.
- You have become sluggish in your self-judgments.
- You are driven to achieve yet continually depleting because you are never filled by any external positivity.
- Your will is getting weaker, but you still want to feel filled by other's words of encouragement.
- You have forgotten to accept yourself first before seeking the approval of others.
- You are distracted easily with regret, lack of love, and false hope.

Hodgkin's Disease

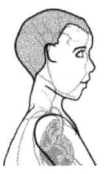

Healing Mindset

Wake up and smell the roses. Even if life has given you a rough road, you can smooth it out with being real with yourself in the moment. Start to appreciate your breath, your ability to think, your ability to care. Whenever you feel down, that means to connect to something of the earth and find beauty therein. When you feel anxious, that means to connect to something of the heavens and send some love to someone who cares.

Allow yourself to feel when love does come your way. The attention you receive may not fill your idyllic needs, because no one knows what they are, so accept whatever the other person can offer. Let each toxic thought turn into positive awareness and action. Find genuine love by being genuine.

Hodgkin's Disease

Affirmations:
- I am attending to my personal heart needs.
- I am paying attention to self-care of my thoughts and feelings.
- I am a good and valuable person.
- I have something valuable to share.
- I take my hurt and turn it into empathy for another.
- I am ready for God to bless me and my family.
- I sense the love of God in my life and my heart.
- I feel that all parts of my body are connecting.
- I am feeling the healing in every cell.
- Today I will be the sunshine in someone's life.

Supporting Foods:
- Citrus fruits
- Berries
- Dark green leafy vegetable
- Apricots
- Cranberries
- Celery
- Sprouts
- Sprouted almonds
- Zucchini
- Broccoli
- Fermented cabbage
- Vegetable broth
- Rice congee

Hyper-Activity

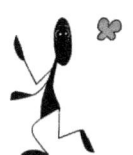

Troubled Mindset

- The demands or stimulation at hand feel beyond what you can handle.
- You fly into distraction as an avoidant pattern not to deal with any pressure.
- It's an ironic twist of overwhelm, fallen into disconnect.
- The pressures of the past left you concerned that you were missing an important detail, so you had to 'catch it all' but couldn't.
- You jump around, seemingly bored with the same old routine and looking for a change.

Healing Mindset

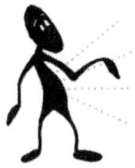

It is fun to be so active, but not so enjoyable for others in your life. You have been skipping out on being real with those who care about you. Avoidance is not joy, but hyperactivity gives you the illusion of thrill. Your boredom is a sign to rest your weary mind. There is so much that you miss when you speed through life. The challenge is to find the amazing in the small and simple things. When you do, you will find "awe" in many things. Your creativity will grow, and your productivity will be the hidden reward. Escape into the quiet several times a day and watch your brain start to work for you instead of driving you.

Hyper-Activity

Affirmations:
- I am quiet for just a moment, several times a day.
- Every once in a while, I choose to be still because the noise is distracting me from the intriguing hidden messages all around me.
- I have so much to experience, and that is the fun of life; to enrich each moment with the wise use of my attention.
- I am clear of distractions.
- Hey life, I am ready for you.
- I so love my mind.
- I so feel my heart.
- I so cherish my wonderful body in supporting my active life.
- I take time for the music that plays only for those who are balanced in their heart and mind.

Supporting Foods:
- Balanced diet of fruits and vegetables
- Only bread, cereals, or crackers made with rice or oats
- Brewer's yeast
- Broccoli
- Carrots
- Bell peppers
- Asparagus
- Avocados
- Bananas
- Green leafy vegetables
- Cantaloup
- Oatmeal
- Sunflower seeds
- Beans
- Salmon

Hypoglycemia

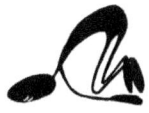 ## Troubled Mindset

- Trust is your most difficult attribute for your heart to express.
- Worry is getting the best of you.
- You over concern yourself with 'too much.'
- You rarely really trust, so you cope with worry, doing, and pleasing.
- You carry the belief that you have to be perfect before you get to enjoy divine love or support.
- You feel your burdens, but you feel the constant urge and need to carry worries about others.
- You run out of energy easily because you burn it up.
- Life's surprises feel jolting, burdensome, and painful.

Healing Mindset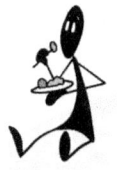

You have the ability to be authentically kind and gracious, but you let your pleasing get in the way. Set your boundaries to not prove yourself, but only communicate what is truly you and not what you think they want to hear. Love can be as abundant and impartial as sunshine or rain. It is available to everyone, including you. Allow yourself to be fueled by the sweetness of every interaction and experience in life as you learn and grow to become a better version of yourself each day.

Hypoglycemia

Affirmations:
- I enjoy life.
- I like the exploration side of seeking answers.
- When things don't work out, I enjoy the opportunity to discover more paths of possibilities.
- I am gracious with myself.
- Life is full of fun.
- I welcome the adventure of life.
- I trust God to bless me and my family.
- I allow God and the universe to assist me.
- I feel my brave heart.
- I trust.
- I am courageous enough to breathe in light and breathe out trust.

Supporting Foods:
- Kohlrabi
- Pumpkin
- Avocados
- Nopal cactus
- Steamed carrots
- Beet greens
- Dark green leafy vegetables
- Micro-greens
- Spirulina
- Salmon
- Grass-fed beef
- Parsnip
- Garbanzo beans
- Psyllium husks
- Crackers
- Flaxseed
- Increase fiber in the diet such as whole fruits and vegetables
- Whole grains
- Popcorn
- Oat bran
- Rice bran

Immune Issues

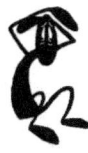

Troubled Mindset

- Your nerves are triggering your immune system to be on alert more than is necessary.
- Your worrisome mind is getting your body to overreact internally.
- It is a good thing that you have systems in place to protect you, but the guards are becoming your enemies, which reflects your mind and heart, thinking that life can not be safe.
- You wish you could control your environment, constantly on edge, while you try to 'force peace.'
- You end up feeling defeated because it doesn't work.
- You've given your all, but still feel blamed and maimed.
- You've fallen into defenseless despair with a 'why try?' kind of attitude.

Immune Issues

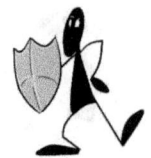

Healing Mindset

Trust in your body's ability to figure it out and that your quest to find answers is for helpful support, not for a twisted anxious control. You can't force your body because that makes your body overreact. If you overthink, you put your body on edge, and inflammation can follow. The best is to rest the mind often, comfort and care for your heart, and bring courage and hope to your body.

Pace yourself, listen, and connect to your body and mind with understanding and compassion. Create a space in which you can feel safe as you learn to let go, relax, and heal. Your physical body is an amazing organic operating machine. Trillions of communications are transpiring every second, so be in appreciation for what it does do. Meditate and connect to the energy of life and work with your body, not against it.

Immune Issues

Affirmations:

- I pace myself.
- I am an opportunity for growth and adventure.
- I am safe and free today.
- I am divine, and I am having a human experience.
- I create friends and family that honor and respect me.
- I listen and connect to others with understanding.
- I trust my body to be strong.
- I work with my body and mind to deal with life.
- I welcome the healing power of my body.
- I easily let go of the attacking nature of the crazy worried self.
- I trust in my body's ability to work things out and to heal all parts of my mind, body, and soul.
- I am safe and free today.
- I pace myself all day long.
- I am grateful for my body, my immune system, and all systems of my life.
- The body is a window into my life and enjoys cleaning the view and letting my body wash away the misconceptions.
- I am an opportunity for growth and adventure.
- My real self is divine, and I enjoy having my human experience.

Immune Issues

Affirmations:
- I create good friends, loving family that honor and respect me.
- I listen and connect to others that bring insightful understanding.
- I flow in trust and strength.
- I am strong and productive.
- I hear and honor the body signals and take time and care to heal my body.
- I feel the strength of mother earth's healing energy.

Supporting Foods:
- Acai berry
- Alfalfa sprouts
- Artichoke
- Asparagus
- Broccoli
- Cauliflower
- Cranberries
- Pineapple
- Fermented foods
  - Sauerkraut
  - Kimchi
- Kale
- Flax seeds soaked
- Lovage
- Cabbage
- Papaya
- Warm soups
- Congee (long cooked grains)
- Garlic
- Slow cooked garlic
- Onions
- Pearl barley
- Kelp
- Green drinks
- Nuts, seeds, grains and other foods high in fiber

Impotence
(Erectile Insufficiency, Libido)

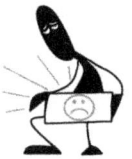

Troubled Mindset

- What is there to prove?
- Why struggle with something that is natural?
- If you worry about what the other person is saying or feeling, then you have the wrong focus.
- Concern yourself about how to perform in the adventure of your relationship. For example, what brings a surprised smile to their face? What causes a warm feeling to come all over them?
- By your actions, your touch, and your caring comments, let them perceive your depth of love, your personal interest, your adventurous personality, and your excitement for life.
- Intimacy is natural, so be natural in your communication and connection. Any fear is just to bring awareness, so cast it to the wind and be on a path of discovery with your heart communications.

Impotence
(Erectile Insufficiency, Libido)

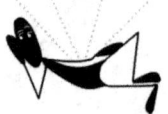

Healing Mindset

You can do this by being your true, natural self. When they complain, they are complaining about their own expectations not being fulfilled. Look and find ways to connect with the adventure of life, and then let the physical connection be "the cherry on top." Listen for their hidden messages of desires, wants, and needs. When you satisfy their heart, you will eventually satisfy their body. Discover your own personal fears as indicators to what your little self needs.

You probably need some kindness and appreciation, and for someone to make you feel attractive and capable. Don't wait for someone else to tell you that you are strong and capable. You practice in other areas of your life with being capable and confident then translate those to your intimate conversations. Life is natural, and so is your physical body. Let go of overcontrol about being out of control and be the curious, adventurous, and fun-loving human that you were born to be.

Impotence
(Erectile Insufficiency, Libido)

Affirmations:
- I love the adventure of love.
- I love being fun and silly with my partner.
- I can be so insightful and tender.
- I appreciate the way my partner cares for me.
- I am amazed at the feeling when I spontaneously care for another.
- I am so grateful for the opportunity to share my heart, mind, touch, and body with another.
- The sensation of natural pleasure is rewarding and invigorating.
- I thank God for the connection I have with another human being in this beautiful way.

Supporting Foods:
- Salmon
- Grass-fed beef
- Asparagus
- Papaya
- Pineapple
- Bananas
- Watermelon
- Raspberries
- Red beets
- Beet greens
- Mussels
- Chicken liver
- Pumpkin seeds
- Walnuts

Incontinence

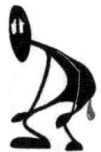

Troubled Mindset

- Most often, fear is behind the problem. Still, there are subtle angry irritations that loom deep because you are afraid to speak your mind. So your heart hides it, and your urinary body expresses it.
- Trying to control things and people hasn't worked, but you keep trying.
- Memories are affecting your physical body too quickly whenever they are triggered by life.
- You believe that if you lose your grasp or control of things, it will all fall apart like it's 'the end of the world.'
- You've kept your emotions and overwhelm in check with great intensity, but you are tired of it. Now your body is giving out under the pressure.
- You are in great need of an emotional release.

Incontinence

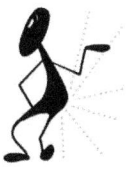

Healing Mindset

Watch when you feel the urge and notice that you are nervous about something. Smile, breathe, relax your muscles, stretch, and try to listen to the subtle chatter that is going on in your head. It is in the background, but it is telling of your discomfort that causes these urges and lack of control.

You can only control one thing, and that is usually nothing. Let go of the constant worry chatter. Try putting on a new article of emotional clothing. Wear the one that has "faith and hope" or another one that has "courage in the wake of the unknown" written on it.

Incontinence

Affirmations:
- I am in a positive state of mind and heart.
- My body wants to release the past, and I am happy to oblige.
- I encourage my muscles and nerves to enjoy the day.
- I am flexible and fluid.
- I am strong and grounded.
- My strength comes in positive self-confidence, and trusting life will work itself out.
- I am relaxed and content. I am courageous anytime, anyway.

Supporting Foods:

- Brewer's yeast
- Soaked nuts
- Sprouts
- Brown rice
- Eggs
- Fish
- Beef
- Chicken
- Legumes
- Peas
- Cheese
- Plain yogurt
- Spinach
- Broccoli
- Avocados
- Asparagus
- Apples
- Apricots
- Bananas
- Garlic
- Grapefruit
- Leafy greens
- Molasses
- Mushrooms
- Whole grains
- Soybeans
- Tofu

Indigestion

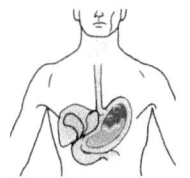

Troubled Mindset

- You think it is too hard to deal with certain people in particular situations, and some issues.
- You think if you can just get over a problem, you can take care of your tummy troubles.
- You are frustrated with too much, and you are irritated with someone or something.
- You take on too much responsibility to deal with the daily crisis.
- Your high hopes or constant expectations are causing deep disappointments.
- Life is difficult to resolve and integrate when your judgments fuel your anger and fears.
- Certain flavors, foods, and dishes just don't blend well. It is the same with life's relationships: certain people, personalities, and emotions clash and cause problems.
- The real issue is you make it too important, instead of enjoying the path of discovery of what and who blends well.
- Everyone has something to offer, so be open and flexible to what works and let go of what doesn't.

Indigestion

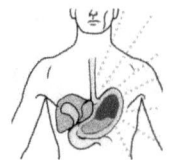

Healing Mindset

Resisting is hurting you. Start to listen and obey your inner intuitive voice. It will guide you on foods, times, and people. How you eat is sometimes more important than what you eat. Enjoy the moment and stop thinking when you are chewing.

The same is true with people: your emotional attitude when conversing with others is more important than what you say. Enjoy the adventure of communication, and you will start to relax your overwhelming internal reactions. You will be able to assimilate life. Rather than trying to 'fix' the outside world, focus inward and living your highest and best self. Recenter, breathe, and enjoy the adventure that life is.

Indigestion

Affirmations:

- I digest my food with ease.
- My body enjoys healthy and vital nourishment.
- My heart enjoys healthy and vital conversations.
- My mind is intrigued by the responses and reactions of others.
- I remember to remember me and my needs.
- I pause and breathe in life before bringing in new food or new thought.
- I catch my cycle of thinking and shift it to enriching and empowering thought patterns.
- I calm my belly and reward it with intentional nutrition.
- I love the personal attention my body gives me, so I mirror the love back with the positivity of thought and feeling.

Supporting Foods:

- Eat fiber rich foods
- Fresh fruits
- Vegetables
- Whole grains
- Fresh papaya
- Fresh pineapple
- Brewer's yeast
- Parsley
- Eggs
- Fish
- Rice bran
- Asparagus
- Broccoli
- Garlic
- Oatmeal
- Seafood
- Kelp
- Spirulina
- Chia seeds
- Flaxseed (buy whole and grind yourself)
- Bran Cereals

Infection

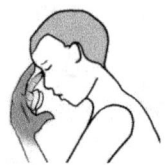

Troubled Mindset

- You opened your door to an invasion.
- You let the enemy in.
- Fear and upset can open you up to outside invaders, which can bring on infections. Why would you do that? Because you were trying to be too much for too many.
- As your mind and heart were trying to fulfill your expectations, others did not, and now you are annoyed and irritated with the results.
- You are upset that life as backfired on you.
- The tension is mounting, and deep chronic resentment has risen its ugly head. But you keep most of this hidden in your body, and you are attempting to pretend that everything is fine.
- This paradox causes a mental gap that the immune system cannot solve. Thus, the body is trying to wage a battle with the physical and emotional enemies of your life, which your inner personal conflict is the worst of them all.

Infection

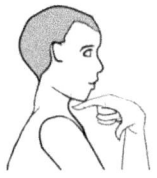

Healing Mindset

Be open to change. Be open to being real with the possibility that you cannot have all your wishes, fantasies, and expectations come true exactly how you want. Be aware of your constant mind chatter that wishes life to be different. Be friendly to your body and your heart by resting all areas of life.

Take the irritability and give it a rest. Take the worry and let the wind blow it away. Enjoy the moment. Inspect your expectations, and you'll find too many dreamy false beliefs. Respect your core self by living your values and loving yourself through life. Let others offer you real kindness and share with how you care. Your body repairs easily when it is not troubled with many things.

Infection

Affirmations:

- I am grateful that my body gives me warnings and that I can respond.
- I open my mind to new insights in supporting and caring for my body.
- I am ready for physical, emotional, and spiritual healing.
- I know my body knows because it is connected to the infinite knowing of the universe.
- I enjoy offering help to myself, and I let go and allow my body to heal.
- I visualize the layers of tissue inside my body, and I see my immune system is strong, capable, and effectual in healing.
- I strengthen all areas of my life, mind, and body.
- I eat and sleep to support my body's quest for health and well being.
- I feel the love of God blessing me.

Infection

Supporting Foods:

- Garlic
- Carrots
- Scallions
- Sprouted whole grains
- Raw nuts
- Seeds
- Dark green vegetables
- Micro-algae
- Millet
- Barley
- Oats
- Quinoa
- Amaranth
- Teff
- Flax seed oil
- Pumpkin seed oil
- Chia-seed oil
- Sprouted beans
- Beets
- String beans
- Black berries
- Raspberries
- Bananas
- Soups, stews and congees

Inflammation

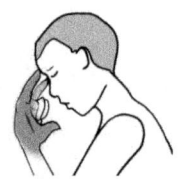

Troubled Mindset

- Water equals emotions, and something has flooded!
- You are irritated and frustrated. However, before the inflamed emotions, your deep feelings and emotions were hurt and not made well.
- Over time, your sadness and self-pity has turned to anger and then to resentment.
- Your body is expressing that which you are unwilling to deal with or communicate.
- An unbalanced emotional and mental life reaps the negative consequences in the physical body.
- Being afraid and holding onto your fears or being frustrated and pushing them way down doesn't help your immune system, it only aggravates it.

Inflammation

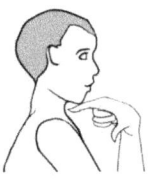

Healing Mindset

You have the opportunity to accept where you are in the present moment. If you don't, your body will remind you of your stubbornness later. Start with what is possible to be and do. Feelings are information, not truth. Choose to be firm in heart and mind concerning what is right while honoring appropriate boundaries. Be flexible and honest. They are like leaves on the wind.

Take your emotions and move through the process of finding much-needed processing and release. Let go of being frustrated with yourself and with others. Your self-judgments aggravate the inner tissues of your body. Stop grating yourself and respect how great you really are.

Inflammation

Affirmations:
- I am safe and secure.
- I move the process of healing along with my appreciation and gratitude for each experience of my life.
- I release the rigid thought and replace it with understanding and insight.
- I cool my inner feelings with wise perspectives.
- I warm myself with good and healthy emotional nourishment.
- I am patient with my learning, and I am responsibly tolerant of their learning.
- I respect my body by eating foods that support my healing.
- I respect my mind by thinking about concepts that transform my life.

Supporting Foods:
- Water/Get hydrated
- Fresh juices
- Herbal teas
- Lots of raw fruits and vegetables
- Dark leafy greens
- Chinese cabbage
- Cereal grasses
- Onion
- Garlic
- Fresh pineapple
- Citrus fruits
- Berries
- Bell peppers
- Broccoli
- Celery
- Figs
- Barley
- Carrots
- Congees
- Potatoes
- Squash
- Sweet potato

Insomnia

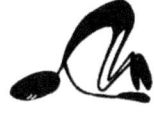 ## Troubled Mindset

- Your mind is racing down a track that doesn't seem to end.
- The frequencies of your brain are trying to do too much and need a rest, but the fears and concerns pop the frequency back to staying awake to be safe.
- Your body is producing biochemistry to fight or flight mode instead of rest and restore mode.
- The complexity of problems is trying to be resolved through the wrong area of the brain.
- The most complex issues are best when they are put to a temporary rest, and the mind allows the body to renew and refuel.

Healing Mindset

Get in the habit during the day of taking 5 minutes every hour to rest and restore your body. You will be more productive and more alive. Being alive in the day allows the body to restore in the night. Journaling, saying positive affirmations, embracing the dark shadows of your fears, and writing down your journey will be a catalyst for productive change. Your conflict is not with the world but within yourself. Literally, it is the conflict of brain waves that keeps you awake. Find a place inside that is quiet and non-combative without the worries. Go to this place often, and you will find hope, assurance, and wisdom.

Insomnia

Affirmations:
- I found myself.
- I enjoy a good story because it relaxes my logical mind.
- My hope is for renewal, and I thank my body for how magically it performs its functions.
- I put to rest the tasks of today because tomorrow I will be at my best.
- My sleep restores my mind, my body, and my soul.
- I thank the good Lord for today, tomorrow, and all the awesome experiences of life.
- I am so appreciative of my opportunity to rest and rejuvenate my precious body.

Supporting Foods:
- Water/Get hydrated
- Bananas
- Oatmeal
- Mulberry
- Oysters
- Sprouted wheat
- Brown rice
- Oats
- Barley gruel
- Cucumber
- Celery
- Mulberries
- Lemon
- Try eating foods high in tryptophan such as turkey
- Yogurt
- Bananas
- Figs
- Dates
- Milk
- Tuna
- Whole grains or Nut butters
- Eat a half of a grapefruit before bed
- Mushrooms for the evening meal

Itching

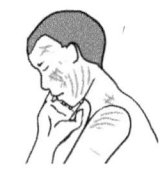

Troubled Mindset

- You have too much going on inside of your head.
- You are irritated or impatient, or both.
- You wish for things that are not possible because they come from pain, suffering, regret, or hurt.
- You are putting value on the wrong things in life.
- You are avoiding a recurring problem.
- Something is bugging you, and this irritation won't go away until you consider your part in the matter.

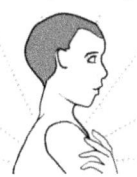

Healing Mindset

Review your life. Take time to settle down and watch how you think about things. You probably review the same thoughts over and over again. Take the moment to write them down and then toss them away. You are being consumed by the junk feelings and junk thoughts in your mind and life. Don't let your circumstances determine your self-worth.

When you feel the itch to get out or run away, breathe yourself back into the present moment. Lovingly empower yourself to rise back into your capacity to face your struggles with strength and peace. Consider the body area for more details.

Itching

Affirmations:

- I am at peace just where I am.
- I accept my good.
- Peace starts with me.
- I am seeing past the confusion of struggle and blame.
- I am embracing my responsibility in all of life's situations.
- I see the value of experience.
- I am grateful for the times that I resist so that I know what I might be upset about or afraid of.
- I move past the silly or petty worries and blame into becoming an empowered, strong, soulful self.
- I ask for forgiveness as I offer gracious understanding to others.

Supporting Foods:

- Asparagus
- Avocados
- Broccoli
- Brussel sprouts
- Cantaloupe
- Citrus fruits
- Mangos
- Bell peppers
- Pineapple
- Berries
- Tomatoes
- Kale
- Spinach
- Carrots
- Garlic
- Fish liver oil
- Yellow squash
- Soybeans
- Sunflower seeds
- Molasses

Jaundice

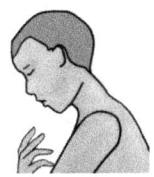

Troubled Mindset

- You are not processing life well.
- It is too difficult to handle the emotions, the feelings, and the physical issues all at the same time. So you resort to being a part-time cynic.
- You are not able to handle the responsibility.
- You are overloaded with unprocessed emotions.
- You don't have the mind to know what to do with all the emotions.
- Since you can't stomach everything you experience, your outward expression is optimistic, but internally you lack the optimism and compassion you need to heal.
- This leaves you with negativity and pessimism.
- You have felt you can't just be yourself and be understood, accepted, or supported.
- You may be carrying fear or anger that has been passed down through the generations.

Jaundice

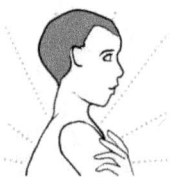

Healing Mindset

Take the first step into the world of surrendering to the natural functions of the body and mind. To be able to move through the mire, you need to first take care of being you and doing what you can do for yourself. Love yourself enough to be you, and let others be themselves too.

Choose to appreciate the purpose and value of all. Do not force life to flow in a certain direction. Instead, flow with life. When overloaded, take one piece of life at a time and carefully process it fully. Take care to be fair to your inner self.

Jaundice

Affirmations:

- I courageously process life, one step at a time.
- I gradually consider all my needs.
- I let the light of the universe shine inside of me.
- My body needs me to be open and free.
- I feel empowered to process energies that are ancient but new to me.
- I can let go of deep-seated emotions with breath, movement, water, and rest.
- I am not my emotions, but I am experimenting with transforming them into light, love, and learning.

Supporting Foods:

- Raw fruits and vegetables
- Aduki bean
- Grape juice
- Turnip
- Watercress
- Beets
- Beet greens
- Fresh lemon juice
- Artichokes
- Carrots
- Cereal grasses
- Garlic
- Cucumber
- Figs
- Celery
- Green drinks
- Beet juice
- Carrot juice

Jaw Problems

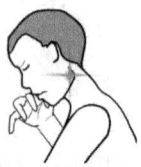

Troubled Mindset

- You chew on ideas but can't seem to find an effective way to implement them.
- This is in part due to your lack of courage in dealing with crucial situations in your life.
- Past trauma or terror in your life may be impacting you.
- You grapple with speaking the truth, often opting to suppress rather than communicate your feelings.
- This may be affecting increasing feelings of tension, frustration, resentment, and rage.
- You are nervous in the night while your subconscious is trying to take control and release your daily conflicts.
- Tightening muscles get their lead from your emotional brain.

Jaw Problems

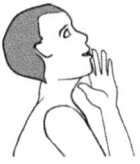

Healing Mindset

Follow your intuition and find the means to express yourself. Trust it above the wave of negative emotions, then release them. Don't give up as you maintain a determination for positive change. You only need a few moments once an hour to practice relaxing your muscles. Your pattern of tightening your muscles can be worked out with the daily practice of release and relax, pause and reflect, and renew and recommit.

Most of your jaw problems are colored by your emotions, so let those feelings lead you to see what is so important that you will cause yourself pain and discomfort. Your little child inside needs some attention, love, appreciation, understanding, and safety. You can change your worry, anger, and controlling thoughts to awareness, appreciation, and trust. Act with calm confidence, and your jaw muscles will stop reacting.

Jaw Problems

Affirmations:

- I speak the truth and listen to my inspiration.
- I release the inner conflicts, so I enjoy freedom from rage and anger.
- I am courage.
- I am complete, with God determination being second nature to me.
- My most focused muscles are attentive to do their job of speaking and chewing, and nothing more.
- I see my day, plan, act, enjoy the rewards, and chuckle at the redos.
- What a great life it is.
- I feel so blessed that I am functionally stable and emotionally clear in the turmoil that is around me.
- There is peace in my soul and fun expressions in my heart.

Supporting Foods:

- Steamed vegetables
- Avocados
- Green leafy vegetables
- Fresh fruits apples
- Apricots
- Bananas
- Grapefruit
- Whole grains
- White fish
- Salmon
- Chicken
- Turkey
- Brown rice
- Homemade soups
- Brewer's yeast
- Dairy products

Joint Pain

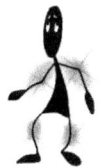

Troubled Mindset

- You don't want to bend to the process of life and the future.
- You don't trust yourself and/or the universe, so fear keeps you rigid and proud in holding on to things as they are, or as you wish them to be.
- You're hanging on to resentment from what has happened. You end up being forceful in your actions rather than moving with gracefulness when trying to avoid unpleasant future outcomes.
- Your rigid nature is not your natural state.
- It happened over time because you tried to control too much, and then you coped with life by thinking and feeling too many negative things about your life and others.
- Bitterness builds up from hopeful expectations that did not come about.
- The gradual accumulation of resentment makes you more inflexible and painful.

Joint Pain

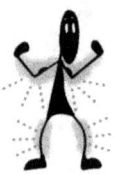

Healing Mindset

You can find a way to become flexible again by taking care of all parts of yourself. You have toxins in the joints, liver, lymph, and more. You have emotional and mental toxins that won't go by putting them in a denial box. The denial boxes are your joints, and they are full of it. You may have thought that if you were sweet enough, kind enough, or even mean enough, then they would change - but it didn't work.

Think a new thought to be kind enough for yourself to be honest in all your communication with your heart, mind, and soul. It is time to release your fantasies and take a step forward with deep feelings of commitment and care. Be true to you. Any negative thought makes you hurt more. Be honest, take the steps necessary to clean up your situations, and then follow through with trusting the universe to support you through the journey.

Joint Pain

Affirmations:

- I find joy in simple acts, simple smiles, simple gestures.
- I find gratitude on my lips, in my heart, and in my actions.
- I find praise in my eyes, in my ears, and in my mouth.
- I find hope in my body, in my soul, and in my health.
- I find flexibility in my thoughts, in my movements, and in my relationships.
- I choose to be kind and honest with myself.
- I detox, one moment, one thought, and one feeling at a time. Releasing it to the earth or the heavens.

Supporting Foods:

- Barley
- Wheatgrass
- Alfalfa sprouts
- Celery
- Black sesame seed
- Mulberry
- Almonds
- Goat's milk
- Herbal teas
- Broths
- Eggs
- Asparagus
- Garlic
- Onions
- Green leafy vegetables
- Brown rice
- Rye
- Whole wheat
- Fish
- Fresh pineapple
- Flaxseeds
- Oat bran
- Rice bran

Kidney Stones

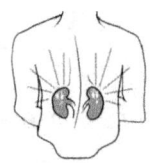

Troubled Mindset

- You are suddenly aware of things happening around you that are out of your control.
- You are afraid that if things don't change that the results of these events will leave you out in the cold.
- You are angry but fear has overtaken you; thus, your kidneys are stuck with dread and anxiety that causes you intense pain and discomfort.
- You think "why do people do what they do? Why can't they just leave things alone and not be difficult and trying?"
- They are changing and demanding too much and too fast.
- You just can't do or be whatever is being demanded.
- Your judgments and inner turmoil are turning you into "stone" while trying to be nice and cooperative.
- Your deep fear and deep resentment are a poor mix for your kidneys.

Kidney Stones

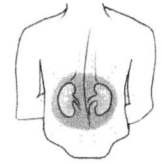

Healing Mindset

It is time to stop and smell the roses. The thorns of life have a purpose but should not consume your thoughts.

Let go of resentments and grudges. When you feel controlled and smothered by the expectations of others it is time to pause and be honest about your real value, purpose, capability, and capacity. Holding onto fear and resentment is harming you, so start to communicate without blame, but with what is real for you.

Learn to be honest with your perception. You might be exaggerating and then holding on too much causing deep dark feelings inside. The way to the light is to stop the blame and build from what is possible for you to deal with. When you catch yourself tightening up start a "flow moment" with breath and movement. Time to love yourself first and then build from there.

Kidney Stones

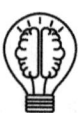

Affirmations:
- I am free to be me in all situations.
- I love my life and I live it by living each moment.
- I soften my hardened emotions by discovering understanding.
- I am curious to see how I will deal with life today.
- I appreciate the opportunity for new experiences.
- I honor my inner core.
- I am coming to know myself.
- I am flowing through the obstacles with strength and intrigue.

Supporting Foods:

- Apples
- Apple juice
- Black beans
- Cardamom
- Celery
- Celery juice
- Celery root
- Chayote (vegetable pear)
- Cucumber
- Grapes
- Grape juice
- Fennel
- Horseradish
- Kiwi
- Lemon and lime
- Parsley
- Pear
- Radish
- Turmeric

Kidneys

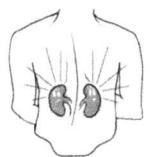

Troubled Mindset

- You don't have an appreciation for your innate worth.
- Life feels heavy and hard to bear. You don't trust in your capacity to take it on.
- You blame others for your feelings rather than dealing with them appropriately and with self-responsibility.
- You end up holding on to experiences and feelings of fear, panic, or loneliness, instead of releasing the negativity of life.
- There is a deep desire for connection, coupled with the feeling of lack in your relationships.
- This constant feeling of concern is putting unnecessary stress on your body.
- All of these block the vitality necessary to living fully.

Kidneys

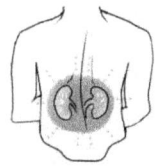

Healing Mindset

Start with creating a healthy relationship with yourself. Let go of the various layers of self-judgment to rise above the waters of doubt and fear. That means when fear comes, acknowledge it and center into the peace and strength that is inside of you. You can use comforting imagery or breathing to support the release of any fear and doubt.

Catch yourself in your self-judgments, stop thoughts such as "I should've," "Why didn't I," or "I'm such a _____ for_____." and transform them into gratitude for experiences that teach you and bring greater wisdom. Choosing the route of maturity may be a challenge. Be consistent as you grow into your best self.

Kidneys

Affirmations:

- I enjoy life.
- I am in awe of the beauties all around me.
- I turn fear into faith and hope.
- I turn dread into hope and courage.
- I turn emotional experiences into wisdom and understanding.
- I take the troubled times of life and create joy.
- I take optimistic action.
- I respect God and the spiritual side of others.
- I am energized with life.
- Peace is natural.
- I open to universal chi.
- I assimilate water.
- I let go of the toxins of life.
- I am faith and trust.

Supporting Foods:

- Water
- Sprouts
- Alfalfa sprouts
- Algae
- Beetroot
- Black beans
- Celery
- Chlorophyll
- Fennel
- Fish
- Globe artichoke
- Greens
- Kidney beans
- Lamb
- Egg
- Mushrooms
- Rhubarb
- Romaine lettuce
- Sesame seeds
- Walnuts
- Watermelon
- Wheat grass

Kleptomania / Stealing

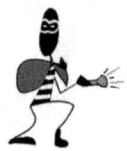

Troubled Mindset

- You are consumed with what you don't have, and with the secret task of getting it. Thus, it is not the object you are missing, but the mature understanding that no physical thing can satisfy the heart or bring peace to the racing mind.

- You feel depressed because you felt overlooked, or ridiculed, or taken advantage of. Now you are secretly harsh on yourself with shame and blame, which worsens the more you take that which is not yours.

- Your quest for better or the spiritual gets clouded by your internal bitterness towards yourself.

Kleptomania / Stealing

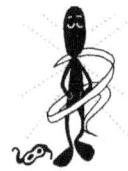

Healing Mindset

The abundance you seek is found within you. Start by offering yourself positive attention to give room to release any shame or guilt. You are not your choices. Choose in a way that honors who you are and have compassion when you fall short.

Your mind needs you to walk your steps carefully when you start the ritual of theft. Because, once your footsteps are on that path, your core mind shuts off and you are a slave to the compulsive mind.

If you want freedom, then you need to start to take a new step, intention-ing towards a new habit that builds your character and connects your real mind then brings positive satisfaction. You can do this, but you will need someone who cares to be firm and supportive with you while you are on your quest for change.

Kleptomania / Stealing

Affirmations:
- I am on the path of change in my mind and my heart.
- My primal brain is listening to my true character of courage.
- Every time I want to hide and take, I take that moment and stretch my body, my breath, walk, and say affirmations of clarity and gratitude.
- I am grateful for my life and all its abundance.
- I have everything I need.
- I share my heart to save my soul.
- I am on the adventure of change.
- I enjoy observing my mind and body as I transform my habits.

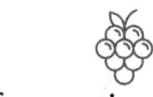

Supporting Foods:

- Eat a well balanced diet of fresh fruits and vegetables
- Whole grains
- Blueberries
- Papaya
- Fresh pineapple

Knee Problems

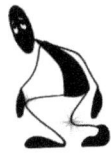

Troubled Mindset

- Your heart and your mind may be pulling you in two different directions. This could be making you quite indecisive.
- You're also feeling stuck because of being unbending or proud about what to do.
- There may be a previous betrayal (including self-betrayal) that you haven't made peace with yet.
- Family troubles may continue to haunt you, unresolved.
- Let go of the past and look forward with interest.
- Make returning to joy your leading priority, with the highest and best good for all in your heart.

Healing Mindset

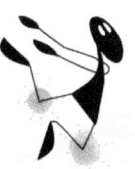

Pain in your left knee, suggests a need to end the resistance to their persistent action or reaction. Be honest with yourself in all your relationships. Transition from blame and regret, to authentic communication, even if, others persist to resist your warm attention. Learn to uplift yourself and others. Focus on aligning your spiritual direction.

Pain in your right knee, suggests a need to transform your awareness. Work on being assertive and balance your relationship with authority figures in your life.

Knee Problems

Affirmations:

- I let go of the past and look forward with enthusiasm.
- I am safe in relationships.
- I create and walk on the path of a great future.
- I solidly walk through life's storms.
- I enjoy uplifting others while supporting my inner needs.
- I gladly release the troubles of those I care about.
- I warmly care what can be safely shared.

Supporting Foods:

- Celery
- Cucumber
- Broccoli
- Brussel sprouts
- Green leafy vegetables
- Sprouts
- Parsley
- Pomegranate

- Watermelon
- Bananas
- Mango
- Papaya
- Pineapple
- Sauerkraut
- Kelp
- Brown rice

- Turkey
- Black beans
- Garlic
- Onions
- Quinoa
- Lamb
- Trout
- Salmon

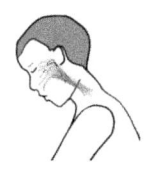

Laryngitis

Troubled Mindset

- You're 'so upset you can hardly speak.' This upset is anger and/or fear, likely toward authority in your life.
- You don't want to share your thoughts or feelings, but you resent that fact.
- You want to speak up for yourself, but guilt or resentment from what happened when you tried to share still cripples you with fear of possible judgment or rejection.
- You believe what you say might be used against you, even if you truly believe it could have helped.
- You believe there is nothing that you can do about it.
- You got lost in resenting that which you could not control.
- Remember that there is no amount of effort that will change what is happening if they are stubborn.

Healing Mindset

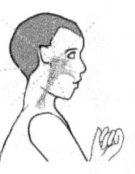

You can let those hidden negative thoughts be indicators that you still want to change your world by changing the world of others. You can have your judgment for a minute, but for the rest of the hour, be productive with your mind by enjoying the transformation of your day instead of thinking of changing theirs. Give yourself a rest from the overwhelm of life, and find a well that is overflowing with insights, peace, and understanding.

Laryngitis

Affirmations:

- I pause to heal my heart.
- I can receive help and share when needed.
- I believe that what I can change is my heart.
- I hold my mind responsible for thinking beyond my fear and being clear about what I can change in my life.
- I speak clearly and effectively.
- I enjoy expressing myself.
- I let those hidden negative thoughts be indicators that I still want to change my world by changing others.
- I am learning to rest my body and my mind.

Supporting Foods:

- Whole grains
- Brewer's yeast
- Eggs
- Fish and other seafood
- Kelp
- Legumes
- Soy beans
- Sunflower seeds
- Apricots
- Berries
- Papayas
- Peaches
- Avocado
- Broccoli
- Cucumber
- Fig
- Radish
- Watercress
- Asparagus
- Onions
- Sweet peppers
- Carrots
- Sweet potatoes
- Yellow squash
- Tomatoes
- Brown rice
- Oats
- Wheat germ
- Drink plenty of water and fresh juices
- Eat a well balanced diet of fresh fruits and vegetables
- Citrus fruits especially lemon and lime
- Dark leafy green vegetables

Leg Problems

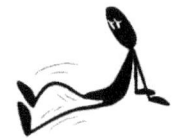

Troubled Mindset

- "Where am I going?" You are resisting your destiny.
- You have many ideas and wants, but you are either avoiding the direction of your purpose and/or a part of you is still immature, not wanting to embrace full responsibility.
- It is confusing to your mind to want something that you keep avoiding or resisting.
- You resist, choosing to deal with the physical pain long before you face up to the feelings and beliefs that hold you back.
- You are still struggling with maintaining a balance in your life.
- You have issues of responsibility in your relationships, including one or more of the following: love, friends, money, work, or living your true purpose.
- Denial is becoming more of your polished traits, rather than developing one of your core talents.
- You aren't enjoying your obligations and carry the attitude of "I'd rather just run away from it all." Fleeing from failure, you end up falling right into it.
- You haven't felt supported in part because you have denied supporting yourself within.

Leg Problems

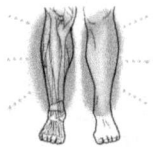

Healing Mindset

Left leg: You feel a lack of support in your life in part because you don't trust it when it is offered, so you turn it down. The left leg has more to do with the struggle to balance the spiritual and feminine aspects of yourself.

Right leg: You are lacking in love support, or you are love avoidant. The right leg has more to do with a struggle to balance the physical and masculine aspects of yourself.

Your legs are speaking loudly but don't speak clearly, so open your intuitive ears, and listen. Observe when they are a problem, and you will notice patterns that will lead you to solve the mystery. You need to become responsible for your patterns of communication with others.

Watch your vulnerability. See how you avoid being really honest with your close friends and loved ones. Take your emotional pain and be real with it and move through that storm. You don't need fear or anger as an excuse to suppress your suffering. Use negative emotions as a path to see what you are resisting. If you don't, the problem could persist.

Leg Problems

Affirmations:
- I am flexible and strong.
- I release the fears into cheers for myself because I am changing my life.
- I appreciate my ability to walk and move.
- I am confident in my ability to act, move, and change the course of my day for the better.
- I am grateful for movement and vitality.
- I enjoy my relationships.
- I love being authentic in all my relationships.
- I observe and learn from any inner resistance so that I can build my character and my strength.
- My energy is building stronger muscles every day.
- I balance life with keen awareness, productive action, and heart-filled confidence.

Supporting Foods:
- Drink lots of water
- Raw nuts and seeds
- Whole grains
- Millet
- Barley
- Tofu
- Mung beans and sprouts
- Fresh fruits & vegetables
- String beans
- Black beans
- Black soybean
- Legumes
- Melons
- Blackberry
- Mulberry
- Water chestnut
- Wheat germ
- Potato
- Seaweeds
- Sardines
- Crab
- Clam
- Eggs
- Cheese

Liver

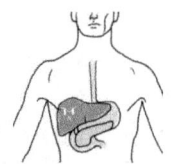

Troubled Mindset

- You may be experiencing strong unresolved emotions of anger, bitterness, excess sadness, or resentment.
- You take much of these excess emotions out on yourself.
You have not understood what has happened, or is happening, that keeps causing hurt feelings.
- You end up complaining, fault finding and being judgmental of yourself and others.
- These attitudes are used as protection from seeing the truth, fearing the truth to be against you.
- Without understanding, you struggle to trust, forgive, and let go.
- The tension in your body makes sleeping, resting, and planning more difficult.

Liver

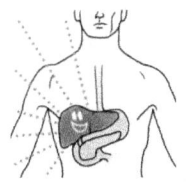

Healing Mindset

The liver has so many functions that it needs the human brain and heart to be more mature and congruent with their feelings and beliefs.

The liver is strong when the mind and heart are together, on the same path, with both firm beliefs and respectful communications with others. Excess emotions hurt the liver. Use your feelings wisely, and your liver will willingly support you.

Seek wisdom and spiritual understanding of this life's experiences. Truth is the highest priority. You can do it, trust yourself. Nourish yourself with appropriate foods to strengthen you in your resolve.

Learn the meaning of true respect. You can't respect others unless you respect yourself. And you can't respect yourself if you have to be right and need to argue. A responsible character doesn't need to use anger, resentment, bitterness, or sadness to prove a point. The responsible emotions from a liver will make sure the body is taken care of, even though it is not given enough nutrients and power to do so.

Liver

Affirmations:
- I transform life to be efficient and powerful.
- I transform anger into productive action.
- I honor and respect leadership abilities.
- I respect my emotions, and I change them for my good.
- I am clean, clear, and focused.
- I can integrate all areas of my life.
- My multitasking is grounded and effective.
- My vision takes root today with clarity.
- I am motivated to start and complete my projects.
- I have the energy to accomplish my goals.
- I can transform the stumbling blocks into stepping stones.
- I trust.
- I lead with God as my guide.
- I release all negative emotions and regrets and frustrations.

Liver

Supporting Foods:

- Apple
- Asparagus
- Avocado
- Barley (sprouted)
- Beet
- Black cherry
- Brussels sprouts
- Carrot
- Celery
- Chia seed
- Fennel
- Garlic
- Globe artichoke
- Grape
- Greens
- Flax seed
- Lemon
- Lime
- Mulberry
- Mung bean
- Pear
- Plum
- Raspberry
- Rye
- Seaweed
- Tomato
- Walnuts
- Wheat grass

Lung Problems

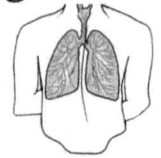

Troubled Mindset

- "I'm so sad I can barely breathe."
- You are experiencing panic or anxiety stemming from a sense of abandonment.
- The grief, shame, loneliness, and hopeless have become overwhelming.
- You may feel confused as you struggle to piece together how to honor your path and purpose, feeling it is against the opinions of others.
- You've suppressed yourself, and you may feel smothered by how others think you should do things.
- Starved for love, you've been unwilling to maintain yourself from one moment to the next, believing you don't even deserve it.

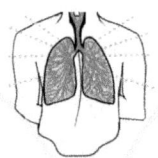

Healing Mindset

Observe your experience as separate from the essence of who you are to make space for healing. Breathe in and out as you use the affirmations to help bring vitality and enthusiasm back into your experience. When flying in an airplane, you have to put the breathing mask on yourself before you turn to help others. Be there for you, rise into you, then you will be able to help others appropriately.

Lung Problems

Affirmations:
- I desire.
- I expand into life.
- I breathe in the gifts of God now.
- I am alive and share.
- I am open.
- I breathe in life abundantly.
- I acknowledge God in all things.
- Everyone is my teacher.
- I reflect with understanding in peace.
- I am thoughtful.

Supporting Foods:

- Apple
- Carrots
- Cauliflower
- Celery
- Chard
- Citrus
- Fennel
- Fenugreek seeds
- Fish
- Garlic
- Greens
- Kelp
- Onions
- Papaya
- Peach
- Pear
- Persimmon
- Pumpkin
- Radish
- Seaweed
- Tomato
- Turkey (for some)
- Yam
- Possibly brown rice
- Chickweed (for some)
- Cantaloupe (for some - if candida or fungus do not use)
- Use garlic & onion to sniff when there is lung congestion.

Lyme Disease

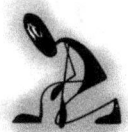

Troubled Mindset

- There is no good time for the problems of Lyme's. However, you can look at some of the overwhelm you have got yourself into.
- There is a lack of boundaries with your relationships, your body, and your time.
- You have worked too hard, too long.
- You give and give and give more, but they are still not there for you.
- You feel not good enough, understood, safe, or trusted.
- You overdue yourself then feel no one is there for you when you collapse from your overextension. You fear them and their emotions anyway, resisting closeness and commitment in relationships.
- You didn't trust them to be responsible for their needs, which is part of why you try to do it all. Still, you feel hurt, frustrated, and unsupported.
- Essentially, you feel stuck between a rock and a hard place.

Lyme Disease

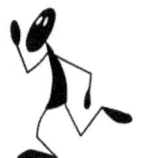

Healing Mindset

Look deeply and realize that most of your problems are the constant conflict inside of what to do and how to do it. Settle the conflict by finding a path of honoring the boundaries of your capacity of energy levels. As you respect your body, your body will respect you.

Choose to watch your negative self-talk or your blame, that will feed the shadows of your problems. Choose to be grateful for learning, for others, for nature, for the gift of trust. Inside the intuition of trust, you will find a gift of awareness that can wisely guide you through your suffering into healing.

Lyme Disease

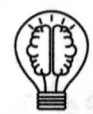

Affirmations:

- I am firm in my faith that I am finding answers for my health.
- I have an abundance of life, and I gradually move it through my body to empower and heal.
- My heart feels my self-care as love.
- I enjoy learning at the pace that my body can turn it into action.
- I trust, and I am healing my body and life one step at a time.
- I have positive boundaries for my body and life.
- I choose to pace my life for rejuvenation of my heart, soul, and body.
- I find the joy in the experience.

Supporting Foods:

- Garlic
- Kelp
- Pineapple
- Brazil nuts
- Brown rice
- Brewer's yeast
- Broccoli
- Chicken
- Molasses
- Citrus fruits
- Organic dairy products
- Liver
- Onions
- Whole grains
- Legumes
- Eggs
- Oatmeal
- Soybeans
- Sweet potatoes
- Wheat germ
- Berries
- Asparagus
- Avocados
- Cantaloupe
- Mangos
- Sweet peppers
- Rose hips
- Tomatoes
- Apricots
- Carrots
- Pumpkin
- Yellow squash
- Green drinks with dark green leafy vegetables

Manic

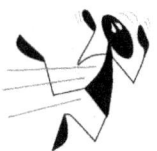

Troubled Mindset

- You have let your fears turn to constant chatter in your head.
- It is as though a fragment piece of you is running the show, and you have chosen to listen to the part that isn't the true core self.
- There are nutritional and emotional needs that are not being met. However, you are sabotaging getting help because you feel out of control, and your mind is narrowing your view of what is real as if you have tunnel vision.
- Your thoughts are speeding up and going into denial.
- The future feels frightening because you base your expectations on past experiences, but it's not realistic.
- Dirty energy fields in your life may be due to trauma and health problems.
- You may sense a darkness within that you wish to be free from, but your intuition has been flawed.

Manic

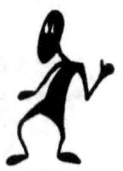

Healing Mindset

You need to practice taking a reality check every hour with breathing and grounding exercises. You need to watch your consumption of sugar and processed food. Slow down and chew your food.

You need to practice opening up your view of life and find new people to converse with so that your narrow focus and tunnel vision is expanded. Notice your body, and anytime you feel the tight shoulders, tight fists, tight gut, stop, pause, breathe, and realize that your body needs attention.

Your body is reacting to your brainstem primal reactions. Your brainstem needs the engagement of your brain's frontal lobes to come online and begin integrating reality, cultivating communication with responsible individuals in alignment with your core values.

Find one person a day to do a random act of kindness that needs no return favor. Speak one gracious statement each day to someone you know. Find one fear you often think and find the way to calm your body and turn it into courage.

Manic

Affirmations:
- I relax and calm my breath, my muscles, and my thoughts.
- I enjoy the moments of seeing the sky, the trees, the flowers.
- When my crazy self is showing, I tuck that part in and chuckle with a deep breath and go forward.
- I relax and visualize my body grounding to the earth.
- I love this very moment.
- I am learning from all parts of myself.
- I open up my view to see the big picture and enjoy breathing it all in.
- I cheer the day and embrace the evening.
- I find quiet moments once an hour to reconnect to my heart and body.
- I am safe and secure.

Supporting Foods:
- Vegetables
- Fruits
- Nuts and seeds
- Beans
- Legumes
- White fish
- Turkey
- Brewer's yeast
- Brown rice
- Carrots
- Asparagus
- Broccoli
- Avocado
- Leafy greens
- Kelp
- Whole grains -except eat those with gluten in moderation.
- Eat foods high in Vit B including

Mast Cell Disease

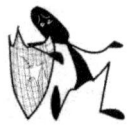

Troubled Mindset

- You have tried and tried but it is in vain, you can't control the outcome of every situation, especially those that matter the most.
- You have used intelligence, perseverance, meditation, tools that you have created and amazing insights of others and your own. But for some reason, it is not going your way now. "But why?" you ask yourself.
- You have the gift of creating and manipulating creation. That is part of the problem.
- While the gift is so useful in helping yourself and others, once you fall out of grace with your inner self the toll can turn on you and actively create emotional problems, mental frustrations, and physical inflammatory states that are difficult to overcome.

Mast Cell Disease

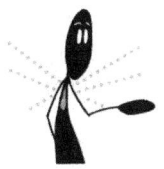

Healing Mindset

It is past due, the moments of not trying to fix everything or everybody. Now is the moment to embrace your pain with a new outlook on your goals. You might even find it necessary to completely shift your objective—strive to experience each role in life with wisdom, humility, boldness, and joy. That task is difficult when life is tough and painful. However, the creation tool can backfire on those who forget to reflect on a possible grander plan.

Even science can't explain the spontaneous organizing events that take place with many microscopic elements. Allow yourself to be a part of the flow of life and watch how life is so forgiving and desirous to work through it naturally and with a resiliency that is beyond our control. Be a part of the mysterious plan of nature instead of forcing your own.

Mast Cell Disease

Affirmations:
- I am ready and open for new insights daily.
- I promise to be patient with the parts of me that are not.
- I have yet to conquer my villain because that part needs love, space and time.
- I hope for a better day while I encourage myself to thoroughly enjoy the amazing moment right in front of me.

Supporting Foods:
- Avocado
- Brazil nuts
- Broccoli (steamed, organic)
- Brussel sprouts
- Cauliflower (steamed, organic)
- Chia seeds (soaked)
- Cucumber
- Jicama
- Moringa
- Peaches
- Salmon
- Squash
- Tuna
- Turmeric
- Yam
- Avoid: Histamine forming foods.

Memory

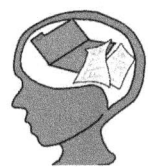

Troubled Mindset

- You are repressing experiences that you fear to see and remember.
- You feel safer with unrealistic fantasies than what is perceived as traumatic realities.
- You may feel that you, or the things you know, are unimportant to others.
- You'd rather not remember than deal with things that have happened.
- You may have a tendency to focus on the negative things in life, making remembering those things abundant and painful.
- You have too much confusion and overwhelm to store everything that is needed for later. So the body chooses to store the survival memories to keep you safe in survival mode.
- Your memory (or memorization) process selects and retains information based on the emotions and feelings associated with the memory or experience.
- Your negative attitude is becoming the storage rather than the facts you need for later.

Memory

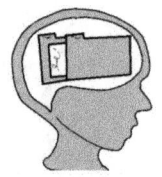

Healing Mindset

You need a change in your emotional attitude. Your beliefs are surrounded by fear. If you change your attitude, you change your memory.

Start with your need for safety. When you are safe to see things as they are, your memories will not need to be suppressed. Your strength to improve will come from truly understanding the nature of the problem, so you can see an appropriate solution.

Allow your heart and mind to work together to guide you. Life is a teacher; learn, integrate, and heal. You have an amazing ability to remember, so choose how you to use it. Thoughts stored with pain and blame will leave their mark. They will, unfortunately, surface later. Feelings and intentions stored with positive insights and wise understandings will responsibly build your memory, and it will offer a happiness that is priceless.

Memory

Affirmations:
- I learn from all life experiences.
- I am intrigued with everything and everyone.
- I am integrating my life experiences into intriguing insights.
- I enjoy the discovery of learning.
- I don't consume my time with arguments and hate but with intrigue, learning, positive communication, and challenging thought.
- I heal my inner child.
- I often visualize the connections of the various areas of life and how interesting how so many things are interrelated.
- I begin each day by simply connecting to my breath, my mind, my heart, and my body.
- I begin each day by letting go of fear, regret, judgment, resentment, and despair.
- I begin each day by reaching out to the negative emotions and calmly turn them around into simple strengths.
- I begin each day by looking at what is possible today.
- I begin each moment with a simple focus and simple action.
- I begin each night with gratitude and appreciation.
- I begin each night by letting my mind and body rest and rejuvenate.

Memory

Supporting Foods:

- Water/Get hydrated
- Eat more raw foods
- Brewer's yeast
- Brown rice
- Millet
- Farm eggs
- Fish
- Legumes
- Nuts
- Sunflower seeds
- Soybeans
- Tofu
- Wheat germ
- Whole grains
- Molasses
- Chicken
- Beef
- Liver
- Avocado
- Carrots
- Bananas
- Beans
- Broccoli
- Cheese
- Potatoes
- Tomatoes

Meningitis

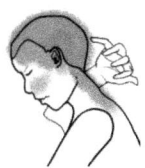

Troubled Mindset

- You may feel 'kicked out' or exiled from your community.
- You felt attacked for being yourself, but you came across as a know it all.
- You feel you have one choice, which means you feel trapped.
- There is no way out, and you can't find the answers you desperately seek.
- You are confused because there is either real danger or perceived. But to your body, it is all the same.
- You are deeply upset and don't understand what to do.
- You are resisting new thoughts or new ideas because how can they help?
- You have forgotten that answers are not always to solve the external problems, but to solve the internal turmoil.
- When you are in turmoil, it is difficult to accurately think and feel.

Meningitis

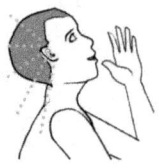

Healing Mindset

You need that which you resist the most, and that is called trust. Trust that there is a purpose to this experience. Don't let the emotions consume you. Breathe through them as you release them. You don't need the negativity in order to gain the insights you desire to heal.

You have a contribution to offer. Don't let your pride prevent you from finding balance while sharing yourself. You have a gift to listen deeply, do it without holding their emotions. You can't save them, so let the listening be the gift, not the holding onto their pain.

Meningitis

Affirmations:

- My heart is feeling safe to heal.
- I listen to my heart and receive the kindness of those who safely share their heart.
- My firm boundaries are good for me and others.
- I bless others to have help from the angels and nature without compromising my needs.
- I am grateful for my immune system that wants to keep up with my emotional life.
- I honor and respect my body by taking care it before I go out into my relationships.
- I understand and support my body in all situations.
- I am secure and grounded in the strength of rebuilding my body and my life.
- I feel blessed to be alive and healthy.

Meningitis

Supporting Foods:

- Eat a well-balanced diet
- Raw fruits and vegetables
- Grains
- Nuts
- Seeds
- Figs
- Fresh pineapple
- Papaya
- Yogurt
- Kefir
- Sauerkraut
- Kimchi
- Garlic
- Onions
- Mushrooms
- Carrots
- Apricots
- Asparagus
- Broccoli
- Cantaloupe
- Sweet peppers
- Spinach
- Sweet potatoes
- Yellow squash
- Berries
- Citrus fruits
- Tomatoes

Menstrual Problems
(Female Period)

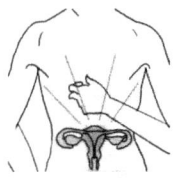

Troubled Mindset

- You're judging your feminine side, believing it to be weak, victimized, or powerless.
- Perhaps you are choosing competition and aggression over unity and compassion.
- You have allowed your runaway emotions to control your mind.
- You are trying to be you, while also trying to be someone that others expect you to be.
- You haven't embraced the power and the gift of the real woman inside.
- You are trying to be loving and kind, tough and strong, and still be nice.
- It is good to be sensitive and strong, but not when you are frustrated, sad, or hurting deeply inside.
- You have to heal first.

Menstrual Problems
(Female Period)

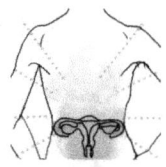

Healing Mindset

Compassion is a positive and deeply needed attribute for all. Embrace the incredible strengths and contributions of your feminine attributes. You have only begun to see and understand the creative abilities that only females carry. Hone in on how you can integrate those strengths into your life and wellbeing.

Be the love that you are, and embrace love above the competition. Learn to be comfortable with your body, your abilities, your heart, and your mind. When others push and shove, use your innate intuitive ability to see past the conflicts. Notice that the bully is only in need of attention but doesn't know how to ask for it. Be firm and kind, but not pleasing nor apologetic. You don't need to have an excuse to be you. Show up to be you and shine your true self with all your amazing gifts.

Menstrual Problems
(Female Period)

Affirmations:
- I thank you, my body, for teaching me to listen and to respect myself.
- I thank you, hormones, for communicating to my body what you think I need.
- I thank you, heart, for wanting to care for my needs with kindness and tenderness.
- I thank you, mind, for thinking positive thoughts and offering positive intentions.
- I thank you, soul, for the depth of wisdom you give me to see and understand how amazing of a woman I am.
- I thank you, my cycle, that goes through my month cleansing and renewing my body.
- I thank you, my relationships, for giving me the opportunity to serve you the way that is best for me and you.
- I thank you, my God, for giving me this female body and all of its amazing wonders and feelings because it is a gift to experience it every day.

Menstrual Problems
(Female Period)

Supporting Foods:

- Alfalfa
- Avocados
- Fish
- Meats (not fried)
- Parsley
- Safflower
- Purple and orange foods
- Legume
- Whole grains
- Cabbage
- Broccoli
- Sprouts
- Rose hip tea
- Green leafy vegetables
- Bell peppers
- Salmon
- Tuna
- Wheat germ
- Nuts and seeds

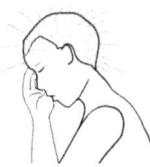

Migraine
Troubled Mindset

- Thinking, "If only they would ____, then I can be happy."
- It's time to wake up and see that running from your problems is not working.
- You are letting conflict rule your life without any insight into what to do about it.
- All you feel is the pressure that mounts inside.
- "Nothing is more important than taking care of the pain." This is a message that is pounding constantly in the background, but you constantly are ignoring the obvious.
- Your determination to keep going without facing some of the facts of what is happening in your life is causing your body to get overwhelmed with dealing with the problem.
- The pressure between what others expect and what you wish is not solved by escaping.
- Pressure from suppressed rage and hidden fears and uncomfortable regrets need resolution.
- You've been indecisive about who you are.
- Do you honor you or your ego?
- Do you honor your feelings or what others tell you to do?
- The pressure of life decisions has now come down to everyday decisions.
- It is now unbearable to control yourself, hoping it will control others' behaviors towards you, but it doesn't work.
- You end up angry, annoyed, and hopeless.
- You suppress your rage and trigger it in your physical body instead.
- All you've wanted is love, but you're looking for it in the wrong places.

Migraine

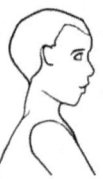

Healing Mindset

Take the time to deal with the cards that life has dealt you. Most of your experiences are a consequence of your expectations not matching the expectations of others. You need to be real and then gradually and consistently become honest and authentic in your communications with others. Choose what is more important, and be true to that. Your troubling pain is determined to get you to stop. So stop, and enjoy life! Do you want to keep the peace or be and enjoy the inner peace?

Don't let your habit of eating your trouble away cloud your vision. Move and breathe through the conflict long before food hits your mouth. Choose to stop eating to run away. Choose to slow down, stop eating too fast.

Choose to be real with what you honestly are thinking, feeling, and doing. Maybe your real enemy is yourself. Maybe you need to take 5 minutes an hour to stop, feel, breathe, be calm, be grounded. Your behavior will not change everyone around you. Choose to do it for you and your wellbeing, honest self-love. Decide to relax the tension before you decide anything else. Laugh at yourself, because most other worrisome activities won't lessen the tension as well as the simple joy of humor.

Migraine

Affirmations:
- I enjoy every minute of every day.
- I let the pressure move me to release it into a passion for living, for experiencing all of life, including self-discovery and then self-care.
- I welcome each experience.
- I welcome the opportunity to spontaneously decide.
- I decide to calm myself first and take care of me.
- I love my life experience.
- My pain is simply a signal to transform my emotions into learning and growth.
- I take the autumn of my emotional memory and allow a new spring of personal growth.
- I take my anger, fear, and grief and change them to courage, insight, and wisdom.
- I flow with life.
- I welcome refreshing relationships.
- I enjoy the variety of experiences from each relationship.

 ### Supporting Foods:

- Almonds
- Almond milk
- Watercress
- Parsley
- Fennel
- Garlic
- Cherries
- Fresh pineapple
- Eat small meals and nutritious snacks between meals to stabilize blood sugar
- Eat a diet low in simple carbohydrates and high in protein

Miscarriage

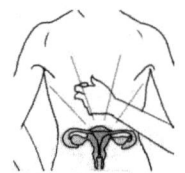

Troubled Mindset

- Your mind and body may be telling you something.
- Perhaps you aren't ready for children, or the timing is 'off.'
- You may fear the responsibility or have some issues in your relationships with your family or partner, that are unresolved.
- Perhaps your body recognized that the fetus wouldn't be able to survive due to underlying issues.

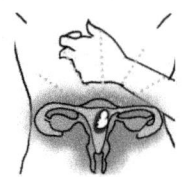

Healing Mindset

Whether the child's body was ready or not, it is important to take this moment and release your grief, sorrow, and unexpected trauma. This is a part of the natural process of nature choosing to give or take depending upon the biochemical and other physical conditions at the time. Although painful, this is the time to dig deep and move through your sadness. It will help you find deeper joy and empathy. This will assist you in building strength and character to be a happier and healthier parent to those who come to you in the future.

Miscarriage

Affirmations:
- I release the sudden pain and sadness with a deep appreciation for the power of creation, for it has the power to give and take at any moment.
- I will prepare myself to be ready for the fullness of God's creation to be expressed through me.
- I accept the grief as a natural process of letting go.
- I appreciate the moments that I did have with the unborn.
- I am ready to renew and prepare for future joy.

Supporting Foods:
- Stay hydrated
- Whole grains
- Eat a well balanced diets including plenty of fruits and vegetables
- Eggs
- Chicken
- Liver
- Millet

Morning Sickness

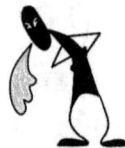

Troubled Mindset

- You are trying to do everything you can, but your body has a different agenda.
- Possibly your busy life is too much for you and the child.
- Being a good mother is both function and connection.
- While you care, taking time to care for yourself helps the child feel that care. It also helps calm the body and the mind.
- Your body may be wanting to get rid of certain thoughts or programming that has been passed down from ancestral struggles.
- There could be a fear of pain, anxiety about being a good mother, or feeling trapped.
- You may have some remorse about not being able to do what you want from now on.
- You have some anxiety about unresolved issues in your relationships.

Morning Sickness

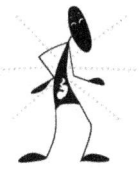

Healing Mindset

The cells of your body will listen if you do. Take care of what is important and then rest and use this time to recharge and renew. Notice your resistance and breathe through it. Learn the resistance just wants you to relook and start with a broader and deeper understanding.

Support your hormonal balance with nourishing foods or herbs as you calm your fears and embrace change. Transitioning from the old way to a new way always brings challenges. These challenges will help you grow, and growth is your friend. As you approach these challenges, release any resistance. Use this time to renew your body and mind. Embrace your fears and upsets and turn them into something of value and purpose.

Morning Sickness

Affirmations:

- I am so blessed.
- I have a body that speaks to me, and I listen.
- I want to receive that which is healthy and strengthening to my body and for the body of my child.
- I am in the spring, and I appreciate my body wanting to be clean.
- I use this time for reflection and renewal.
- Fears easily transform into something of value and purpose in my life.

Supporting Foods:

- Water/Get hydrated
- Raspberry tea
- Ginger tea
- Lemon tea
- Wheat germ
- Whole grains
- Grapefruit (small amount)
- Millet congee
- Brewer's yeast
- Sunflower seeds
- Brown rice
- Bananas
- Squash
- Eggs
- Carrots
- Avocado
- Ginger
- Foods high in Vit. B-6
- Non-dairy coconut yogurt
- Possibly small amounts of baking soda in water.

Motion Sickness

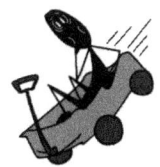

Troubled Mindset

- You feel lost in a sea of commotion.
- Ask yourself, "Why can't I feel safe when there is no reason to try to over-control my situation?"
- You want to try to find answers to your problems, but there seems to be none.
- You have been pushing through your fears for too long, and your body is trying to unwind.
- The process to stay balanced in the conflicting world around you requires too much.
- Your body wants you to listen.
- Your fears are coming true, and it is difficult to stop trying to stay in control.

Healing Mindset

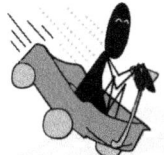

Find the truth that is real and not wished for. Find the inner peace that has nothing to do with your expectations of others. Breathe while you can, when your body lets you. Let each breath take you to the center through the warmth of mother earth. Let go of your fear of being guilty and of overwhelm.

Let the consequences of other's actions be less important and only live and breathe what you truly can. Breathe through your fears and open to new insights. Control is an illusion. Embrace the adventure of life.

Motion Sickness

Affirmations:
- I find peace in the simple.
- I find hope in the present.
- I find truth in being true.
- Despite the storm, I breathe through the conflict with calm confidence that my heart, mind, body, and soul can and will be stronger.
- I am safe.
- What more can I ask than to enjoy my life as it is?
- I enjoy my life as it is.

Supporting Foods:
- Pumpkin seeds
- Squash seeds
- Olives
- Ginger or peppermint tea before a trip
- Foods high in magnesium & Vit. B-6
- Apples
- Apricots
- Green leafy vegetables
- Avocados
- Bananas
- Brewer's yeast
- Brown rice
- Cantaloupe
- Millet
- Nuts
- Salmon
- Sesame seeds
- Whole grains
- Dairy
- Carrots
- Chicken
- Eggs
- Meat
- Spinach
- Wheat germ
- Walnuts

Mouth

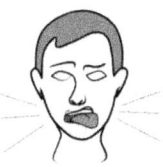

Troubled Mindset

- You've made up your mind, and you don't want to talk about it.
- Effectively you are maintaining a closed mind and mouth.
- You are conflicted about sharing your thoughts.
- Part of you wants to flow freely, but it is too uncomfortable and vulnerable.
- You don't want to risk revealing your secrets or allowing nourishing support or new ideas in. You don't trust it.
- When you blame, you think it is truth, not realizing the negative energy is pointing right back at yourself.
- You don't want to be frustrated or negative, so you mask it with other activities or words, but the feelings fester.

Mouth

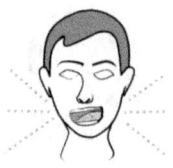

Healing Mindset

Not flowing is not growing. Start with your breath. Cherish the gift of experience as you give through breathing out, and receive through breathing in. Gently allow yourself to open and release any tension as you prepare to engage with life in a balanced way.

Be aware of your thoughts and notice what they do to the jaw muscles. Be aware of your communication and notice if it carries negative feelings. Be aware of your judgments and notice if they are hiding your fears and other emotions.

You are not your emotions and your beliefs, so stop letting them control you. Life may not be fair, but it can be an amazing experience of learning and growth. Let go of the need to be right and embrace the opportunity of inner expressions of learning, light, and love.

Mouth

Affirmations:

- I choose to open my mind to new ideas and to trusting others.
- I am safe to share my heart.
- I allow myself to be nourished by my life's experiences.
- I learn from all of life.
- I am grateful for the gift of personal expression.
- I share my expression of gratitude often.
- I let go of personal judgments and make room for wisdom, insight, and action.

Supporting Foods:

- Water/ Get hydrated
- Eat a variety of fresh fruits
- High fiber foods such as whole grains
- Vegetables and legumes
- Green leafy vegetables
- Sprouted almonds
- Pumpkin seeds
- Garbanzo beans
- Pomegranate
- Bell peppers
- Oranges
- Lemons
- Grapefruit
- Spicy peppers
- Black beans
- Spinach
- Jicama
- Lentils
- Millet
- Tofu
- Salmon
- Meat

Multiple Sclerosis

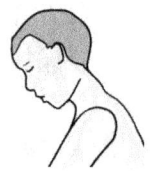

Troubled Mindset

- Your mind thinks that your nerve-racking life experiences come from everyone else, and your heart feels stubborn and inflexible to your enemy.
- You plead with others to see your side, but you are running from your core values and true feelings.
- You push yourself too hard to compensate for not maintaining sufficient communication with others.
- The body is in so much conflict that hardened feelings, desperation, and guilt is fueling your thoughts.
- You are stuck in a mental rut and a physical conundrum.
- Your will is pushing your body to eat away that which is protecting you.

Multiple Sclerosis

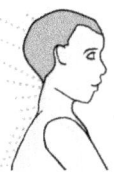

Healing Mindset

You have the opportunity to live free by listening to your core self. You first need to find it. Write your values. Write the negative thoughts and feelings that come all the time and then write what each one is trying to teach you. Be sure every day to flow through that path so that you become automatic in your thoughts of transitioning from the negative to the positive understandings. Then find ways to bring caring to your heart and body without all the drama.

Find ways to calm the stubbornness, even if you see the hard-headedness of others; you are mirroring that in your body. Bring fluidity into your life. Find ways to bring emotional protection to your nervous system. That protection includes a positive shield from your negative thoughts. Start with accepting yourself. Relate to yourself the way you would a young child. They are valued just for existing. Allow positive will into your daily life, moving with joy and inspiration towards a natural and appropriate goal. As you relate to your true self and stop running from your true feelings, you will be able to integrate living in a new paradigm of experience.

Multiple Sclerosis

Affirmations:
- I begin each day with simply connecting to my breath, my mind, my heart, and my body.
- I begin each day with letting go of fear, regret, judgment, resentment, and despair.
- I begin each day by reaching out to the negative emotions and calmly turn them around into simple strengths.
- I begin each day by looking at what is possible today.
- I begin each moment with simple focus and simple action.
- I begin each night with gratitude and appreciation.
- I begin each night with letting my mind and body and rest and rejuvenate.

Supporting Foods:
- Increase water intake
- Organic eggs
- Fruits
- Vegetables
- Gluten-free grains
- Raw nuts and seeds
- Foods high in fiber
- Cold pressed vegetable oils
- Raw sprouts
- Alfalfa
- Dark green leafy greens
- Green drinks
- Sour foods:
  - Sauerkraut
  - Kimchi
  - Dill pickles

Nausea

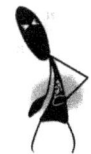

Troubled Mindset

- "I wish that never happened!"
- You actively don't want to digest an experience that is real or an imagined future outcome possibility.
- You may have confronted something that causes flashbacks to a traumatic memory.
- You feel like something wrong or immoral has happened, and you deeply reject it.
- You fear possible consequences.
- You have regret and disgust about your current situation.
- You are blocking the forces of nature because your body can't distinguish who the enemy really is, so your body blocks energy from everything and everyone.
- You are afraid of the negative potential of your life experience.
- You wonder if you had done something differently in the past, would things be different now?

Nausea

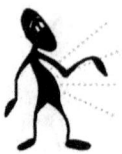

Healing Mindset

We can't change the past, but we can learn from it. When we fully integrate our experiences, we can be strengthened with conviction and understanding to do what we believe is truly good. The past doesn't need to plague the future. Trust that there is a positive purpose behind this experience.

You have an opportunity to notice your life, just do it without holding your breath. Notice your belly and chest. Relax them by focusing the energy on your feet and into the earth. Notice your inner feelings of disgust and discomfort, take those and gradually move them to down your body to the earth. Allow some help to assist you in dissolving the blocks. Those blocks are trying to protect you, so find responsible ways to deal with your life issues without over-reacting.

Nausea

Affirmations:
- I live in the moment by simply connecting to my breath.
- I sense and feel my feet.
- I sense my energy moving down my spine, into my legs down to my toes and then deeply into the earth.
- My courage is growing to face my life and those around me.
- I am hopeful and strong.
- I begin each moment with a simple focus and a simple action.
- I accept life's dramas as opportunities of intrigue and growth.
- I am learning to ride the wave of experience.
- I begin each night with gratitude and appreciation.
- I begin my sleep with rest and rejuvenation of my mind, body and soul.

Supporting Foods:
- Bananas
- Applesauce
- Non-dairy foods
- Coconut
- Yogurt
- Squash
- Zucchini
- Foods high in Vit. B-6
- Brewer's yeast
- Eggs
- Carrots
- Avocado
- Sunflower seeds
- Pumpkin seeds
- Wheat germ
- Brown rice
- Whole grains
- Brown rice congee
- Ginger tea
- Peppermint tea

Neck Problems

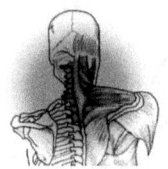

Troubled Mindset

- "Stiff neckedness."
- You may believe something or someone is "a huge pain in the neck."
- Your mental judgments and rigid perspectives are blocking out any heartfelt connections to yourself and/or others.
- You struggle to express or translate your honest feelings into understandable thoughts or concepts.
- You feel a need to be perfect.
- You don't want any negative feelings to be acknowledged, but it is strangling your authenticity.
- You hold a lot of shame for any 'impure' feeling or expression.
- You end up trying to control everything while losing touch with the heart of the issue.
- It may become so frustrating that you do not even want to keep living. But the fear of death, disgrace, misfortune, or any type of perceived failure motivates you to keep trying.
- Your current situation is challenging your inflexible convictions and perspectives of the way things "should" be.

Neck Problems

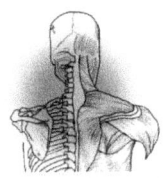

Healing Mindset

You are here to feel. Every feeling is meant to be a part of this life's experience, but only in passing. When we attempt to resist or deny the honest feelings within ourselves, we end up chronically stuck in that state.

The situation that is challenging you is meant to help your heart expand with love. That is only possible as you allow yourself to pass through the inevitable pains, sorrows, and frustrations that come with letting go of the old and embracing something new. One great thing about feelings is that they don't need to be "right," they just are. It's an experience, an observation of the heart. On the other side of your question is wisdom.

Neck Problems

Affirmations:
- I am here to feel.
- I feel and express honestly.
- I speak with clarity of mind and heart.
- I love myself through any mistakes.
- I feel the courage to speak my passion.
- I lovingly speak with no attachment to the outcome.
- I honor what is.
- I feel loved and honored by myself, god, and my loved ones.
- I release any blocks to God and embrace strength with passion and openness.
- I enjoy a natural flow of energy from my heart to my mind, and back again.

Supporting Foods:
- Drink plenty of water
- Sprouted grains
- Beans and seeds
- Fresh fruits and vegetables
- Cabbage
- Turnips
- Kohlrabi
- Cauliflower
- Broccoli
- Brussel sprouts
- Strawberries
- Peach
- Cherries
- Pine nuts
- Sweet brown rice

Nerve Problems

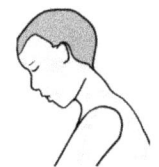

Troubled Mindset

- You have excess information and not enough capacity to deal with it.
- Your body is trying endlessly to take care of passing on the information but it is exacerbating the problem.
- You "can't compute..." all that is going on.
- You are overreacting to something physical or emotional.
- You are holding back some key information.
- You may not be saying enough because of fear of retribution or reactions.
- You may be saying too much because you feel you are not heard nor respected.
- The excess reaction inside is deflecting additional insights.

Nerve Problems

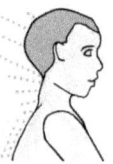

Healing Mindset

You need to slow down to a still neutral point where your body, heart, and mind are not so scattered and reactive. You need to recognize when you react to any suggestion so that you can breathe through it. Any reaction feeds the fire no matter what the reason. Learning to bring yourself back home to a safe, grounded place is so important—more important than being right.

Discover your true intrinsic core values and build your life on those first. Remember focusing on the thought that "no one understands me" will propagate the problem of what seems like "random nerve problems". Change your thoughts to "I am gradually starting to understand myself, and I will express my thoughts and feelings so that others can understand me at the pace that I can handle."

Nerve Problems

Affirmations:
- I center myself to a still and quiet place that lies between thoughts.
- I feel grounded and supported by the roots of mother earth.
- I am discovering the unique ways that I can express myself safely to others and maintain my personal integrity.
- Although others are still discovering who I am, I am enjoying the path of expressing myself freely, openly, and safely.
- What a day this is, a day to discover and feel fully.
- I appreciate my nerves for reminding me about life and function.
- I visualize and see the nerves relaxing and expressing themselves as it is beneficial for me and my body.
- I feel blessed to have expression.

Supporting Foods:
- Drink plenty of water
- Eat a diet of fruits and vegetables esp. Celery
- Vit. E rich fats such as unrefined oils
- Fresh nuts and seeds
- Legumes
- Whole grains
- Foods high in B vitamins

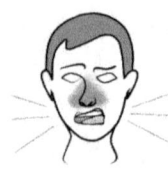

Nose

Troubled Mindset

- You want to be noticed, respected, acknowledged, appreciated, and loved by others.
- You have unmet desires, but not sure how to act on them.
- You are intelligent but you have difficulty announcing it to the world.
- You feel an inner disgust and distrust towards yourself, which leads you away from your true power, authority, and responsibility.
- You don't trust your ability to distinguish or recognize the real issue.

Healing Mindset

Trust comes with building an inner strength so that you can protect your sensitive heart. You need to take the time and effort to build that inner self-confidence that did not come naturally. Don't use your inner fears to bully yourself or others, find a use for the scary parts to indicate where and with whom you can learn to build your character.

Learning to love yourself and enjoy life would do you a world of good. Don't worry about what others think because their thoughts are filters of their problems, not yours. It is time to focus on just being yourself. Expand your intelligence, pursue your dreams, strengthen your abilities, and grow caring love safely.

Nose

Affirmations:
- I am fun to be with.
- I enjoy the path of discovery and adventure.
- I am strong in my mind and my heart.
- I take care of my body.
- I see where I am going and I clearly pursue my dreams.
- I am passionate about life and my dreams.
- I openly share my unique perspective with intrigue and joy.
- I accept the wisdom of the past and the hope of tomorrow.

Supporting Foods:
- Water/Get hydrated
- For dry nose: soy products
- Spinach
- Asparagus
- Millet
- Barley
- Salt
- Seaweed
- Apples
- Tangerine
- Persimmon
- Pears
- Pine nuts
- Honey
- Oysters
- Clams

Nosebleeds

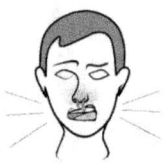

Troubled Mindset

- "Losing love."
- You don't trust yourself, or you don't feel validated.
- You're feeling emotionally undernourished and don't know how to cope with the hurt feelings.
- You end up blaming and become angry about not getting the attention you want.
- You are covering the feelings of shame and low self-worth.
- You may be hoping that someone else will compensate you for your withdrawn attempts to be noticed.
- There may be an unconscious shock from a past trauma.

Nosebleeds

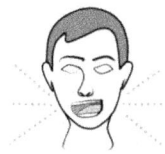

Healing Mindset

Face your needs honestly, and don't place the burden of blame on others. Be present with yourself. Become aware of how to value yourself. Discover the many parts of your personality that make a difference in the lives of others. Build inner courage and strength to make contributions.

Get appropriate nourishment to help with the blood and gut balance. You may lack protein, which might signify you need to build courage. You make lack iron, which indicates you need grit and some toughness in life.

You might be confused about what will happen to you, then find the will to get answers and do the things to bring stability in your life, your body, and your mind. Because your thinking is randomly confused and worried, start enjoying the simple things and moments of simple peace, with your feet firmly planted on the earth.

Nosebleeds

Affirmations:
- I am firmly planted in my goals and actions.
- I am safely moving through life.
- I have the courage to communicate my feelings and ideas.
- I am brave when others fear.
- I am clear when others are confused.
- I filter the clutter and see my purpose clearly.
- I am ready to take productive and significant action.

Supporting Foods:
- Water/Get hydrated
- Eat foods high in Vitamin K
- Alfalfa
- Kale
- Dark green leafy vegetables
- Spinach
- Kelp
- Broccoli
- Brussel sprouts
- Asparagus
- Cabbage
- Cauliflower
- Eggs
- Oatmeal
- Rye
- Soybeans
- Wheat
- Liver

Numbness

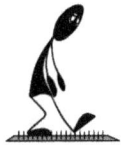

Troubled Mindset

- You are suppressing your feelings because they are overwhelming to you.
- You don't want to deal with these emotions so you do not want to feel them.
- You are withholding love or rejecting a part of yourself that you believe to be truly unacceptable.
- You genuinely distrust your environment, believing that if you express or follow through with your feelings, it will backfire.
- You're convinced it is safer to detach from feeling any sensations in your heart or body because the shock, overwhelm, and pain is too much.

Numbness

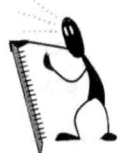

Healing Mindset

Look at the source of your numbness and it isn't the shock and overwhelms. It is the sensitive part of yourself just trying to protect you. Deal with your past and your inability to deal with the crazy parts of other people and the pain they gave you.

Gradually work at opening your heart and mind at the pace that is safe for you. You can do this. Be honest with yourself, and others. If you feel attacked, then find mature ways to let the negative energy pass around you. Their upset is their problem. You are to be you, not their false imagination of you. Let them deal with their feelings. For you, be lovingly honest to yourself, and safely open so that mature communication can take place. Find the way to follow through with your best intentions for the highest and best good for all.

Numbness

Affirmations:

- I sense the simplest of things in life.
- I enjoy the refreshing sunrise, the beautiful day, and the gorgeous sunset.
- I enjoy checking in with my physical body and easily sense areas of the body.
- I respect when I need to be quiet so that I can renew my energy and my mind.
- I honor my heart by slowly letting others into my life experience.
- I am learning to cherish people in my life, passions on my quest, and discoveries in my mind.
- I feel deeply, and I let my heart and gut sense those feelings.
- I am fear no emotion for each one is a gift for my learning and growth.

Supporting Foods:

- Fermented foods
- Sauerkraut
- Kimchi
- Soy sauce
- Pickles
- Sourdough
- Eat lots of vegetables
- Sprouts
- Leafy greens
- Seaweed
- Spirulina
- Whole grains
- Legumes
- Liver
- Figs

Osteoporosis

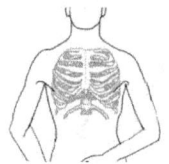

Troubled Mindset

- You feel that unless you keep a strong stance that you will be crushed or manipulated.
- You are overthinking and over-controlling but pretending not to. You are just trying to cover your bases.
- There are smart people around you and you need to stay on your toes to keep ahead of them.
- Others think they know a lot about everything, but you can't let them control you anymore.
- You doubt yourself too much and your self-critic makes you overcompensate by doing more than you should.
- You don't like being surprised, especially when it comes to the unexpected, such as being embarrassed, encountering non-integrous behaviors from a partner, or being put in compromising situations.
- It was difficult to stand up for yourself and setting things straight, but now you make sure you have your way even when it is challenging.
- You want to be loved and cherished but often you feel the other person is insincere in their promises and communication.
- You can't quite trust them with your heart completely, so you reserve a part of you just in case.

Osteoporosis

Healing Mindset

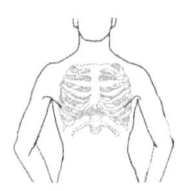

Since you can't stand unexpected changes or events, practice mindful moments every day where you connect to nature and watch the simple movements of the leaves when the wind blows, or the flight of birds and butterflies.

Your apprehension of what could happen or what does happen directs your path and causes reactions to those who should have your back. You have to remain strong in most situations and it is wearing on you. It is time to find your own peace, your own truth that is valid for you.

Look inside and find the real self. Find and write down what is important to you. Be honest with yourself and be true to what is true to you. Keep your values, stand up for yourself without force or bitterness. Replace inner resentment with peace. Let the heaviness of life be the burden of the angels or the universe.

Why carry the past as if you could change by trying? The past can be your teacher if you let life be an experience and a discovery. Real strength never comes from anger or wishing. True strength comes by first being strong with loving yourself enough to honor and respect you first and then serve others only at the level that is within your capacity to do so. Everyday grow a little stronger.

Osteoperosis

Affirmations:
- I am loved.
- I am strong.
- I stand up for myself.
- I love simply.
- I watch the movements of nature to remind me to be free in my expressions.
- I am free to be me.
- My heart wants to express the newness of life.
- I listen to my inner voice.
- I know what is true for me.
- I feel strength coming up from the earth.
- I feel inner peace spreading throughout my body.

Supporting Foods:
- Asparagus
- Bamboo
- Beets
- Broccoli organic
- Carrots with celery
- Cauliflower organic
- Celery juice
- Dulce
- Green leafy vegetables
- Halibut
- Kelp
- Noni
- Nutritional yeast
- Phytoplankton
- Seaweed
- Salmon
- Spinach
- Trout
- Yam

Overweight / Weight Issues

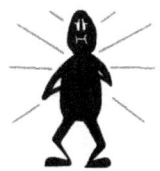

Troubled Mindset

- You are craving love and attention, and you're angry, perhaps even hateful, for not having it.
- You are filling a void in your soul with comfort foods.
- Your precious foods cover your sadness, regret, and any other feeling that bothers you.
- Your eating style compensates for what you wish you could receive from other people.
- You use the excess as a protection and method of keeping your emotions stuffed.
- You wish you could have it all without letting go of hidden anger that is not serving you.
- You are a good person, but you are afraid of letting people see the real you.
- You have given up and think, "why try?"
- After a while, you forget and try another idea, only to fail, thus causing the feelings of self-failure and personal regret.

Overweight / Weight Issues

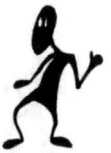

Healing Mindset

Failure comes too easy when you do the yo-yo dieting. The only way to conquer yourself is to not conquer but work with all the parts of yourself in a consistent daily manner. Consistent daily exercise, positive mind resets, doing simple challenges, and taking one step at a time is all part of creating success.

You are not a failure. You are a human learning how to cooperate with all parts of yourself. Be your best friend by treating your mind with positive affirmations, discovering new friendships, exploring new thoughts. Be good to your heart by eating slowly, caring for your emotional self, releasing the pain with your breath, meditation, exercise, and emotional balancing.

Forgive yourself and others. Breathe as you release the fear of your emotions. Trust there is safety in being yourself without the need to compensate or blame for hurtful experiences. Grow from life's challenges and rise back into your highest and best self.

Overweight / Weight Issues

Affirmations:

- I love my body and my body loves me.
- I am peaceful and clear inside when I eat quality food.
- I am strong, with a trim and slim body.
- I release the need to hold onto past pain and suffering.
- I release the need to hold onto cravings and false expectations.
- I release the need to be resentful of others.
- I release the clutter in my life, in my body, in my mind, in my surroundings.
- I give myself permission to be slim and trim.
- I give myself permission to look beautiful.
- I eat with healthy feelings.
- I can let go of my favorite food.
- I enjoy eating to live.
- I love myself.
- I can respect my body by eating what is great for me.
- I am the best I can be.
- I nurture myself today with 100% love and caring.

Overweight / Weight Issues

Supporting Foods:

- Eat fresh fruits and lots of raw vegetables.
- If vegetables are cooked- bake or lightly steam.
- Broccoli
- Cauliflower
- Celery
- Cucumbers
- Green beans
- Kale
- Lettuce
- Onions
- Radishes
- Spinach
- Turnips
- Apples
- Cantaloupe
- Grapefruit
- Strawberries
- Watermelon
- Eat complex carbohydrates such as tofu
- Lentils
- Plain baked potatoes
- Sesame seeds
- Beans
- Brown rice
- Whole grains
- Skinless turkey or chicken breast
- Fish

Pancreas

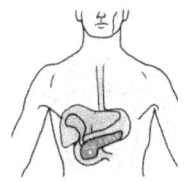

Troubled Mindset

- The many stressful emotions are building up inside.
- You might feel betrayed, controlled, or have felt the anger from others.
- You have suppressed bitterness.
- You have cyclic thoughts that are self-critical and critical of others.
- You drive yourself, placate, or seek to please others.
- Worry is consuming you whether you are happy or not.
- You are struggling to see the good, the point, or the purpose.
- You are easily affected by others' thoughts or feelings.
- You may carry shame and bitterness because you do not think that you have reached a level of success that you should have by this point.

Pancreas

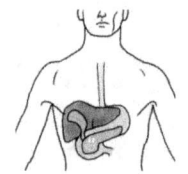

Healing Mindset

You need to be honest with yourself. You don't have all the resources you need if you continue being secretly frustrated and openly nice. You need boundaries not only in your behavior but also mental and emotional boundaries too.

The bursts of anger are a sign that you can now start to use meditation, mindfulness, and exercise to move your emotions out. You can start eating with positive feelings and eating balanced meals. You need to cherish life's moments because they only happen once. You can release those worries because they are troubling to your heart and soul.

Pancreas

Affirmations:
- I turn the corner of trouble into hope of dealing with life one step at a time.
- My anger is in the past.
- My grief is long gone.
- My fear is but a whisp in the wind.
- My faith, my hope, my love goes to the individual parts of myself including my cells. They deserve my attention.
- I am grateful for my body and all my cells for doing the very best that they can during all my stressful moments.
- I let worry change now to trusting each moment that God will provide pathways of change and transformation.
- I am building my new character of integrity, intelligence, caring, creativity, and joy.
- I trust God fully so that I can be an instrument in God's hands.
- I relax and do my best.

Supporting Foods:
- Eating a healthy balance of vegetables and protein.
- Eating too many carbs increases the problem.
- Eating too many fats and too many meats will cause pain and constipation.
- Eat the variety.

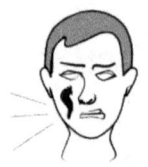

Parasites

Troubled Mindset

- You are being taken advantage of.
- You have given away your personal power.
- You may not be the driver of your personal destiny.
- You have offered too much so that you can have favor, approval, or safety. It didn't work, and it is draining your vitality as you give in to the demands of others.
- Your feeling and emotions have a mind of their own, as you have taken a back seat.
- The chaos you are experiencing seems beyond your control, and it is if you fail to do something about it.
- You have betrayed or deserted your true self.

Healing Mindset

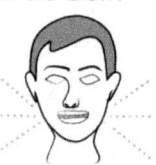

Start with identifying the self-betrayal. People can only take advantage as far as you let them. However, you need to learn more about yourself because the betrayal can happen at any level of thought or belief. Become aware of your thinking patterns and see if they are supportive of your true agenda if you are living your principles and not theirs, and if you are comfortable being in your skin. Breathe clearly and calmly in stressful situations. Re-identify your true self one step at a time until you pull and integrate all the pieces of yourself back together. Take charge of your life and with your decisions. Be decisive. Nourish your body with healthy food and healthy thoughts.

Parasites

Affirmations:
- I discern what is me and what is not me.
- I feed my body parts and none other.
- I take the fragments of my life and clear them through the filters of my core values and goals.
- I release the need to hold onto the past and embrace my positive future.
- I am secure in my personal relationships.
- I let go of co-dependent and destructive relationships and engage with supportive people.
- I appreciate the wakeup call from my body so that I can take proactive action.
- I am grateful for past issues because I am growing up and taking care of my body, heart, and mind.
- I feel the intriguing difference in the feelings of my body when I let myself authentically connect to my inner core self.

Supporting Foods:
- Black walnut
- Pumpkin seeds
- Cabbage
- Carrots
- Cucumber
- Lemon/lime
- Garlic
- Onions
- Oregano
- Ginger
- Papaya juice
- Pineapple
- Pomegranate
- Coconut oil
- Kefir
- Sauerkraut
- Yogurt

Parkinson's Disease

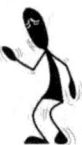

Troubled Mindset

- You overdid it and there are consequences to your body and mind.
- You went too far in trying to do everything while emotionally being full of fear, upset, and denial.
- You may avoid trying to recognize the real cause of why you are afraid.
- You don't trust yourself enough to act or share appropriately.
- You feel guilty about not contributing enough or too much.
- There is an old trauma that has not been dealt with and needs releasing.
- The old stuck emotions and cyclic beliefs keep you from trusting yourself.
- In the past, you have been avoidant of your feelings and focused on maintaining hands-on control. Now you are left with feeling unlovable, unsuccessful, fruitless, or broken.
- You feel there is no hope in changing your life or the behavior of others.

Parkinson's Disease

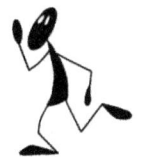

Healing Mindset

Trust in a higher source and a higher power. Trust in your higher purpose in your life and in the life of those around you. Consider that you are only a part of the massive plan and actions that take place in the universe. Trust to enjoy the path of how things play out in life and society. You have a contribution, but it is not up to you to save the day, thank heaven! This is a blessing that permits you to live without the need to 'fix' whatever ails the world.

Get the appropriate professional assistance to help you process the trauma that you have experienced. Have faith in yourself and your experience. Become flexible in your thinking and actions. Remember every movement is the body trying to adjust to all the messages it receives, thus slow the pace of the mind and soul and calmly go into the stillness of peace.

Parkinson's Disease

Affirmations:
- I am peacefully aware of those around me.
- I am calmly considering my role this day.
- I enjoy what I can do and happily surrender what I can't.
- My nervous system easily filters the worries and only responds to what is truly necessary to act upon.
- Life is a perfectly wonderful gift.
- I calmly release my perfect self and happily change into my enjoyable self.
- I am flexible with whatever comes my way.

Supporting Foods:
- Grains
- Raw oats
- Sprouted wheat
- Brown rice
- Raw goat's milk
- Green drinks
- Tomatoes
- Green leafy vegetables
- Foods high in vitamins c
- Eat a diet high in raw foods
- Include foods with phenylalanine
- Limit protein, especially meat & poultry.
- Only eat protein in the evening and eat other sources such as barley, tofu, yogurt, & beans
- Broccoli
- Bell peppers
- Asparagus
- Avocado
- Berries
- Citrus fruits
- Pineapple
- Papaya
- Lentils
- Seeds
- Nuts
- Almonds
- Brazil nuts
- Fish
- Pecans
- Pumpkin
- Sesame seeds
- Lima beans
- Chickpeas

Phobias

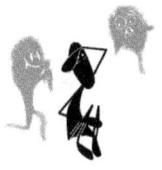

Troubled Mindset

- You experienced a traumatic event as a young child, possibly while in the womb, that is still affecting you in your adult life.
- These struggles limited your ability to mature, or self-soothe through the mind's attempt to resolve deep traumatic conflicts.
- The fear of the unknown is too great.
- You could have a childhood fear of being trapped, confined, or manipulated.
- The false experience is real to you because your body thinks that it will protect you with these fake beliefs and excess fear-based feelings.
- Once the body and mind are stable and congruent, the experience can change.

Phobias

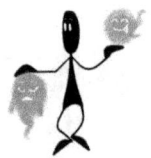

Healing Mindset

The phobia type of fears are rooting from the survival primal brain, thus are difficult to clear by simple techniques. However, if you learn to bridge the gap between your logical brain, emotional brain, and your primal brain, you can eventually become safer when these phobias re-appear. Bridging this gap is learning to integrate the many parts of your mind, heart, and body.

Learn breathing and self-soothing techniques. Learn to do brain integration exercises. Become aware when you are in the phobia and pace yourself through the process of connecting all parts of yourself into a congruent functional person.

Remember, there is a purpose in your fears, and gaining wisdom from the experience helps mature and bring healing to the mind. You are more than a mind or a heart. You are a soul with physical, emotional, nutritional, mental, and energy needs. Trust that as you learn and grow, you can begin to re-orient your perspective from a place of survival-based fears to a place of trust and joy.

Phobias

Affirmations:

- I feel a strong sense of courage and confidence filling my body.
- I encourage myself to face my obstacles with opportunities to grow and experience.
- I can't wait to discover what will happen next.
- I really enjoy the adventure of life.
- The past is but a leaf in the wind, the future is hardly a twig in the forest, and in the present, I am solidly rooted in my positive emotional experience.
- I appreciate the awareness of my senses which I tone down with my breath, thought and wisdom.
- I change the scary walk along a tight rope into a stroll along a wide and confident path.

Supporting Foods:

- Eat a well-balanced diet including
- Apricots
- Asparagus
- Avocados
- Bananas
- Brewer's yeast
- Brown rice
- Dried fruits
- Figs
- Fish
- Garlic
- Green leafy vegetables
- Legumes
- Raw nuts and seeds
- Soy products
- Whole grains
- Yogurt
- Wheat germ

Pneumonia

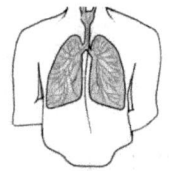

Troubled Mindset

- Feelings of abandonment loom over your mind and body.
- Desperation and sadness are turning into doom and gloom.
- "Why try?" Thoughts of giving up bring a flood of negative thoughts and feelings.
- Now you have lost your ability to stay above your negative thoughts and feelings.
- It has been too long in the making of suppressing your negative thoughts, feelings, and grievances.
- You wish and long for support, but it doesn't happen the way you want.
- You feel emotionally abandoned with no opportunity to heal your grief.
- You tried to take charge of your situation by pushing yourself or demanding of someone, but it doesn't work.
- Grief doesn't lead to solutions, but you forgot how to work the sadness out.

Pneumonia

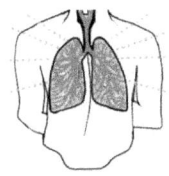

Healing Mindset

It is time to get your head on straight. Sadness never was happiness or productivity. Pity and desperation lead nowhere but to congested feelings of the heart and confused thoughts of the mind.

Nourish your wounds by taking small actions that honor your mind and body. Allow the love and compassion of others that they can offer to be yours to receive. And for the rest of the love your body needs, you offer it fully and completely.

Set your ego aside as you give yourself permission to embrace your humanness and appreciate flowing through all of the experiences that have helped you grow. Let go of that which is no longer serving you and regain an adventurous outlook on life.

Pneumonia

Affirmations:
- I strongly feel the need to take each breath with a positive outlook on life.
- I firmly feel the desire to quiet my mind and nourish my soul.
- I warmly feel the lower part of my body connect to mother earth and to my inner self.
- I respectfully honor my immune system and calmly support its efforts.
- I sensibly sense the feelings of hope as I warmly send healing energy throughout my body.
- The bubbles of fear, regret, and betrayal are popping, and I feel faith, wisdom, trust, and hope fill my heart and soul.

Supporting Foods:
- Water/Get hydrated
- Apple
- Carrots
- Cauliflower
- Celery
- Chard
- Chickweed (for some)
- Turkey (for some)
- Citrus
- Fennel
- Fenugreek seeds
- Fish
- Garlic
- Greens
- Kelp
- Onions
- Papaya
- Peach
- Pear
- Persimmon
- Pumpkin
- Radish
- Seaweed
- Tomato
- Yam
- Possibly brown rice
- Drink fresh juices and green drinks
- Cantaloupe (for some - if candida or fungus do not use)
- Use garlic & onion to sniff when there is lung congestion.

Post-Nasal Drip

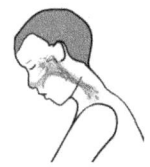

Troubled Mindset

- The fears, tears, and regrets are slowly dripping in the night and quietly in the day.
- Hiding behind your fears and self-pity is making life worse for you. Pretending that it will go away is only adding to the infection of self-denial and negative self-talk.
- You can't be honest with yourself when, to others, you pretend there is nothing wrong.
- You have unresolved grief and frustration that you have chosen not to face.
- You are becoming cold and mean, or sugary sweet; neither will release you from the negative thoughts drip.

Post-Nasal Drip

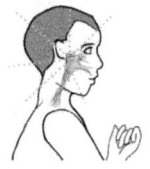

Healing Mindset

You can stop the inner torture of your situation by being completely honest and not blaming yourself or another person for 24 hours. You will come to see how often you go to negative thoughts and unproductive wishful thinking.

You are the cause of your suffering because you have chosen to hide, so stop the inner escape and begin to deal with those emotions. Understand your grief and subsequent anger from a higher perspective. Cherish the lessons and release that the unproductive parts of your thinking. Embrace responsible kindness from someone who won't enable you but encourage you to be real in your life.

Post-Nasal Drip

Affirmations:
- I respect those who bring clarity to my thinking.
- I appreciate those who responsibly bring healing to my heart.
- I surrender grief and regret in exchange for the emotions of courage and strength.
- I envision a better future.
- I speak honestly to myself and to all others.
- I take charge of my day and do what I say I am going to do.
- I let the clutter go, and the clarity come.
- I enjoy a healthy portion of self-respect, self-confidence, and self-awareness.

Supporting Foods:
- Water/Get hydrated
- Fresh vegetable and fruit juices
- Herbal teas
- Soups (esp. with cayenne, or raw onion)
- A little salt water
- Ginger tea
- Lemon
- Grapefruit
- Okra steamed
- Zucchini steamed with a little salt
- Figs

Premenstrual Syndrome (PMS)

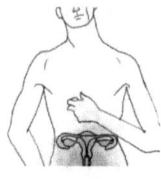

Troubled Mindset

- What happened? One day you just grew up, and then you had to be responsible, perfect, beautiful, sweet, wonderful, gorgeous, smart, and capable. And you have been internally repeating self-judging thoughts ever since.
- You've stuffed your expressions and emotions all month long, now the cork has popped, and it's all coming out.
- You have believed that you will not be heard or that what you say will be rejected.
- A part of you accepted the false belief that you are "less than" as a female. The other part of you venomously rejects it.
- The part that accepts it judges your feminine side as weak and tries to compensate by being more masculine, not appreciating the true nature of feminine power.
- The frustration from feeling disrespected from men is flowing out.
- You may use this time as an excuse to be a little reckless with your emotions.
- You are not living life to the full extent because you have fears of being judged if you express your authentic, specifically feminine self.
- You are not responsible for everyone and everything at the expense of your body, mind, and soul.

Premenstrual Syndrome (PMS)

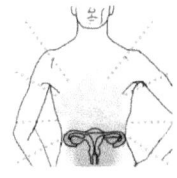

Healing Mindset

Rediscover your true capacity and value. Do not give others power over you. Flow with your emotions in a positive and empowering way throughout the entire month, so there is not a blow-up of emotion each cycle.

It may seem easier to ignore the potential conflicts, but you're paying a price. Learn from your past experiences with men and cherish the lessons learned, then let go of that which no longer serves you.

Finding the true meaning of beauty is part of the adventure of your life. Beauty is not satisfying the needs of others at the loss of yours; it is living your life in the integrity of being true to your core values of truth, empathy, courage, and growth. Be aware of how you take your fears and upsets and act them out physically and emotionally. Become emotionally intelligent so that you can process and clear unwanted judgments, fears, and resentments. Become the beauty and the love that you really are.

Premenstrual Syndrome (PMS)

Affirmations:
- I find my personal power in my inner core values of strength, truth, sharing, empathy, and confidence.
- My beauty is the combination of self-love, self-awareness, self-confidence, and connection to the self-love of others.
- I ignore the external false messages by filtering them through my inner truths and values.
- I am beautiful, courageous, and strong.
- The false energies and judgments of others are small breezes that I toss to the wind.
- I don't reflect the fears and control of others, instead, I reflect my faith in myself, in the divine, and the goodness of others to the world.
- I am at peace with the role I choose and I enjoy being honest with all parts of myself.
- My body is amazing and I am honored to be a part of its releasing and changing.
- The monthly cycle is a gift to release unwanted energies.
- I am mentally, emotionally, and physically changing for the better.
- I am enthusiastic and focused as I spiritually reconnect to my core each and every month.

Premenstrual Syndrome (PMS)

Supporting Foods:

- Drink water/Get hydrated
- Eat fresh fruits and vegetables
- Whole-grain cereals and breads
- Beans
- Peas
- Lentils
- Nuts and seeds
- Broiled chicken
- Turkey
- Alfalfa
- Avocados
- Fish
- Meats (not fried)
- Parsley
- Safflower
- Soybeans
- Wheat grass
- Drink mainly fresh juices and spirulina for several days before menstruation to help PMS symptoms

Prostate

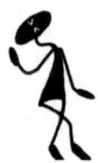

Troubled Mindset

- You have this image that you are strong, tough, capable, and responsible. Illusions of grandeur combined with the reality of stupid mistakes and mishaps are causing a conflict with your inner, male self.
- You are talented in some areas, but not all.
- You want to satisfy the image that you perceive society places upon you, and it is not working.
- You feel insufficient as a male.
- You carry shame and feel stuck.
- You suppress yourself and give away your power to determine your value and personal role.
- You keep a protective barrier to hide sexual conflicts, guilt, and fear of aging.
- You are conflicted when you try to let go of old, dogmatic, critical thinking.

Prostate

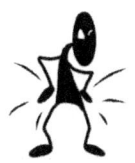

Healing Mindset

It's more about becoming the true you than performance or power. Seek spiritual growth and understanding to appreciate the purpose of what has happened and help find and be your authentic self.

If you are fighting the critical women in your life, it is a sign you are battling with your own self-worth and ability to speak from a self-confident and courageous place. End the blame game to yourself and others because it makes you an inner victim and an embittered companion. You can choose how you react to life, don't let your reactive and defensive win the day.

Learn the ability to discover your truth, your values, your inner strengths, and natural gifts. Shutting down or bursting pain out doesn't prove anything or help you progress. Others will be unpredictable, so you find your own predictable place by finding your core strength in the spiritual, mental, and emotional set point of being you. Enjoy expressing yourself to those who reflect back to you honestly and with care. Your strength is not in proving, but in the being.

Prostate

Affirmations:
- I enjoy being a man and living from my core truth.
- I am courageous when others are not.
- I forgive myself for any real or perceived self-blame.
- I am able to find strength in my daily adventure.
- I deeply care, I wisely share, I appropriately support, and I perceptively guide.
- My strength is not in 'the proving' but in 'the being.'
- When pushed or shoved, I will always maintain my personal power.
- I often open my guarded heart when I can safely share.
- I deeply enjoy and feel empowered when I make a positive difference in the lives of others.
- I am uniquely creative, curiously intelligent, and naturally strong.

 ### Supporting Foods:

- Increase water intake
- Wheat grass
- Whole grains
- Kelp
- Garlic
- Raw nuts and seeds
- Cruciferous vegetables
- Yellow and orange vegetable
- Fresh fruit & vegetable juices esp. carrot & cabbage juice
- Legumes
- Brown rice
- Millet
- Wheat
- Oats
- Bran
- Berries
- Foods high in zinc
- Mushrooms
- Pumpkin seeds
- Seafood
- Spinach
- Sunflower seeds

Receding Gums

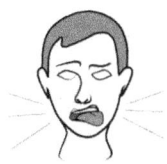

Troubled Mindset

- The demands of life exceed your capacity.
- You are overcommitting and deny it with excuses and justifications. But you keep putting expectations on yourself and others.
- You are using up valuable energy and resources to accomplish your goals and tasks.
- You are too nice and internally whisper the blame to others and shame to yourself.
- You want acknowledgement and respect but the way you go about it is costing you.
- You wish you could follow through with all that is asked of you and what you ask of yourself. But you are getting exposed to what is possible, and you don't like it, it doesn't feel good.
- Life is unfair but you try not to show it.
- You get discriminated against and you have something to prove but you keep that under wraps while you go forward.

Receding Gums

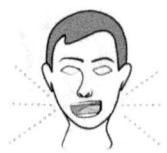

Healing Mindset

When you feel that life is getting away from you and you're losing your grip, then it is time to let go of the beliefs that are spinning you out of control and worry.

Eat slowly and methodically. Act as if you have all the time in the world because you do. Chew and pause when you eat and when you think.

Life is meant to be an adventure of experience not a test or obstacle. You are not failing, you are experimenting. When you overcommit, commit to keeping life simple. Sometimes you are escaping something else when you are getting overwhelmed.

If your inner sadness is causing frowns and worry, then you can open your heart in a simple way to a simple person with a single focus of bringing a smile to someone. Share your thoughts and feelings with those who will respect you as a person more than anything you do or say. Breathe and take care of yourself today, tomorrow, and from now on.

Receding Gums

Affirmations:

- I have nothing to hide, I just express my whole self to respecting souls.
- I have nothing to prove, because I am good enough as I am.
- I am at peace with what is.
- I find it encouraging to express new thoughts to those who want to discover.
- I nip in the bud, any negative thought and plant a new seed of positivity.
- Life is an opportunity just waiting for me to experience it.
- I commit to being true to my truth.
- I am honest with myself.
- I love connecting to caring people.

Supporting Foods:

- Green leafy vegetables
- Seaweed or dulce
- Sunflower seeds
- Lemons and limes
- Green beans
- Apples
- Celery
- Carrots
- Grapes
- Kiwi
- Oranges
- Papaya
- Peas
- Pineapple
- Salmon

Restless Leg Syndrome

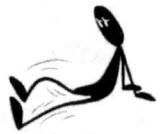

Troubled Mindset

- "Am I going the right way?" or "Am I making the right choice?" You are anxious and resistant to your direction in life.
- If it is your right leg, then it's more of your mental and physical direction.
- If it is your left leg, then it's about your biochemical and spiritual direction.
- You have felt that you have to figure it all out on your own.
- You believe if you don't get it right the first time, all will be lost.
- You think too much and don't want to hurt other people's feelings.
- You don't have a chance of permanently changing the other person because they are unpredictable and confused about their own situation.
- Your legs are trying to think for you.
- You are sorting through the cluttered messages, and you are confused with what to do with all of the problematic possibilities.
- You have a belief that there is no escape.

Restless Leg Syndrome

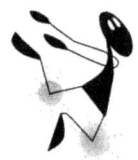

Healing Mindset

To make mistakes is human. To learn from them is sublime. Breathe yourself into a calm state, then make a decision. Honor your decision as you progress forward in your direction, embracing any learning it offers. As you do, the peace will expand and nourish as you follow a path that is appropriate for you. If it is not the path meant for you, then you can learn, grow, and adjust as you redirect.

Stop letting your legs think for you. Gradually and consistently let down your body's high alert. Notice when your body wants to run away while another wants to solve the problem and get it over with. The emotional and mental gap between two internal agendas is causing you to be restless, so calm the inner conflict and give your nerves a chance to relax. Learn to toss out the constant thoughts about the outcome and clearly focus on what you can do and let the rest go. Trusting in the value of allowing others to learn from their mistakes will remind you to trust and embrace your own learning journey.

Restless Leg Syndrome

Affirmations:
- My adventure today starts with bended knee, courageous heart, honest voice, and a clear mind.
- I listen for an inner voice of calm, clarity, and peace.
- I let the daily worries fade as I honor and respect my core values.
- I put my mind at ease with daily reminders that others will find their way; it is not mine to choose.
- I find the core place inside that can bring me the ability to trust in my path of learning and growth.
- There is an escape from my false fears; it is enjoying the discovery of my unique daily adventure.

Supporting Foods:
- Dairy foods
- Legumes
- Sunflower seeds
- Sesame seeds
- Oats
- Almonds
- Pecans
- Green leafy vegetables
- Tofu
- Soy
- Apricots
- Apples
- Avocados
- Bananas
- Brewers yeast
- Brown rice
- Yams
- Fish
- Seafood
- Poultry
- Figs
- Garlic
- Whole grains
- Citrus fruits
- Egg yolks
- Mushrooms
- Eat a well balanced diet including foods rich in calcium, potassium, magnesium and zinc

Rheumatism

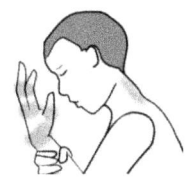

Troubled Mindset

- You've got a collection of resentments that keep you bitter and ready for attack.
- You are convinced your pain is everyone else's fault.
- You want love but set up a self-fulfilling prophecy ensuring you never get it when you send out negative thoughts and feelings to others.
- You can hardly move without pain because you are running out of options emotionally.
- You are holding onto old expectations that now deliver sadness, regret, and subtle resentments.
- It is as if you are drowning in the pain because there is nowhere to move it to.
- You pushed away your loved ones because you couldn't handle the manipulation.
- Even if you don't see them as manipulative, your body is responding with a wall that won't let in the love and wisdom of others.
- You don't trust them, or the universe to offer safe love.
- You've been inflexible or unbending in your opinions, with the belief that you can't change.

Rheumatism

Healing Mindset

Learn to open the door to others slowly and methodically. They may not change, but you can learn to be safe with them. Teach your mind and heart how to deal with their agendas and judgments. You may feel that they are trying to control you. See how the control of others comes from their insecurities. Learn to detect their insecurities so that you can breathe and move easier when they are acting out.

Change doesn't happen overnight, but it does happen. It takes determination and a refusal to give up. Believe that healing is possible and heal from the inside out. Your joints and life need a chance to accept the simple things, the simple love, the simple experience, the simple thoughts. The complexities of life are difficult but are sought by many because they are afraid of the quiet and calm.

Notice, are you afraid of the stillness? Your body is forcing you to be still. Take the opportunity of your restrictions to find the bliss in sharing and caring. Be open to let your heart release that deep and old sadness. You have tried your whole life to care; however, you forgot to express your own emotional pain, while taking care of the pain of others. Make room for the love by releasing everything that is not light and love, and you will be more receptive to the healing of the universe.

Rheumatism

Affirmations:

- I gradually and carefully share my feelings with those who care enough to be there for me.
- I end the self-sacrifice and replace it self-care, self-love, and self-share with my heart and soul.
- I meditate on creating more pathways of releasing my fears and my trauma so that I can heal.
- I am grateful for every movement that I can make.
- I appreciate every drop of love that the divine sends me.
- I discover the old burdens, release the expectations that I had on myself and others.
- I am happy to be responsible for only what I am capable of.
- I blissfully acknowledge that everyone will be okay without my superhero showing up today.
- I feel blessed to learn so much and even more blessed to trust in allowing others to serve me.

Supporting Foods:

- Almonds
- Black sesame
- Black soybean
- Carrots
- Celery
- Drink water/Get hydrated
- Fruits and vegetables and their juices
- Cereal grasses
- Papaya
- Cherry grapes
- Mackerel
- Trout
- Salmon
- Tuna
- Kombu
- Kelp
- Whole grains
- Legumes
- Sprouts

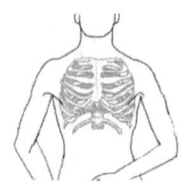

Ribs

Troubled Mindset

- "My protection is gone!"
- You feel emotionally exposed and delicate.
- Perhaps you were expected to follow a family pattern that you resist, but it still persists.
- You struggle with self-doubts that are based on limiting beliefs and fears.
- Your fears are penetrating your lungs, ribs, and chest because you worry too much and question your actions.
- You don't trust others but pretend that you do.
- You fear the possibility of betrayal, but you are stuck in how to deal with your situation.
- You feel a cold wind coming from the personalities of an important person that you know.
- You are not being devoted to your true self but to your worries.
- You want to accomplish and be successful but fear the consequences.
- On your left side, there is a conflict with the sabotages of emotional and spiritual accomplishment.
- The internal conflict associated with physical and mental accomplishments is more on the right side.
- Shielding yourself is helpful until it blocks your heart from experiencing love and life, or if it blocks your mind from creating positive, productive actions.

Ribs

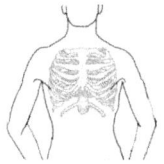

Healing Mindset

Learn to flexible with your thoughts and emotions. Rigidity comes from fear, false beliefs, and compensation of scattered objectives. You have a great mind and a good heart. You need to bring them back to the same home with the same agenda. Recenter and realign with your genuine core self.

Perhaps there is something that needs a resolution from your past so you can free yourself up again. Identify the limiting beliefs that are destructive and cumbersome. Learning to breathe out the past fears and breathe in the new possibilities is a positive daily action to take. Learn to commit to what you believe from your heart and soul, then from there, make conscious and clear decisions. Explore any reasons for doubt in order to uncover the wisdom or insight that your body is trying to help you see. Learn to accept yourself in any environment.

Ribs

Affirmations:

- I imagine my flexible body, chest, shoulders, and neck.
- I am fluid with the energy that flows through me.
- I feel the energy pour into my soul with courage and joy.
- I gladly change resistance into the consistency of positive thoughts and flexible actions.
- My shield is my joy and my core truth.
- I am grateful for my strong and flexible body.
- I share my heart with care.
- I accept all of me: from the top to the bottom.
- I feel great.
- I breathe in the love that nature freely gives me each and every moment.
- I am never alone because I am aligned with my body, heart, soul, and the angels.

Supporting Foods:

- Acorn squash
- Avocado
- Black beans
- Brazil nut
- Butternut squash
- Carrot
- Cauliflower
- Celery
- Cucumber
- Greens
- Green pepper steamed (stuffed)
- Kelp
- Oats
- Papaya
- Salmon
- Turkey
- Wild rice with natural butter
- Yam

Sciatica

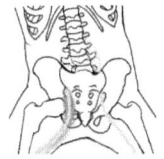

Troubled Mindset

- You fear the next step, your next move, their reaction, and possible outcomes of your decisions.
- Making decisions is difficult because your future seems frightful and scary.
- You fear the attacks from others or your own self-shame if you make another major mistake.
- You are living too much in survival mode.
- You fear whether you will be able to pay the bills, have a financial loss, or what the future might bring. It all feels so heavy.
- You are troubled by the direction you are going, and you'd like to disregard it.
- You either felt you had to figure it all out on your own, or you felt like you'd never be able to figure it out.
- You're thinking and worrying about your relationships with others.
- You are often people-pleasing and easily influenced.
- You worry that if you are open with your intentions that you will no longer be liked or accepted.
- If you are pregnant, your concern with the baby's needs over your own.
- Facing your enemy or your internal monster is overwhelming, so you let your body take the consequences and burden.

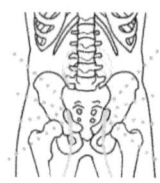

Sciatica

Healing Mindset

Fear is your own enemy. Calm the fear. We can't control outcomes, but we can recenter and balance the tension within ourselves. Focus on living in the 'now' and be present with today's needs. Then orient your attention with trust in what you can appropriately do for the future. Let go of your negative beliefs and fears because they are causing you to be so reactive that it is attracting more problems than you had before. Fearing the reactions of anger by an authority figure makes you into a victim who is just waiting to be taken advantage of. Fearing financial doom affects your mind so that you will make poor decisions.

Find those excessive worries and concerns that you carry on your hips and notice how they are causing you to walk in too many directions at once. Take the fears of what will happen and pick one. Worry about that one and let the others go, because not all your fears will happen anyway. Your focus on one will help your nerves have a chance at releasing the constant reactions. Notice your compensations in your relationships and allow yourself to calm the excess action, reaction, and worry to be given to somebody else because your body can't take the burden anymore. It is time to empower yourself to do what you can do, instead of picking on yourself for what you can't do. Stress is waiting for your permission to leave your body.

Sciatica

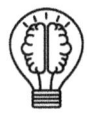

Affirmations:
- I let go of the past and make room for a great future.
- I consistently learn from my eventful life.
- Life is a great adventure.
- I let others be and learn from their experiences while I let myself be true to me.
- I give myself permission to gratefully release negative beliefs and concerns.
- I clear my cluttered path in order to make positive clear decisions.
- I am financially safe as I consistently take care of fiscal matters with faith and action.
- I fear no evil because the dark is just a reflection of my own inner conflict.
- The heavy burdens are no longer mine because they were really never mine, to begin with.
- I am free to move, breathe, feel, and live.
- I hope for a better future while living a peaceful one now.

Supporting Foods:
- Eggplant
- Carrots
- Orange pepper
- Drink water/Get hydrated
- Purple or orange colored foods
- Black beans
- Black sesame seeds
- Grass-fed beef
- Red beets
- Carrot juice
- Celery juice
- Watermelon

Scoliosis:
Curvature of the Spine

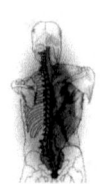

Troubled Mindset

- You are being pulled apart from all different directions.
- You have the responsibilities of family, friends, work and they all need more than you can give.
- The real problem is that you have forgotten about your needs, and your body is trying to muscle through every problem through constant muscle contraction. The push and the pull are always there.
- It feels that if one part of you gives up, then it is hell to pay. So, you keep pushing every day just to get through the pain with no gain.
- You fight the dreams and wishes of your younger self.
- It is as if you didn't want to grow up and deal with all the problems that life forces you to deal with.
- A part of you is rebelling against having to be mature, and another part is too responsible by always being supportive of others.
- You compensate for your perfectionistic tendencies while continuing to refuse to trust wisdom, help, and support.
- You withhold your true feelings because you fear your vulnerability.
- You keep many of your thoughts and feelings hidden behind the complex door of your heart.
- You may express feelings, but you replace them faster than you release them.
- At times the heart wall leaves you feeling disappointed, depressed, limited, and hopeless.

Scoliosis:
Curvature of the Spine

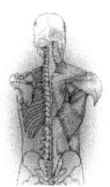

Healing Mindset

Straighten up your life by dealing with the tears coming from the deep pain inside your heart that never seems to dry up. Take time to resolve childhood sorrows and judgments that burden your life. Face your pain and find what you gained.

Learn to appreciate the growth. Your logical mind is going one direction, and your emotional heart is going the other way. You can bring the two together if you understand the positive intention of each part. You are a human with both a head and a heart, thoughts, and feelings. Ignoring your inner self and all its crazy parts will only add to your problem.

Be honest and take time to be sincere with yourself. It is good to have passion about something unless it is driving you into pain, suffering, and setbacks. Life is a journey that is worth taking if you truly believe that each step is a progression to discovery, growth, and wisdom. Find your spiritual truths that honor all parts of yourself and be faithful to those core values. Learn through meditation how to sense and release the physical reactions of your body and mind.

Scoliosis:
Curvature of the Spine

Affirmations:
- I take pride in finding the gain from the burdensome pain.
- Each step I take is another step towards a better me.
- I have the opportunity to deeply connect to my body through my muscles.
- I am a friend to my inner self that struggles with making life work perfectly.
- My inner self-friendship is discovering what I really need and what I can be in order to relax and enjoy the moment.
- I trust that my family is learning from their experiences.
- I connect my mind and body to my heart and soul.
- I take comfort in the understanding that I don't need to please and change others.
- I find it interesting how my body reacts to my thoughts and feelings.
- I love the adventure of self-discovery and self-healing.
- I am grateful for my body's desire to do everything it can to satisfy my spontaneous inner directives.
- I give my body permission to ignore my fears and pay attention to my joy and fun.
- I give all my muscles peace of mind and bliss of heart.

Scoliosis:
Curvature of the Spine

Supporting Foods:

- Water/Get hydrated
- Applesauce
- Asparagus
- Avocado
- Broccoli steamed
- Butter, clarified
- Butternut squash
- Carrot, steamed
- Cauliflower
- Chicken
- Slowly cooked delicata squash
- Eggs hard boiled
- Garbanzo beans
- Green beans
- Golden beets
- Hummus
- Parsnip
- Pumpkin
- Red beets
- Rice noodles
- Salmon
- Squash
- Vegetables dark leafy greens
- Vegetables, steamed

Shin

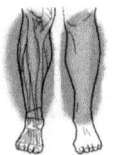

Troubled Mindset

- You want to give up.
- You have tried too much, and the difficulties make you feel that it isn't worth it.
- You wondering if your push and drive are working.
- You are playing by the rules, but others seem to get ahead who don't have high values or principles.
- You resist making all the changes you need to in order to manifest what you desire.
- You think working without wisdom is good enough.
- You have had a judgment that change always indicates that life will get worse, so you avoid real change.
- Your right shin indicates you struggle to trust supportive methods and resources, even though they point you in the right direction.
- You have this low lying belief that things won't work out anyway.
- The left shin indicates fear or paranoia about which direction to take.
- Your body is pushing you to be yourself, but you resist it.
- You are not being true to yourself, your values, and ideals. You are holding onto feelings because you are upset, angry, or betrayed.

Shin

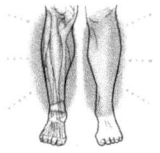

Healing Mindset

You need to step back and relax. Observe and identify what changes are needed. Write them down. Look at them and notice a pattern of acting and reacting. See how you resist in certain areas of your life and see that it is holding you back.

Discover the limitations that keep you from making those mental, emotional, and spiritual changes that will enrich your life. Progress starts by working through your limitations gradually, consistently, and productivity one by one. Release those limiting beliefs by looking into the fears behind them. Your resistance is shielding a fearful side, and that is the part of you that needs attention and understanding. Use your breath to calm yourself as you face your fears and pains.

Shin

Affirmations:
- I stand tall and true to my inner core values and truth.
- I take the time to be grounded and firm with my ideals.
- I pursue my goals with full purpose, clarity, understanding, and wisdom.
- I appreciate any inner resistance because it shines a light on what to deal with next.
- I enjoy the path of discovery and change.
- I can do this, and I can make a difference.
- I am focused as I go forward with strength and courage.

Supporting Foods:

- Sprouted almonds
- Delicata squash
- Butternut squash
- Asparagus
- Egg boiled
- Avocado
- Black beans
- Broccoli
- Cucumber
- Lentils
- Kiwi
- Mango
- Papaya
- Salmon
- Sweet potato
- Yam

Shingles

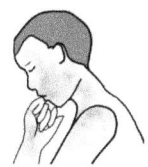

Troubled Mindset

- Life is full of surprises and you can't handle one more.
- You are holding your breath in pain and resistance which leads to more of the same.
- You are a mix of fear of surprise and anger at those around you that can spring one on you.
- Also, you may feel a deep fear of abandonment; as if someone is going to leave you. So you try to please and be nice and over-extended yourself but it is not working.
- You have not been taking care of the most important person - you.
- Your energy has plummeted to an all time low and there is little left.
- It is difficult to deal with your emotions of hidden resentment, hidden fear, apprehensive of possible surprises and still keep a happy smiling face.

Shingles

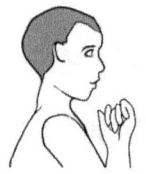

Healing Mindset

Look for hidden agendas and hidden hopes and dreams that you assume others will support but don't. Find patterns in your ancestors of feeling rejected, lost hope, but struggled to keep going anyway. As you see a pattern, take the time to release the frustrations and fears that have become too important.

Emotions are indicators of the weather inside, they are not supposed to be your masters. Discover the value in the adventure and let go of the hidden resistance that makes you hold on to way to much stuck energy. Also, it is time to start taking care of yourself like you take care of others. You are important and it is time to be true to you every morning, every afternoon and every evening.

Shingles

Affirmations:
- I love myself.
- I am a wonderful person that cares.
- I stopped carrying and now I care.
- I discover each day and enjoy fun surprises.
- I appreciate what I learn each and every day.
- When people are clueless, I am insightful.
- When people are careless, I still am careful.
- I softly release pain and flow new life through my veins.
- I calmly breathe out the suffering and let in healing.

Supporting Foods:
- Apple
- Applesauce
- Cauliflower
- Carrots
- Celery
- Chickpeas
- Cucumber
- Garlic
- Lemon
- Lentils (small amounts)
- Kidney Beans
- Papaya
- Peach
- Pear
- Pineapple
- Quinoa
- Rice (brown, with quinoa)
- Avoid: All sugars, chocolate, fried foods, peanuts, white flour, white rice

Shortness of Breath

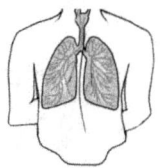

Troubled Mindset

- You are confusing what is important, what is urgent, and what is not necessary.
- You get mixed up between your senses and your emotions.
- You overreact to the fears and overwhelms of your life. It is time to separate what is real and what is over-reaction.
- You are holding on for "dear life."
- You are chronically hasty and scattered.
- You resist living calmly because of past trauma or drama.
- You are slow to trust others and participate in life because you feel anxiety from all your perceived vulnerabilities.
- Your fear prevents you from living life to its fullest.
- The issue may be caused by trauma during your fetal or infancy stage or what you learned from your relationships.

Shortness of Breath

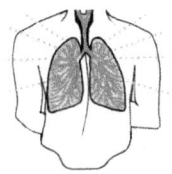

Healing Mindset

Surrendering to a more peaceful life may seem scary, so start simply by finding the difference between holding your breath and a true fearful moment. Learn to pause your breath instead of holding it and then gradually let it out. Learn to do interval breathing and interval walking.

Learn to embrace each moment of life with joy and gratitude. Do deep breathing exercises to help you integrate a new habit and way of living into your daily life.

Your body only does what it is asked to do, so find those inner switches that turn on the body's reactions. Life is as joyful or scary as you make it, even in the emotional storms.

Shortness of Breath

Affirmations:

- I trust that I can connect to my body and soul.
- I take time each day to ground my energy to mother earth.
- I take time to pause my thoughts and breathe in the fresh air, fresh thinking, and friendly affirmations.
- I take time to make time for self-care and self share.
- I take time to share my heart with someone I love.
- I stretch my body every day and stretch my mind often.
- I am safely walking on the planet earth.
- I am courageous to talk my walk, and walk my talk.
- I can be relaxed by slowly breathing and sensing my muscles relax.

Supporting Foods:

- To strengthen the lungs, eat small meals of primarily cooked foods
- Brown rice
- Oats
- Carrots
- Sweet potato
- Yam
- Ginger
- Garlic
- Soups
- Congees of millet
- Barley or brown rice

Shoulder Pain / Tension

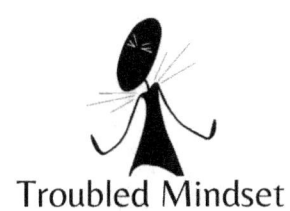

Troubled Mindset

- Burden.
- How do you relate to the responsibilities in life? Do you go about them joyfully? Or do you feel resentments, discouragements, fears, guilt, or exhaustion from excess responsibility?
- It's an attitude that 'life is weighing down on my shoulders' or 'life feels so heavy.'
- You may believe that what you do should not be your responsibility.
- You carry a conflict about success and what it means to be successful in life or with intimate relationships.
- You have ambivalence about how to express your needs.
- Though you want to feel support, you resist it, believing, 'I won't get what I want anyway.'
- Instead of making life fun, you support your burden and of those around you.
- You may feel stuck between doing all that is needed to take care of your wants and still attend to others.
- There are excess physical and emotional toxins.
- The left shoulder is about a more spiritual/emotional burden. Insecurity with your emotional/mental capacity or struggling to be yourself.
- The right shoulder has to do with physical stress. You are not enjoying or rejoicing in your progress.

Shoulder Pain / Tension

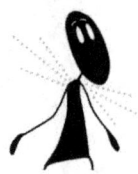

Healing Mindset

Be honest with yourself. What part of your load is worth keeping? It is better to let it go. Pay attention to the emotional burden you carry. Take a step back. Assess what is important and what is not.

Behind your need for a burden is a worry or fear that if you don't over-concern yourself that something harmful might happen. Negative emotionally based beliefs about the future become the problem instead of the real problem. Your body is carrying all the negative possibilities.

It is time to focus on what you can think, want to feel, and beneficially do. Seek to do your responsibilities with joy. Let go of any belief, attitude, or emotion that limits your happiness. Balance what you choose to take on and practice sharing the load. Express your need and desire. Be aware of how you respond.

Dance! Enjoy the journey.

Shoulder Pain / Tension

Affirmations:
- I enjoy the journey of life with all its adventures.
- I love my family and friends; they are so interesting and amazing.
- I encourage others to learn from their life experiences.
- I responsibly share only what I can do and let the rest be theirs to learn from.
- I trust that God and angels are deeply supporting those around me.
- As I awake today, I am prepared to be relaxed, share to be fulfilled, and surrender to be uplifted.
- I am on track to be completely relaxed on my focus of this day.
- Life is smooth sailing on any rough or calm sea.

Supporting Foods:
- Water/Get hydrated
- Apples
- Asparagus
- Bananas
- Barley
- Beans
- Beets
- Cabbage
- Carrots
- Celery
- Citrus fruits
- Fibrous foods
- Fish
- Greens
- Meats(moderate amounts and not fried)
- Green beans
- Green peppers
- Kale
- Millet
- Okra
- Rice
- Romaine lettuce
- Watermelon

Sinuses

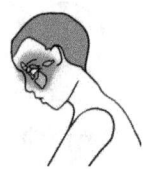

Troubled Mindset

- You are angry and struggling to learn from your experience.
- You are searching, but not grounded in your evaluations.
- You've become angry with yourself amidst self-pity and self-hate.
- You regret and blame yourself for what has happened.
- You felt rejected or hurt from a loved one, but haven't allowed yourself to process the range of emotions.
- Now you are left depressed, lonely, stuck, or worried.
- You may try to replace the old relationship with new people or things to fill the void.
- It isn't supporting real healing.
- You withhold taking action on your irritations, hoping to get validation, but it attracts excess judgments instead.
- Your right sinus deals with external disappointments or irritations.
- Your left sinus shows stress when there are internal self-rejections.

Sinuses

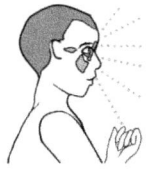

Healing Mindset

Have love and compassion for yourself. Ground yourself through breathing exercises as you seek to make peace with your emotional hurts from the past. Grow in wisdom and understanding through insights. Make peace with who you are and embrace the ever-present love from nature and the divine. Consider that any self-pity, hatred of yourself and others, and wishing life would be different won't change a thing except make your sinuses worse.

Notice any post-nasal drip, clearing your throat constantly, slight or constant frontal headaches are signs that the sinuses are accumulating inflammation. Take note to deal with your conflicts that are right in front of your face. You need to face the fear of being honest and speaking out your truthful feelings. You need to release that deep anger that surfaces as mucus, pain, fatigue, cloudy thinking, and self-pity. It is time to be clear, and be your real self in public and to yourself in private. Love you, yourself, and life.

Sinuses

Affirmations:
- I know who I am, and I live my principles and values in all areas of life.
- I stop the self-sacrifice of my heart, and I care for me now, today and tomorrow.
- I enjoy opportunities for growth that allow me to explore and still rest and renew.
- I am clear about my choices and choose to be true to self-empowerment.
- I barely notice any negative self-talk, and gladly focus on clear positive thought patterns.
- I enjoy taking action.
- When I rest, I rest; when I work, I work; and when I recreate, I recreate.
- I believe in healing, confident in myself, courageous in my adventure, and trust in divine support.

Supporting Foods:
- Water/Get hydrated
- Fresh vegetable and fruit juices
- Herbal teas
- Soups (esp. with cayenne, or raw onion)
- A little salt water
- Ginger tea
- Lemon
- Grapefruit
- Okra, steamed
- Zucchini, steamed with a little salt
- Figs

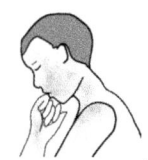

Skin: Cancer

Troubled Mindset

- You are in self-attack.
- You are destroying yourself because you believe you are unworthy.
- You don't feel supported.
- Sometimes you think that you don't have what it takes to push through, but you keep trying until you can accomplish everything that you need to do.
- You were surprised and somewhat shocked by someone who you thought was a friend.
- They turned on you in the most subtle ways. You didn't want to see it.
- It was betrayal right in front of your face, but it was so subtle and smooth that you were fooled.
- You don't think they fully intended to harm, but then again, it seems their jealousy leaked into your friendship, and their side jabs of criticism eventually caused a hurt that went more than skin deep.
- The pain of the betrayal seems to go deeper because the other person is transferring their story so hard and strong and constant on you that it feels you are being pulled into their world of self-pity and blame.
- That criticism sends the message and energy that you are the cause of their problems.
- You hate what is happening.
- You catch your mind thinking negative thoughts about them and justifying these judgments because of this or that.
- You can tell it is making you sick inside, and you work hard not to be physically and emotionally upset.
- You overcompensate and bend over backward to make sure the relationship lasts. But the last straw was broken.
- You went frustrated, numb, and fed up.
- You don't want to deal with them anymore.

Skin: Cancer

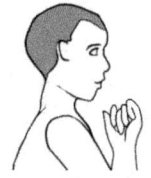

Healing Mindset

You must realize that any negative talk in your head about a very close and dear friend affects some part of your body. Even if you were in so much denial about the events, the skin is showing you clearly that there is a problem. Embrace the reality that this friend is two-sided. If you continue the relationship, you need to know how to communicate and deal with both sides of that person. Or, let go of the destructive relationship. Find ways to release the grief and inner pain of losing a friend. The truth is, you were losing the friendship for a while. It is time to embrace your inner emotions of feeling betrayed and the justified hatred you send back to your old friend/new enemy. It is not worth your time, and especially not good for your skin.

Their sadness and suffering is no longer your responsibility. It is time to enjoy and embrace your life, heal your story, grow up a lot, find new empowering relationships, and forgive those teachers of life that gave you a temporary obstacle. Release the pressure that the negative people give you. You are in charge of your own life.

Skin: Cancer

Affirmations:

- I honor and respect my values.
- I am loyal to the true friend in myself.
- I make sure I take care of myself, my heart, and my body.
- I clear my mind of negative thought and flow into a progressive thought pattern of enjoying every day, every moment.
- I feel blessed to be here and sharing my life.
- I see and clear the seeds of destructive patterns.
- I plant and nourish the seeds of spontaneous and enjoyable experiences.
- I transform the pressure into an adventure of change, clarity, and peace.
- I feel a new hope.

Supporting Foods:

- Eat a diet high in antioxidants
- Low in fat
- Garlic
- Carrots
- Sweet potatoes
- Squash
- Spinach
- Broccoli
- Brussel sprouts
- Cabbage
- Kale
- Turnips
- Citrus fruits
- Blueberries
- Foods high in Vit. E may protect the skin.
- Asparagus
- Green leafy vegetables
- Raw nuts
- Wheat germ
- Cold pressed vegetable oils
- Fish oils

Skin: Dry / Irritations

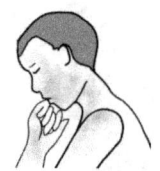

Troubled Mindset

- You are resisting the uncomfortable moments of life.
- You suppress your frustration and try harder to handle life anyway.
- You fear what others may think, and you deny that opportunity to enjoy your mistakes as learning opportunities.
- You try to share but often feel misunderstood, leaving you feeling shoved aside and unimportant.
- Feeling inadequate is a natural form of growth and can be used as a positive challenge.
- Holding onto the past is a form of lack of confidence and leads to internal turmoil and drying up of life's experiences.
- Letting go of the pain of the past is counterintuitive to the fearful side, but essential to the healing side.
- You're not sure how to share your true self and think there might be something wrong with you when you don't easily relate.
- You feel inept as you focus on trying to be the best in things that are not for you, while simultaneously being frustrated that you can't focus on what you enjoy and are good at.
- Start with dealing with those feelings and thoughts that overly ruminate then percolate through the body into the gut, which inflames the insides.
- It then dries up your insides while drying your protective skin.

Skin: Dry / Irritations

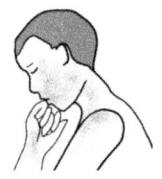

Healing Mindset

You are unique. You are wanted. You are safe. Stop pulling inward and let your real self shine. You've withdrawn your energy as a protection, but it's drying you out. Stop being overly protective. Try being safe in your environment.

You have a spiritual capacity that you may not fully understand how to communicate yet, and it may not even be the appropriate time to share the things you long for. Have patience with yourself and others as you develop into your highest self.

Let go of the painful moments that have gotten under your skin and honor the learning and growth you gain from experience. This will allow you to return to the love that you are and release the resistance towards the love that you seek. Most of all, enjoy the day. Show some warmth and understanding toward your heart and the hearts of others. Fully enjoying each other brings so much fun and happiness. It is a natural form of healing.

Skin: Dry / Irritations

Affirmations:
- I lovingly protect myself with thoughts of joy and peace.
- The past is forgiven and forgotten, and I am free in this moment.
- I honor my true self as I maintain patience through growth.
- I am patient with myself.
- I am forgiving of those around me who don't quite understand my needs.
- Although I want to wash away everything that is uncomfortable, I am learning to appreciate life as a safe and rewarding experience.
- Each relationship can enrich my life.
- I am protected by being enriching and encouraging to myself and others.
- I fill my mind and heart with thoughts of peace and joy.
- I am honorable to myself by being safe and calm in the moment.
- I am free and safe.

Skin: Dry / Irritations

Supporting foods:

- Apples
- Asparagus
- Bananas
- Barley
- Beans
- Beets
- Cabbage
- Carrots
- Celery
- Citrus fruits
- Fibrous foods
- Meats (moderate amounts and not fried)
- Figs
- Fish
- Green beans
- Green peppers
- Kale
- Millet
- Oats
- Buckwheat
- Okra
- Rice
- Romaine lettuce
- Watermelon

Skin: Eczema

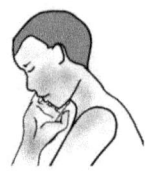

Troubled Mindset

- You're avoiding yourself, and you attack yourself to beat others to the punch.
- You fear that you might ruin everything if you share your genuine self.
- You feel powerless and frustrated to correct what has happened or is happening.
- You feel restrained from acting on what you think should be done.
- You want to have a contribution, but you've allowed others to dominate, not knowing how to promote positive cooperation.
- You resent this, and your body reacts through skin outbursts to compensate for repressed mental outbursts. Though you still erupt when you don't get what you want.
- Your sense of inadequacy leads you to resist love, isolate yourself, and direct frustrations inward.
- Your external manifestation of resentment, blame and intrapersonal discord is showing.

Skin: Eczema

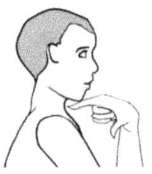

Healing Mindset

It is difficult to let go of these old patterns. Begin the process of change by lovingly nourishing your sense of worth in the darkest times. During the moments when you feel the least for yourself, show love and kindness to yourself.

Take your feelings of inadequacy and use them to find your true inner values. Your desire to hide your feelings in isolation is a sign to find yourself. You have the greatest influence for positive change as you patiently nourish and rise into your authentic self.

Skin: Eczema

Affirmations:
- I am calm in the storm, strong in the fray, patient in the quest.
- I completely wash the pain and the blame away from my skin and body.
- I feel a sense of freedom from any upset or concern.
- I know that I am healing my story because I don't have to be right that they were wrong.
- I feel the caring of others that is all around me.

Supporting Foods:
- Drink at least 2 quarts of water every day
- Eat a balanced diet
- Raw vegetables
- Fruits
- Millet
- Brown rice
- Seeds and nuts
- Garlic
- Onions
- Eggs
- Asparagus
- Bell peppers
- Yellow and orange vegetables like carrots and yellow squash
- Apples
- Citrus fruits
- Tomatoes
- Grapes
- Blackberries

Skin: Issues

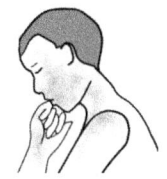

Troubled Mindset

- "It's getting under my skin!"
- Your skin is your boundary and protection.
- You have irritations from not maintaining your mental, emotional, or physical space.
- You are not in your true feelings and overly concerned with others' thoughts and feelings about you.
- You feel misunderstood.
- Your lack of security with who you are makes you behave in ways that are not true to you.
- You resent or hate that, but you suppress your anger and cover your embarrassment.
- You end up irritable and overly critical of others, and feeling guilty about it.
- You don't like the negative emotions but are afraid to live in your true feelings.
- You try to focus your efforts on things that you are not particularly good at. Yet, you are irritated you can't share your gifts.
- You wish for love, approval, or to be valued, but feel unworthy of it.
- There is a fear that if you seek out these needs, you'll get burned.
- Sometimes you may use the skin issue as an excuse to keep away.

Skin: Issues

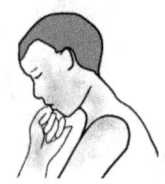

Troubled Mindset
(Continued)

- Skin Rashes:
    - You are itching to do something.
    - Suppressed rage or hatred.
    - Fear or panic of going forward, living, or speaking the truth.
- Skin Peeling:
    - You want to believe in yourself and your worth, but you aren't doing anything about it.
- Dry Skin:
    - You've plugged up your feelings, and you are holding onto something precious or secret.
- Skin Cancer:
    - It's a self-attack.
    - You are destroying yourself because you believe you are unworthy or imperfect.

Skin: Issues

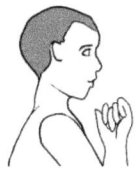

Healing Mindset

You have a great capacity to be sensitive to the energies of your environment. When you desire and then seek spiritual awareness, take the time to share some of your insights. Finding safety in being honest with your wisdom and insights. It is okay to have an opinion. When others criticize, it is because they are afraid to see their own troubles. Let others have their own problems, and you enjoy seeing past the obvious.

Start to release the anger about yourself and others. Remember, you can make a difference, but if you question yourself and resent others, the positive change that you could make diminishes quickly. Don't judge yourself or others for not understanding yet. Embrace the adventure of discovery for all. You are capable, and your gifts are needed. Become the light that you are and grow into your true self.

Skin: Issues

Affirmations:
- I am ready to be the best of me without pushing myself too far.
- I am feeling the care inside for me without the cares of the outside getting in the way.
- I am full of purpose, and I follow that purpose with wisdom and passion.
- I am excited to be me wherever I go and whomever I meet.
- I hope for the best, and let God take care of the rest.
- I am satisfied with the results of the day because I was good to me and myself.
- I am grateful for the cleansing of my body, and I help it with good sleep and healthy eating.
- I flow with my desires and goals.
- I take my time and enjoy life.
- I let go of resentments to all people.
- I am true to me, others, and my truth.
- I trust life.

Supporting Foods:
- Apples
- Asparagus
- Bananas
- Barley
- Beans
- Beets
- Cabbage
- Carrots
- Celery
- Citrus fruits
- Watermelon
- Fibrous foods
- Romaine lettuce
- Green beans
- Green peppers
- Greens
- Kale
- Millet
- Okra
- Rice
- Fish
- Figs
- Meats (moderate amounts and not fried)

Skin: Rashes

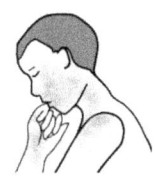

Troubled Mindset

- "What am I worth anyway?"
- Your boundary is weak, and your value is affected by others.
- Feeling attacked, irritated, or shamed, you are easily irritable and angry with life.
- You try to ignore or push your emotions away, but they are reemerging through your skin.
- Your rash decisions are internally burning you up.
- You are trying to be there for everyone, yet you are angry about it.
- You are upset that your condition isn't changing, so your body is pushing out the negativity.
- There are emotional toxins that are building up.
- You have let it happen because a part of you felt trapped by your situation.
- You have been wallowing in the "what if's" and "if only's" too long.
- This has been festering your insides until it is coming out in all the wrong places.

Skin: Rashes

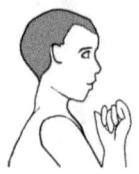

Healing Mindset

Start by identifying your negative thoughts about others and yourself. What you don't know is troubling, and what you think you know is bothersome. So, take those crazy feelings, dump them down the drain and start over. Those old negative feelings of loneliness, pity, resentment, and shock have little room in your home.

Start by discovering your innate value. Don't over-inflate or depress the truth. Your limitations are self-imposed. The power is within you to regain your confidence and personal identity.

There is no way that re-cycling your thoughts is going to solve your problems. Observe every thought and learn from it. Your mind is trying to help you, but if it is worried and negative, then it is not speaking your true core language. Your core language is built on courage, faith, support, and encouragement. Simmering emotions can't help you anymore, so it is time to filter them through until you responsibly become self-motivating, self-empowered, and self-directive.

Skin: Rashes

Affirmations:

- I carefully approach each day with wisdom and understanding.
- I articulate my thoughts with little concern about the opinion of others.
- I calmly sense the needs of my body and relax the worry and the frustration.
- I release the old festering feelings and make room for beneficial beliefs and positive experiences.
- I find a way to be truthful, courageous, and bold in my relationships.
- I defuse the spite with lively emotional conversations.
- I release my judgments and hidden agendas so that I can enrich the lives of others.

Supporting Foods:

- Drink plenty of water/ stay hydrated
- Eat a well-balanced diet including fresh fruits and vegetables
- Whole grains
- Legumes

Sleep Apnea

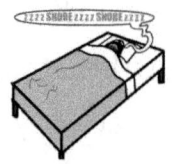

Troubled Mindset

- Your daily life is being played out on the stage of your nocturnal mind.
- If you don't resolve your conflicts by day, they will be role played in your mind while you sleep in the night.
- You have conflict that is often unresolvable, so your mind is pushing you to deal with the conflict until you hold your breath long enough to get your attention concerning the problem.
- Holding your breath is activating the sympathetic nervous system to make sure you do not relax too much.
- The subconscious may be wanting you to stay alert in case trouble looms.
- Your worries are more important than your rest.

Sleep Apnea

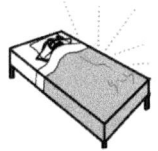

Healing Mindset

Why trouble yourself with concerns that you have little control over? Why over think feelings? Why over feel chaotic thoughts? It is as if the mind of your child self has more sway in your reactions to life than your adult self.

Take moments every hour to pause your mind, calm your heart, relax your body. Practice daily mindfulness so you can sleep at night in restfulness. Create a habit and a routine to start the process of calming your mind early in the evening, every night. When the wind blows and the dog bites and you are feeling sad it is time to take time to heal your heart and unwind the mind. Learn to listen to your fears as warning that you let worries become too important.

Pierce through the emotional whirlwind and in the middle of it all you will find tiny bits of wisdom that are trying to get through to your conscious mind. Find the character-building traits that are waiting to be acknowledged and supported so that you can feel confident in the day and quietly settled in the night.

Sleep Apnea

Affirmations:
- I am ready to live fully then and ready to relax completely.
- I enjoy taking time to observe and unwind.
- I pause during the day so I can sleep at night.
- I reflect and see the wonders of my life.
- I am grateful for the moments of quiet contemplation.
- There is nothing too difficult that the divine or universe can't calm and soothe.

Supporting Foods:
- Acorn squash
- Almonds
- Asparagus
- Avocado
- Bananas
- Celery
- Celery juice
- Cucumber
- Delicata squash
- Dragonfruit
- Eggplant
- Jicama
- Radish
- Salmon
- Tuna
- Walnuts
- Yogurt (unsweetened, greek)
- Avoid: Eating past 7 or 8 pm. Excess sugar or sweets.

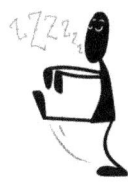

Sleepwalking

Troubled Mindset

- You are lost somewhere inside.
- Your subconscious is desperately seeking answers during the day and night. But no matter how far your sleepy dreams take you, they don't have the solutions.
- Your mind and body are pushing to walk into the solution or escape from the inner drama.
- The need for control to deal with the dramas of life is causing this act of non-conscious movements.
- Every night the mind processes the day. It organizes and releases what is not needed or necessary. However, when there is too much emotion attached to the events, the biochemistry is challenged, and the brain needs more conscious processing. And when this is not enough, the muscles are activated in order to move away or escape from the perceived fears of the day.
- The chaos of your life is overwhelming your subconscious, which mirrors your past or present.
- The fear and distrust of the environment are overriding a peaceful sleep.
- For a child, they fear that they will be judged or rejected if they share their real feelings.
- If it is an adult, it is a replay of past childhood trauma and dramas that formed deep-seated beliefs that still need to be resolved.

Sleepwalking

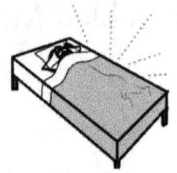

Healing Mindset

Do something spontaneous every day with fun and excitement. Reach inside of yourself and find the parts that want to bear the burdens of the past. Write, talk, meditate, process the big little fears until they are your friends and teachers.

Flow with the spontaneous happenings of life. Observe your surroundings with a sense of adventure and discovery. Take appropriate breaks to recenter as things play out throughout the day. Consider creating a habit of journaling at the end of each day to help process your experiences. Clean up your act of eating, thinking, and caring. Get some healthy exercise even when you don't feel like it.

Sleepwalking

Affirmations:
- My heart cares deeply for those around me, and I care about my heart even more.
- I feel much, so I move a lot.
- I release my daily concerns at the foot of my bed so that I can deeply rest my head.
- Escape the past is ancient, avoid the pain is gone, embrace the learning is now, and find my heart is best.
- I hope for the best in my nightly rest.
- I release the expectations of the past and receive the gifts of the day.
- I find fears and squeeze them with love, and they become my friend.

Supporting Foods:
- Stay hydrated
- Raw nuts
- Seeds
- Legumes
- Whole grains
- Apples
- Asparagus
- Avocados
- Beets
- Leafy greens
- Carrots
- Celery
- Fennel
- Garlic
- Lemon
- Limes
- Pears
- Tomatoes
- Eat a high fiber diet with lots of fresh fruits and vegetables.

Sneezing

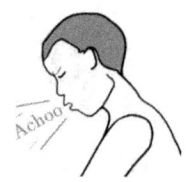

Troubled Mindset

- You had a surprise that you were not ready for.
- Even though you didn't think you were scared, your hesitation stems from deeper fears.
- You are too sensitive to surprises.
- You hate making agreements against your inner will.
- You really dislike and fear pathogens, bacteria, viruses, or another possible enemy.
- You fear secrets or what others are saying, as well as seeing what is real.
- You are harboring resentment towards a person or situation, but you suppress your anger.
- If you sneeze while putting on mascara, it may be related to the resentment of the extra time and effort you take to look a particular way.
- There's not enough time to do the extra work and not have positive acknowledgment.
- There are issues with your significant other.
- Sneezing often has to do with believing that whatever brings joy into your life will be lost.

Sneezing

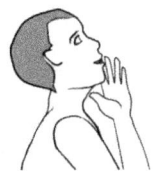

Healing Mindset

You need to become aware of the subtle conflicts that could get blown out of proportion. Release beliefs that are not serving you. Rather than fearing your way through life, put trust in yourself, faith in your capacity, and hope in your growth through experience.

Choose to find the difference between your real needs and wishful needs. Choose to create methods of dealing with those feelings that get pushed under the rug and out of sight. Choose to be who you are. Take the time to focus on loving the tender you, the sensitive self without expectation and without dependency on outside validation. Hold gratitude for all the good that comes into your life.

Sneezing

Affirmations:
- I am open to the light that allows me to see and release my hidden fears and tears.
- Dare to be bold when others back off.
- Dare to be sincere when others placate or please.
- Dare to be true when dealing with hidden frustration.
- Dare to be a bearer of strength and courage.
- Moving hesitation over, I welcome the spontaneous serendipitous life.

Supporting Foods:

- Water/Get hydrated
- A little salt water
- Fresh vegetable and fruit juices
- Herbal teas
- Soups (esp. with cayenne, or raw onion)
- Ginger tea
- Lemon
- Grapefruit
- Okra steamed
- Zucchini steamed with a little salt
- Figs

Snoring

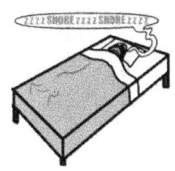

Troubled Mindset

- You are stubborn about too many things in your life, but you don't let most people know.
- You appear to go along with others, but inside you harbor a different point of view with a few extra feelings.
- You are stuck in an old mindset and not accepting positive changes that will bring appropriate growth into your life.
- You try to accomplish everything all on your own and take responsibility for anything that happens.
- You're not trusting others or the universe to support you in mind and heart.
- You cannot become your best self when you stay stuck in the past.
- You are trying to process the day without dealing with the troubles of the previous day.
- You are allowing your problems to grow and grow without a real and final solution.
- You don't think you can deal with everything.
- You have taken on too much responsibility.

Snoring

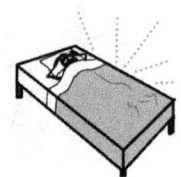

Healing Mindset

You need to face the daily challenge of dealing with the conflicting inputs from those around you. You need to deal with the way you communicate. You need to be more honest, and to do that, you need to be more introspective about your wants, desires, goals, and the realities of achieving them.

You can deal with your fear of telling your truth by being authentic with yourself first. If not, you will take your discomfort of the day with you and will try to breathe it out in the night. You must realize that the input from others is appropriate and necessary for your success. The intention is not for you to solve everything by yourself. Humans are meant to be together and to work and help one another. Let go of old beliefs that keep you back from sharing your ambitions and accepting change.

Snoring

Affirmations:

- I take my troubles and set them aside for the night, and if they are there in the morning, I can pick them up again for another ride.
- I find comfort in calming the discomfort of daily conflicts.
- I release my need to solve everyone's problems.
- I accept myself as I am, and as I will be.
- I am a conscious breather and a subconscious achiever.
- I maintain my personal integrity while being flexible with others.
- I breathe the full cycle of creation and completion.
- I feel energized in the day and rested in the night.
- My kidneys love the joys I seek and live every day.
- My jaw appreciates the moments of laughter, intriguing conversation, and caring love.

Supporting Foods:

- Water/ Get hydrated
- Eat a low diet diet with lots of fresh fruits and vegetables
- Raw nuts
- Seeds
- Legumes
- Whole grains
- Fish

Spleen

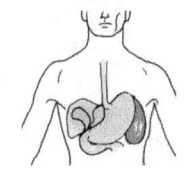

Troubled Mindset

- Your spleen filters your blood, or in other words, your love.
- You haven't loved yourself or others, nor do you believe you deserve to be loved, so you've become bitter.
- You have excess frustration, worry, and obsessive thoughts.
- You are easily influenced because you are sensitive and feel a need to please others.
- You have a thin boundary to maintain your personal identity, and you are skeptical to compensate for being uncertain of yourself.
- You fear to lose your close relationships, so you act possessive, needy, pushy, controlling, and insecure. This behavior drives them away and creates a self-fulfilling prophecy.
- You can be critical.
- You'd rather correct others than deal with your own problems.
- You have tended to be catastrophic and focus on the most negative possible outcomes.
- You end up unhappy, irritable, and uncaring about others.

Spleen

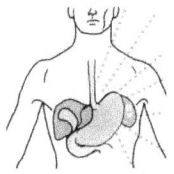

Healing Mindset

Allow yourself to offer and receive deep, sincere love. Reconnect to the gentle, positive, and nourishing energy within you. You can have strong compassion with healthy boundaries and courage as you do so.

You are very driven with a desire to excel in life. Direct your drive towards healing and spiritual growth. Let go of hate, blame, perfectionism, and over-thinking everything. Your cyclic thoughts betray and harm you, so notice them and find ways to redirect them to a positive and productive path. Be aware and be appreciative.

Spleen

Affirmations:

- I release the belief and feelings that my image is more important than my soul.
- I safely create nourishing relationships.
- I easily bond with family and friends.
- My faith is deeper and richer than my mind.
- I have a strong mind and a courageous will.
- I breathe in the abundance of life and peace of mind.
- I feel the balance of my mind and heart, body, and soul.
- I am authentic with myself.
- I filter what is not mine and share what is.
- I am aware of my thoughts and let them be for my benefit.
- I find comfort in being true to my body's life force and connect with it inside my body.
- My past efforts bring fruits to my life today.
- I am grateful for my strong immune system, healthy digestive system, and mindful awareness system.
- I reciprocate positive emotions and beneficial energy to others.

Spleen

Supporting Foods:

- Alfalfa sprouts
- Algae
- Asparagus
- Barley
- Bee foods
- Beef
- Brown rice
- Carrots
- Cauliflower
- Celery
- Cherries
- Chlorophyll
- Fennel
- Fish
- Green peppers
- Greens
- Honey (small amounts)
- Millet
- Molasses
- Oats
- Oranges
- Papaya
- Peas
- Potato
- Proteins
- Red lentils
- Rice
- Romain lettuce
- Royal jelly
- Spinach
- Spirulina
- Strawberries
- Sweet potato
- Sweet vegetables
- Tofu
- Vegetables (lightly cooked)
- Wheat grass
- Yam
- Yellow squash
- Warm foods

Sprains

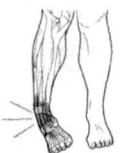

Troubled Mindset

- The pressure you felt makes it difficult to go forward, but you are compelled to do so anyway.
- You fight a battle inside of not wanting to listen to the control of others and the desire to be nice and get along with them.
- You resist any change that you think will hurt or cause you harm, but you don't want to make any "waves" that would result in personal conflicts with them.
- You are ignoring an authority or your own higher wisdom.
- It makes you angry inside when you can't have it or do it your way.
- You feel that you have always done it alone and somehow figured things out in the past.
- You don't want to have any interference now.
- You end up with feelings that are out of your control.
- Your mind is scattered.
- You hesitate too much, and yet you take too many risks.

Sprains

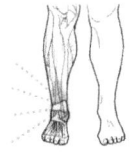

Healing Mindset

Slow down because you are going to fast without thinking of the consequences. You can calm the chaos with breathing and meditating. Bring yourself back to your body and create a feeling of peace and safety.

Everyone has trust issues with authorities, but being double-minded when dealing with them has caused you problems. Take the time to be clear about where you are going and where you want to be. Be clear about the consequences of your decisions before taking action.

Try not to 'please' to solve your issues with authority figures or significant people in your life. Be true to your core self. Find the core values that are more important than external and shallow wishes. Listen to your inner wisdom because it will offer the clearest path to satisfaction and happiness.

Sprains

Affirmations:

- I take the time to look at my situation before making decisions.
- I am grateful for my intuition, and I take the time to listen to that inner voice.
- I respect my body and all its functions.
- It is remarkable to experience the healing power of my body.
- I am grateful for the divine gift of self-healing of the body, mind, and spirit.
- I am in awe when I listen to the wisdom from my spiritual side of myself and others.
- I respect my body when healing from injuries.
- I understand the value of the signs given to me by my body and apply wisdom in my life.
- I am slowing the pace and take time to enjoy life.

Sprains

Supporting Foods:

- Stay hydrated
- Drink plenty of juices made from fresh raw vegetables including beets, garlic, & radishes
- Foods rich in calcium, potassium, magnesium, zinc, and Vit. C
- Dairy foods
- Green leafy vegetables
- Legumes
- Tofu
- Soy
- Oats
- Almonds
- Pecans
- Sunflower seeds
- Sesame seeds
- Apricots
- Apples
- Avocados
- Bananas
- Brewers yeast
- Brown rice
- Yams
- Fish
- Seafood
- Poultry
- Figs
- Garlic
- Whole grains
- Egg yolks
- Mushrooms
- Broccoli
- Bell peppers
- Citrus fruits

Stiffness

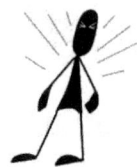

Troubled Mindset

- Your stiff attitude is getting the best of you.
- The emotional stiffness can be stubbornness towards others or to yourself. It also is a resistance to dealing with life events.
- Furthermore, you may not realize that your stiff muscles are trying to keep you aware of other problems in the body and the fear of dealing with all your issues.
- Fear, worry, and frustration eventually wear the body down until the muscles stiffen up.
- When you become stiff and inflexible, you use it as a protection.
- Sometimes you may not realize what you are protecting yourself from. The reason for this ignorance is that you have allowed your unconscious body to take over the role of being your protector.
- You don't feel safe.
- You are not sure what to do next, feeling like there are high stakes involved.
- You are harsh on yourself or others about mistakes.
- Fear keeps you resisting any change, but you come across as a know it all.
- Check this app for the specific body area for more details.

Stiffness

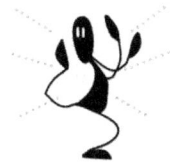

Healing Mindset

Start with stretching your body slowly and for several minutes. Breathe deeply and slowly. Your determination is good, but your stubbornness is not.

Learn to be firm and not tight. Learn to be focused, not obsessive. Learn to be honest with expressing your feelings and not suppressing them. Learn the difference between the ego and the core self. The ego is demanding and stubborn. The core self is confident and proactive. Connect to your true core self in order to strengthen your ability to be flexible, directed, productive, and motivated.

Be forgiving of your mistakes because the resistance to experimenting with life will tighten you up. Life happens and so flow with the learning and growth. Find joy in the journey, lead by example, and find a sense of adventure in your experiences.

Stiffness

Affirmations:
- I listen to my body, take a breath, and relax.
- I am secure in my life and confidently move forward.
- My intention to get through the day is better when I inhale trust and exhale hope.
- I communicate well and appreciate often.
- When I allocate my time, I am gladly flexible with my family, friends, and my personal needs.
- I enjoy taking care of my body.
- When I find my heart in all the right places, my body relaxes, and my mind is clear.
- I peacefully turn my fear into calm focus.
- I am grateful for the amazing challenges of my life.

Supporting Foods:
- Dairy foods
- Green leafy vegetables
- Legumes
- Tofu
- Soy
- Oats
- Almonds
- Pecans
- Sunflower seeds
- Sesame seeds
- Apricots
- Apples
- Avocados
- Bananas
- Brewers yeast
- Brown rice
- Yams
- Fish
- Seafood
- Poultry
- Figs
- Garlic
- Whole grains
- Citrus fruits
- Egg yolks
- Mushrooms
- Drink plenty of water/stay hydrated
- Eat a well balanced diet including foods rich in calcium, potassium, magnesium and zinc

Stomach Problems (Digestive)

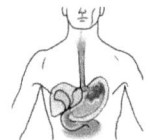

Troubled Mindset

- You are sensitive to everything and everyone.
- You are empathic to other people's feelings and add your own worries.
- You tend to mix up the emotions of those around you with your fears and concerns. The 'feelings soup' doesn't sit well in your stomach.
- Your sensitivities are worse when you can't control the personal attacks on your character or when you see the overwhelming problems of your family or friends.
- You want to release your frustrations, but you hold them in because you don't want to make things worse or deal with the consequences.
- The impending doom causes you to hesitate to make permanent changes.
- Your overwhelm makes it difficult to digest more information and new concepts.
- You would rather keep doing things your way.
- You may be demanding of others, but you have the agenda that it is good for them.
- Your personal power is often challenged.
- You back down to some and explode on others.
- When you are attacked, you struggle to express yourself.
- Like a "punch in the gut," you consistently restrain yourself.
- Out of fear, you deny yourself the opportunity to expand your awareness and consciousness.
- You end up confused, angry, bitter, hateful, resentful, and very sad.

Stomach Problems (Digestive)

Troubled Mindset (Continued)

- You can't digest these toxic emotions.
- You reject the energy and qualities of the gender opposite to you.
- You feel you don't deserve love.
- You resist support by being inflexible to the caring of others, but you wish others would be flexible with you.
- You have a hidden agenda that blocks real love and fosters self-rejection and self-blame.

Healing Mindset

You have the ability to sense and feel deeply, but it is time to make boundaries for yourself. Your excess empathy is good for understanding and caring, but not good for your digestive tract. Your worry does not match the problem. Your concern does not equal the solution. You easily lose your power with fear, worry, upset, and blame.

Reclaim your power by being true to your core self. Find that core self with time along and nourishing yourself in every way but food. When you nourish your heart with food, it hurts your stomach, and it makes matters worse. Food is for nourishment but not for fixing and hiding problems. Sadness makes your stomach sluggish. Anger makes your stomach hurt. Fear makes your stomach ache. Your power could be in conscious living by heart and mind. Allow your mind and heart to work together. Seek harmony in living whole and human. Take time to truly heal the pain and "hurts" from the past. Learn compassion by first wisely caring for yourself.

Stomach Problems (Digestive)

Affirmations:
- I am grateful for every moment of life.
- I discover the joy in my experience.
- I respect myself and my gifts.
- I stand up for myself first, and then I can courageously stand up for them.
- I assimilate what is needed and discard the rest.
- I pass through life with ease and comfort.
- I have all I need in order to live in a fulfilling way.
- I enjoy eating my food slowly and methodically.
- Life is safe and beneficial to me.
- I trust myself.
- I honor myself with healthy food, positive thoughts, and warm feelings.
- I respect and trust others at the level of their honest capacity.
- I am safe with allowing others to learn from their mistakes.
- It is safe to let people see me for who I am.
- I relax and do my best.
- I feel courage from within.
- I feel comfortably satisfied.
- I enjoy feeling compassion for others.

Stomach Problems (Digestive)

Supporting Foods:

- Chew your food
- Squash
- Zucchini
- Minerals: calcium, iron, magnesium, phosphorus, potassium, sodium & zinc
- Alfalfa sprouts
- Algae
- Bamboo shoots
- Bananas
- Basil
- Beef
- Bell pepper
- Brown rice
- Buckwheat
- Cabbage
- Celery
- Chlorophyll
- Cinnamon
- Ginger
- Grapefruit
- Grapes
- Greens
- Kale
- Mango
- Millet
- Molasses
- Papaya
- Parsley
- Peas
- Peppermint
- Potato
- Pumpkin
- Rye
- Soy
- Spirulina
- Sweet potato
- Tofu
- Wheat grass
- Yam

Stroke

Troubled Mindset

- You are impatient with yourself and with those who stand in your way.
- You want to be helpful, but you question the motives of others.
- You are afraid that what you do harms others.
- You tend towards being too hard on yourself.
- You think that you could do more, be better, and not make any mistakes.
- You hold onto the past with an intense demand on yourself to change the future.
- You are afraid that you might not have the answers you need.
- You are having difficulty sorting things out.
- Sometimes you just don't know, and it is frustrating.
- Your impatience with the path to healing is compounding your issue.
- You are less interested in the way, or the journey, and overly concerned with the destination.
- You are having a lost sense of purpose in life.
- Love has become a bitter feeling.
- You genuinely believe no one cares.
- You are frustrated with yourself for not being able to figure things out.
- It's gotten so much so that you'd rather give up and 'go home' than stay and truly change. You are resisting spiritual growth.

Stroke

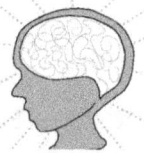

Healing Mindset

Remember when life was easier and more functional. Find the path to bring clarity, functionality, and joy back into your life. Reconnect with a deep and purposeful way of living. Find your real value and purpose. Inner growth and change can manifest your desires in ways you never believed possible.

Seek spiritual growth and transformation to allow your inner light to shine once again. Notice your impatience, then communicate to the immature side of yourself to find any fears and upsets. Calm the fears with your breath, walking, clean eating, clear thinking, and sincere gratitude. Practice sorting the simple things of life, so that you can organize the more complex things. Count your blessings, and you will find a hidden treasure behind one of them.

Stroke

Affirmations:
- I am grateful for every moment and every breath.
- I appreciate my body for all the amazing things it can do.
- I enjoy life when my heart and my mind are on the same team.
- I validate that I am going through my struggles, and I validate my progress.
- I clearly communicate to connect and make a difference.
- I feel validated by others and by my own mind.

Supporting Foods:
- Eat a high fiber, low fat diet
- Eat mainly fruits, vegetables and whole grains
- Foods high in Vitamin E
- Dark green leafy vegetables
- Use only cold pressed olive oil or omega-3 oils
- Rye
- Eggplant
- Legumes
- Nuts
- Seeds
- Soybeans
- Wheat germ

Stuttering

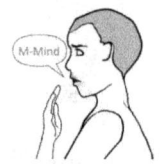

Troubled Mindset

- You have been made to believe that you are inferior or inadequate.
- The belief is false, but you are making it true by your fearful actions.
- You feel unworthy to speak, and you 'know' others will ridicule your words.
- Your intentions are to be accepted, but the emotional brain is being fueled by the primal brain, and it overrides your good intentions.
- You have a contribution and a message, but fear inhibits you from sharing.
- You don't want to upset the authority figures in your life.
- You desperately dread mistakes, which brings about a pattern of anxiety and repeating your perceived errors.
- You have forgotten that this life is an experiment, not a test.
- Those who believe in perfectionism live in fearful delusions or angry control.
- You have given your power away to another person and to your terrified self.
- Your mind is racing faster than the mouth.

Stuttering

Healing Mindset

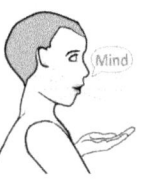

Stop believing the false beliefs like 'I am no good,' 'I am not good enough,' 'I don't know anything,' 'I am not lovable,' or 'I can't say it right.' These negative beliefs are only there because your subconscious wants to protect you from my ridicule if you tried to be accepted. However, it is a false protection because you are hurting yourself.

Believe in the path of adventure, learning, and discovery. Believe in the part of you that wants to express and be a part of life. Take a chance at being embarrassed and moving through it without taking it personally.

Breathe deeply and realize the judgments of others are the reflections of their fears forced upon you. Let their fears be like a breeze, and let your mind and heart connect to the only person that really matters, and that is you. Listen to you and your deep passions for being alive, communicative, sharing, caring, and living a meaningful life.

Allow strength to rise and bring you courage. When you are ready, open up while maintaining a calm state. Embrace your mistakes, forgive yourself frankly, every time. Make a game of your learning and growing as you embrace your authentic voice. Reclaim your personal power.

Stuttering

Affirmations:
- I reclaim my personal power.
- I hear words and intentions that are for my highest good.
- I speak my truth with clarity and focus.
- I speak to the heart of the other person.
- I am grateful for this experience because I am empathetic and understanding of others.
- My heart is good, my mind is good, my friends are good, and life is good.
- Opportunities for growth and learning amazingly show up every day.
- I am expressive, and I am meticulously sharing my thoughts with clarity and joy.
- I realize true power comes from within.
- Today I will find at least one person that will share my heart's deep feelings.
- I know my mind is faster than my mouth, so I choose to slow the process, to bring clarity into the words that I speak.

Supporting Foods:
- Black beans
- Blueberries
- Carrots
- Cauliflower
- Celery
- Cucumber
- Millet
- Pumpkin
- Quinoa
- Salmon
- Salt (small amount)
- Watercress
- Yam
- Yellow squash
- Zucchini

Suicidal

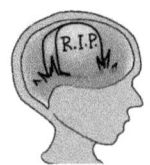

Troubled Mindset

- You are being bothered by the overwhelm of the conflicts of your life.
- The dramas are now traumas.
- You forgot that you are human, not a movie or a stage.
- Humans are meant to learn flexibility and to grow. Movies have to follow a script, and you have got lost in the script that is taking you down a dark path.
- You know you can't figure this out, and you think that you are the problem. But are you the problem? Or is it the voice in your head that is guiding you wrong?
- You feel like you can't manage life and all its crazy overwhelming problems.
- The same pain that drives you to think strangely keeps coming back because there is a fear to really find a valid and true solution.
- Sometimes you try to be heroic and make a difference in someone's life, but the results don't always work out, and you have lost hope.
- You think they will be better off, but that is a big lie that only makes you turn off real logic and truth.
- You feel like a burden and wish to escape.
- The part of you that wishes to escape wants to take away that horrible feeling.
- The horribleness is not you; it is just a stuck piece of emotional and mental furniture that needs some major cleanup.

Suicidal

Healing Mindset

Get help, and be honest with your professional assistant. The goal is more than stopping the problem. The goal is to find the reason the pain doesn't move out and change. The pain is a sign that might point you to the problem, but chances are that it is guessing. Pain doesn't speak English, Spanish, or any other cognitive language. It only knows how to speak the language of pain.

Look at what you are escaping from, and you will see a door to some of the answers you seek. Faith doesn't come from fear. Faith comes from trusting that, in the dark, you will trust that you can learn and develop character. This is taking responsibility. This is learning how to choose. When you learn to choose, you will create the freedom that you seek. Then you can start putting value into your own heart, your own life, and the experience of this life.

Saving others or saving yourself is not the key, but the sign that you really do care deeply. Before saving, start by finding yourself, and by finding your heart. Let others love and care for you for a change. Life doesn't need fixing; it needs caring. Focus on becoming you, your awesome self. Be the one who has something to share within your unique capacity. Change takes time, go at your own pace. That is the only way to go. Strengthen yourself to become strong against the dark beliefs so that you can wake up and smell the roses. Life is a daily challenge with a lot of sunshine to boost us along.

Suicidal

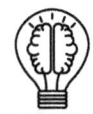

Affirmations:

- Here comes the sunshine of my soul.
- I am empowered to be tough on any darkness I sense.
- I am grateful for this day, this moment, and this thought.
- I am responsible to breathe, to eat, to move, and to smile at someone who could use one.
- If I fear, I let it guide me to the part of myself that needs direction and love.
- If I hate, I let it guide me to the part of myself that needs understanding and hope.
- I am not the painful darkness, but I am the will to win the day.
- I push and shove my way through the horrible until I see the light of day and feel the warmth of heart.

Supporting Foods:

- Water/Get hydrated
- Whole grains
- Soybeans
- Soy products
- Brown rice
- Eat a well balanced diet including raw fruits and vegetables
- Millet
- Legumes
- Salmon
- White fish
- Turkey
- Cucumbers
- Apples
- Watermelon
- Cabbage
- Micro-algae
- Apple cider vinegar

Swelling / Edema

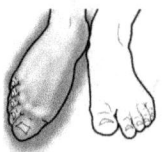

Troubled Mindset

- Your emotions are getting the best and worst of you.
- You are being flooded with past memories that are confusing current problems.
- You are trapped in your pain and your beliefs.
- You have deep-seated anger and some hatred.
- You went through some trauma that scared you deeply.
- Your feelings are hurt, so now your cells are resisting any help.
- Your body is exhibiting physical protection to compensate for holding on to the unnecessary emotional hurts.
- You tend to keep your emotions bottled up while hiding from any confrontations.
- You resist the flow of emotions, which are meant to come and go.
- Right now, you'd rather stay put and find a reason not to move forward.
- You can look in the app for the specific body area for more details.

Swelling / Edema

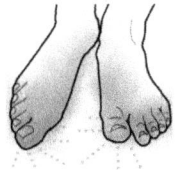

Healing Mindset

Begin by eating slowly and consuming healthy foods. Junk food will feed your self-pity and cause your cells to block the needed hydration and nutrients. The same goes for your emotions. Chew on your emotions slowly and honestly. Assimilate healthy thoughts and emotions; the rest is just junk. Your cyclic thoughts are embedding the problem, and they will "pit" your heart and soul with more problems.

Blame only hurts you deeply. As you face your beliefs and emotions, start to release the silly judgments and breathe through your emotional feelings. Your body is telling you to let it go and move forward. It's not worth holding on to anymore. Listen. The wounds can heal without any additional trauma. Trust your body, your heart, and your mind as you let go and heal. Create a pattern of accepting the flow of emotion in your life.

Swelling / Edema

Affirmations:

- All the little cells of my body are ready and accepting good nourishment.
- I see my cells resisting, and so I meditate to open them to love and kindness.
- I move my mind and body to create open spaces in my life.
- I already have all that I need, so I release the clutter from my heart.
- I have so much to offer.
- I am free to be only me and nothing else.
- I love the challenge of learning to release the struggles of the past.
- I sense my true power is listening to my inner voice of self-love.
- The voice I hear from within is one of respect and gratitude.
- My strength is not in food or doubt, but encouragement and intrigue.
- My kindness is not in pleasing or junk thoughts, but empathy and applause.
- I am a force for good in the world.

Supporting Foods:

- Lettuce
- Celery
- Turnip
- Kohlrabi
- Rye
- Amaranth
- Aduki beans
- Asparagus
- Alfalfa
- Pumpkin
- Papaya

Tailbone

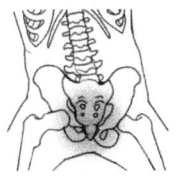

Troubled Mindset

- Your orientation is off.
- You fell into something that you didn't agree with, and now you are struggling to get out or deal with it somehow.
- You are going into survival mode too often.
- You can't get what you want, and it's not fair.
- You have become too preoccupied with material goods to enjoy life.
- You are holding on to old shame and pain, believing that you 'deserve' it. This may manifest as sexual shame.
- You are stuck with the past.
- You are fighting to keep your own ground but don't feel solid nor firm enough in your relationships.
- You want resolution, and sometimes you feel that you have to be angry when the fear and anxiety rise.

Tailbone

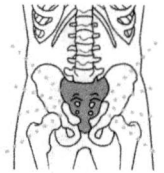

Healing Mindset

You are resisting so much it is difficult to know how to be flexible enough to change. You need to consider that the nervous self works the brain and the tailbone the same. When you worry and fret, you will tighten your mind as well as the muscles that affect the tailbone. When you try to control the outcomes of your life, you make your thinking rigid, and the muscles that affect your tailbone rigid.

Don't blame yourself. Learn from what has happened and breathe out the past hurts. Wake up and value each moment with mindfulness. Understand your experiences and find bounty within to allow room and space for balanced abundance around you. Stretch your muscles and your mind to receive help from the universe and your angels. You can relax and find a way through your excessive control by being open to learning from your experiences and your reactions. Your subconscious is only trying to do its best, but it is running on the past fears and not the current maturity. It is time to grow up and be an empowered version of yourself.

Tailbone

Affirmations:

- I am flexible with my thoughts and my feelings.
- I find opportunities for growth in all my experiences.
- I open my mind to the possibility that I am safe and growing.
- I observe my mind through my challenges, and I choose to relax my thoughts and muscles in response.
- I peacefully breathe life into my body and soul.
- I release any "shoulds" because, really, I am good.

Supporting Foods:

- Whole grains
- Kelp
- Soy products
- Dairy
- Eggs
- Fish
- Oatmeal
- Sweet potatoes
- Brewer's yeast
- Green leafy vegetables
- Almonds
- Asparagus
- Broccoli
- Cabbage
- Figs
- Apricots
- Cantaloup
- Papayas
- Carrots
- Garlic
- Red peppers
- Yellow squash
- Water/Get hydrated
- Eat a well balanced diet including fresh vegetables and fruits.

Teeth Grinding

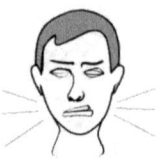

Troubled Mindset

- You are forcing change in your life, but the problem is you are doing it while you sleep.
- The movie your mind dreams up every night is pushing your limits, and your jaw is responding with grinding you to a halt.
- It is effecting your teeth, your breathing, your muscles, and your spiritual self.
- Your subconscious is giving in to the angry and fearful parts of your survival mind.
- You are refusing to communicate your anger and upset so your body is taking the punishment out on yourself.
- Your inner logic is off and damaging.
- You want to make a change, but your efforts are failing.
- The hurts of the past have been so sore and deep that you've angrily created an intense subconscious barrier as protection.
- You have blocked the door of creation, of authentic expression, and any true solution to your problems.
- A wall of mistrust and anger doesn't solve a thing.
- Your mistrust of others blocks the appropriate insight or direction for your life.
- Your soul has fear about following through with your true life's path.

Teeth Grinding

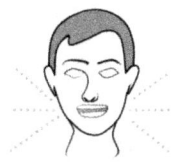

Healing Mindset

Your compassion should be your passion, but instead, it is being right, being upset, and keeping it tied up in knots. Release the entangled knots of your heart and mind. Process the logic with the understanding that being right is not being happy nor productive.

Your heart can only handle so much anger, so give yourself the opportunity to heal your life and your jaw. Have compassion for your sensitive heart, and patience with your soul's plan.

Release your anger; it is not serving you. You have a contribution, but it needs to be offered on a foundation of love, instead of power or control. Trust your deeper intuition. Open your heart to others and patiently bring about positive change in yourself that will have a positive impact on the world around you.

Teeth Grinding

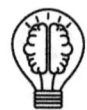

Affirmations:
- I am putting up with a lot, so I will put it somewhere else tonight.
- I can't help myself; I just want to celebrate another day of letting the light into my mind, heart, and life.
- I want to be really happy, so I often open my mouth and release whatever is stuck in there.
- My head is meeting my heart tonight, so I can get some sleep.
- I really want you to know that I forgive you for anything and everything.
- Tonight, I love myself so much that I write all my worries down and toss them away.
- I love a good challenge; all the rest I give back to God.

Supporting Foods:
- Foods high in calcium
- Eat a diet high in fiber and protein and include plenty of fresh vegetables and high fiber fruits
- Eat starchy vegetables and very sweet fruits in moderation.
- Eat 6-8 small meals spread throughout the day
- Legumes
- Raw nuts
- Raw seeds
- Chicken
- Turkey
- Fish
- Whole grains

Tendon

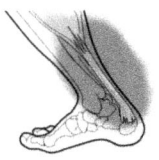

Troubled Mindset

- Your connection to your core self is through your ego, pride, and control.
- The authentic side of you is getting lost in your self-demanding world.
- You cope with your fears and vulnerability with rigid self-control and intense emotions.
- You may blame yourself for the pains, sorrows, and troubles of your past, but you still demand to push forward anyway.
- You can't just let your self stop the cycle, not for one moment.

Tendon

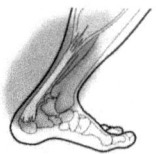

Healing Mindset

Wake up and smell the roses. The roses have thorns and flowers. That is the beauty of life. It is to grow from the experience and turn the struggle into positive, inner character building. Forgive, and have compassion for yourself. Imagine that your experiences are intended to help you grow to become more loving and even stronger than before.

If you are taking the blame, it is a part of yourself that is trying to motivate you to change. Unfortunately, self-blame makes it worse, not better. Consider a new, different perspective—one rooted in self-love and self-discovery. Choose to empower yourself with wisdom and insights from your experiences. Practice flexibility both in your approach to yourself and others, all while honoring your true intentions.

Tendon

Affirmations:
- I flex my mental muscles to expand my mind and creativity daily.
- I plan, I create, I act, and I motivate.
- I responsibly go forward in life while respecting every part of my body and mind.
- I am not easy on myself; I am respectful and caring to myself.
- I respect my capacity; while maturely challenging myself forward.
- I act and do from a place of self-discovery and self-respect.
- I take a chance at occasional vulnerability in order to open the door of spontaneous authenticity.
- I am experimenting with becoming intimately connected with my inner self.

Tendon

Supporting Foods:

- Drink water/ Stay hydrated
- Dairy foods
- Legumes
- Tofu
- Soy
- Oats
- Almonds
- Pecans
- Sunflower seeds
- Sesame seeds
- Whole grains
- Egg yolks
- Mushrooms
- Bell peppers
- Citrus fruits
- Green leafy vegetables
- Yellow squash
- Brewers yeast
- Brown rice
- Sweet potatoes
- Wheat germ
- Avocados
- Asparagus
- Garlic
- Apricots
- Apples
- Carrots
- Broccoli
- Yams
- Fish
- Seafood
- Poultry
- Figs
- Eat a well balanced diet including foods rich in calcium, magnesium, zinc, Vit. A, Vit. C, and Vit. E.

Throat Problems

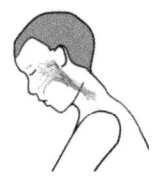

Troubled Mindset

- You have one problem, and that is your need to hold back while pushing forward.
- You think that the whole world might implode if you speak what you are thinking.
- You suppress your voice because of fear and anger.
- You don't want to accept things the way they are, but you don't feel you have a right to speak up about it either.
- The conflict has shut you down.
- You are resisting inner change.
- Your fear of critique towards anything you say, or how you say it, is intense and personal.
- You fear any efforts to articulate yourself. This self-sabotage angers you.
- You have stuffed the emotional pains while refusing to feel or express the truth of what has hurt you.
- You essentially refuse to stand up for yourself, due to insecurity and a belief that perhaps you are better off seen, and not heard.
- You want to be understood so much that you swallow your pride and your resentment.
- With suppression, you hurt inside while the outside world has not a clue of your inner struggles.

Throat Problems

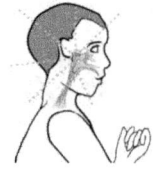

Healing Mindset

You can start by nourishing your heart and your mind with self-worth, self-care, and positive self-talk. Authentic self-worth is beyond logic. All humans, animals, plants, and the earth have a worth that comes from the universe and the divine. How you express that worth is what is troubling. If a person believes they lack confidence and courage, that doesn't translate to worth, that translates to the capacity to act or react in a given situation. It is a false pride that causes you to belittle yourself. Begin by finding people that you can share a part of your passion, heart, talents, interests with. Release the false pride that compensates for the insecurity.

Real confidence comes from being aligned and true to your values, acting on them, and honoring yourself more than what others say about you. Remember, inner resentments to yourself or others are an excuse to not change. Stop the madness of blame and resentment and turn the pages over to self-forgiveness, self-acceptance, honesty, integrity, and respect for yourself and others. You can find the courage to end the attachments to the lies you have told yourself and create an honest place of expressing the authentic real you to the world.

Throat Problems

Affirmations:

- I speak my truth with confidence and heart.
- My heart wants to cry out, "I am free to be me; can't you see?"
- My body wants to shout out, "I am so alive; I can just be!"
- My mind wants to boldly think, "I am clear, I understand, and I am understood."
- There is a place for me in the world, and that place is called Me, Myself, and I.
- I deliver my passion and purpose boldly and graciously.
- I express my love, affectionately.
- I offer my wisdom curiously.
- I conserve my vital energy while abundantly sharing universal energy.

Supporting Foods:

- Drink plenty of liquids
- Fresh juices
- Herbal teas
- Broths
- Garlic
- Strawberries
- Watercress
- Apricots
- Foods high in Vit. C such as lemon & limes

Throat Problems: Specific

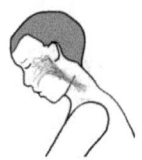

Troubled Mindset

- If you have lost your voice, it may be because you don't want to waste your time trying to get your message across. With pride, you feel you know what you are talking about, but you are not confident it will be heard or understood anyway.

- With throat phlegm, you are blocking your emotions to keep you from relating to another person's experience. There is irritation or discomfort about having empathy, perhaps due to a lack of an appropriate boundary.

- If you have a sore throat, you are 'fired up' about not having your perspective heard or understood.

- With a tickle in your throat, you may be judging yourself because of something you have done or said.

- If you find yourself constantly clearing your throat, it has to do with an intense fear of how others will interpret what you are saying. You feel that a lot is weighing on what you are sharing, and you fear the possible repercussions and implications.

Throat Problems: Specific

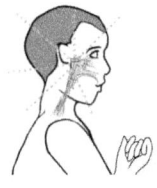

Healing Mindset

The true voice doesn't come from fear or resentment. The real sound of your core self doesn't come from manipulating yourself or others. If there is irritation or discomfort, the change starts inside. Be responsible for any and all thoughts and feelings that flash across your mind and pierce your heart. If you blame others for your problems, you will recycle them over and over again with other people.

Find your appropriate boundaries for your mind, for your emotions, and for your communications with others. Change the beliefs that you are not good enough or that they are bad to "I am capable, and I can learn from anyone, even an enemy." To move through the tickle in the throat, you really need to deal with your self-pity and resentment. If you continue to wallow in stuck emotions, they will continue to "drip" down the throat and irritate your body. Wake up and be yourself. Self-pity and resentment don't represent you; it represents the symptoms of your fear and judgment. It is time to be honest with yourself, take care of your heart, and heal your life.

Throat Problems: Specific

Affirmations:
- I see the truth, and I am ready to be set free by expressing it honestly.
- I clear my life of those pestering fears that hold me back.
- I clear my heart of emotional blocks and open to be my true self.
- I express myself with joy and gratitude in every way possible.
- My personality is attractive and charismatic.
- I catch any thought of resentment and turn it into responsible communication and action.
- I am honest with myself.
- I want to see the truth.
- I respect my energy capacity.

Supporting Foods:
- Drink plenty of liquids
- Fresh juices
- Herbal teas
- Broths
- Garlic
- Foods high in Vit. C

Thymus Gland

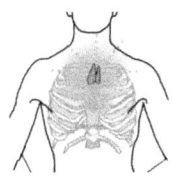

Troubled Mindset

- You think, "Life is so hard!"
- You have become passive and lazy in dealing with your responsibilities.
- You don't know what to do when you are in too much stress.
- The problem stems from losing your core identity and not being connected to yourself.
- You have set your integrity aside and convinced yourself to believe in falsehoods.
- "Whoa is me."
- You have been unstable emotionally and feeling pestered and victimized, continually.
- The thymus keeps your immunity/protection balanced, but both are failing. In this state of feeling vulnerable and unprotected, you feel that you are under attack by others.
- You feel that you have no choice in the matter, nor the power to change it.
- You think you deserve the punishment.

Thymus Gland

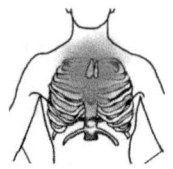

Healing Mindset

Define who you are and what you are not. Stand up and fight like a courageous human for your real self and real purpose. Get some passion flowing in your veins. Immunity and strength need a little or a lot of personal fire and positive pride.

Seek to nourish your body with great nutrition, positive mindfulness, and inspiring spirituality. Be proactive in your thinking and actions. Start the day with a new positive outlook, each and every day. With dedication, you can change your mind and life. Return again and again to the pathway that brings joy and happiness.

Thymus Gland

Affirmations:

- I'm okay, you're okay, we're okay, and it's great that life is good.
- I am clear on who I am and where I am going.
- Every once in a while, I like drifting with my thoughts; it catches any low flying new ideas.
- I clearly identify the problem and have the will to do something about it.
- I am ready to take action now.
- I love to walk with my spiritual soul on this earthy terrain.

Supporting Foods:

- Foods high in Vit. A, Vit C, Vit. E, and zinc
- Asparagus
- Avocado
- Cantaloup
- Carrots
- Green leafy vegetables
- Yellow squash
- Berries
- Citrus fruits
- Sweet potatoes
- Onions
- Garlic
- Brown rice
- Egg yolks
- Fish
- Whole grains
- Nuts and seeds
- Poultry
- Soybeans

Thyroid

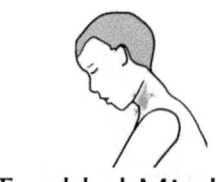

Troubled Mindset

- You are pre-occupied with the "doing" of life and less attentive to the "being."
- You had the will to push forward, but you continued to use more energy than your body wanted to give. You eventually collapsed, but still, you then forced it more. Then you finally gave up when there was little 'steam' left. This 'up and down' energy was confusing to the body and mind. It gave rise to the 'up and down' type of communication with people. You can't be totally honest with them because you want it to be a certain way, but sometimes your body and mind go in different ways.
- With inner conflict about your communication with others, you now want to speak your truth. However, you worry that others will judge or criticize you, so you modify your conversations: always adjusting and silently suffering.
- Towards those who don't want this crazy, 'in and out, back and forth' way of communicating, you have become convinced that you are right, and some bitter feelings rise up against those who question or doubt you. Now, you are desperate from sensing an unmet need, and you are feeling powerless to change it.

Thyroid

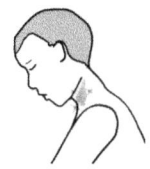

Troubled Mindset
(Continued)

- Your actions are now a pattern of negative self-talk that leads you to believe either you are a victim to your circumstances, or that you are above the rules. They don't apply to you but don't know what you want. If this shows up with food, your body and heart will suffer.
- You feel it isn't fair that others get what they want, but you don't.
- You think that you work really hard at life, diets, projects, but it doesn't go your way. Subtle jealousy makes it even more difficult to get up and take action.
- You are in a disastrous negative self-talk cycle that is spinning you down into feeling ostracized and resentful. It is leading your body into a defensive state of protection and leads to physical sluggishness that reflects this shielding against emotions.
- You wonder, 'why has everyone else figured out life and why do happiness, success, and love come to them so easily?'
- You are sinking with embarrassment and screaming to be heard by those who you remain convinced have no respect or interest in you. This behavior elicits negative responses, which then reinforces those same feelings and beliefs. A vicious cycle ensues.

Thyroid

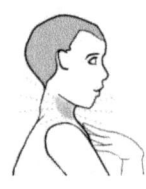

Healing Mindset

The core self, residing deep within, needs honesty about life. Write down your feelings and beliefs. Pay attention to your daily thoughts and actions. You'll notice that you're only harming yourself with your thoughts, feelings, and actions. It's not everyone else causing your problems.

Now, take a look at yourself. You tend to blame yourself more than others, but recognize the truth that you're not the problem. What you need is some guidance on how to grow, follow through, clear the "dirty" air of negative thoughts, and embrace discovery and adventure instead of desperation and resentment.

Any desperate or resentful feelings you experience are indicators that you're listening to the wrong boss inside your head and heart. Your true core self desires the best for you, reminding you to prioritize self-care rather than being scattered, harboring resentment, or shutting down. You're amazing. Connect with that part of yourself, even if it's a gradual process. Begin by slowly creating new patterns of thought and action. Humans are entirely capable of change, but if you're stubborn, inflexible, and burdened with regrets, change becomes more difficult.

Thyroid

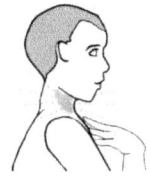

Healing Mindset
(Continued)

It is time to see things differently, even if it is hard to understand. You think the false belief that they have to understand you and change for you to move forward. That will get you nowhere. Rethink and challenge the beliefs that you are a victim, or that you are above the rules.

The same air is offered to all, so breathe it fully without filtering it with misbeliefs and harmful feelings. Open your mind and eyes to observe your gradual change daily until it is a fundamental part of you.

Treat yourself and others gently, with a full understanding that your body, and the bodies of others, are human and deserve respect, kindness, and not resentful judgment. As you do this, trust that the riddle of love, success, and happiness will be apparent to you. Your opportunity to share your insights will come.

Thyroid

Affirmations:
- I enjoy the beauty of nature; my heart feels it and it fills my soul with bliss.
- I am grateful for the energy to live my life with strength and vitality.
- I appreciate the gift of being nurtured by nature, and I receive it graciously.
- I recognize any emotional weight as a sign to be clear with my thoughts and actions.
- I recognize any mental negativity as a sign to nurture myself with exercise, healthy food, and love.
- I recognize any sluggish body feelings as a sign to breathe, meditate, and share my soul with someone in need.
- I trust my heart to be gracious to myself and others.
- I respect my body with foods that build health and thoughts that build character.
- I speak truth, and I am honest.
- I enjoy people and the events in my life.
- I balance my hopes with actions and my desires with clarity.

Supporting Foods:
- Apples
- Avocados
- Bananas
- Leafy greens
- Raw potato
- Kelp
- Seaweed
- Sprouted wheat
- Brewer's yeast

Tinnitus (Ringing in the Ear)

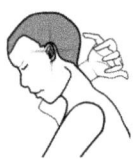

Troubled Mindset

- "I don't want to hear it!"
- A part of you is resisting information that the other part of you wishes to know.
- Your expectations of your situation don't match your reality.
- Your irritation towards what you want versus what is happening is causing internal conflict and discomfort.
- You may have a subtle refusal to listen to truth, yet be constantly seeking it.
- The inner voice is drowned out by wishes and actions.

Healing Mindset

You might consider what is real, and what is not. Take time to deeply feel and sense the truth that comes for others, which includes the signals and sensations your own body provides.

Take care of yourself by eating less sugar, getting more sleep, and forgiving yourself. Yes, the world has mistreated you sometimes, but you have been too open to your environment without taking care of your body's and spirit's needs. You are not to blame yourself for your juvenile dreams. Calm down your quest, then follow your path with honoring your body, mind, and heart, all together.

Tinnitus (Ringing in the Ear)

Affirmations:
- I love my true self, but first I honor my inner child and listen to my simple needs.
- I gradually let go of the need for sugar and replace it with enjoying the simple things of life.
- I listen to my body's needs and to the truths of others while honoring my truth.
- I let stubbornness turn into positive firmness with balanced empathy for me, my body, and others.

Supporting Foods:
- Carrots
- Parsley
- Citrus seed extract
- Millet
- Barley
- Tofu
- String beans
- Mung bean sprouts
- Kidney beans
- Black beans
- Watermelon and other melons
- Blackberry
- Blueberry
- Wheat germ
- Seaweeds
- Spirulina
- Crab
- Eggs

Toes

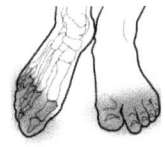

Troubled Mindset

- You push forward with determination and will, but you have regret, misdirection, confusion, and anger.
- You focus on the details, but the insecurities in your heart make them overwhelming.
- The toes are trying to maintain balance on a path that may seem more dangerous in your mind, mainly because you've perceived it this way.
- You fear rejection, lack of control, the outcomes of life, judgment, abandonment, and betrayal.
- You compensate your body in favor of fearfully pushing forward.
- You hope it will work out but frustrated all the while.
- Your obsessive focus clouds your clarity, your purpose, your direction, and who you are.
- You tend to lose reasonable thought in favor of frustration at your situation or to the mindlessness of daydreams of idealistic possibilities.
- The mindless path leads to unstable ground and a lack of understanding of how to manifest your needs and desires. In other words you don't understand how to manifest or make things happen after you dream it.
- You fear you are are not capable and then get annoyed at the whole process of too many details and tasks to accomplish your vision.
- You have become emotionally drained with anxiety about the future and its details.

Toes

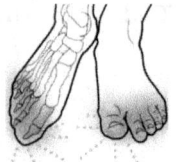

Healing Mindset

You need a double-check with your heart and those deep-seated emotions that have become so embedded and stuck they are pushing you into trouble. Ground yourself with your breath. Breathe deeply and slowly to help you pull your energy and focus back to earth. You may do this multiple times throughout your day as you observe yourself drifting off into your daydreams. There is nothing wrong with having a vision, but you want that vision to be based in reality for it to have strength. As you do this, you will strengthen yourself to face your real fear of not achieving acceptance and approval.

Be kind to yourself. Offer yourself the compassion and forgiveness you seek as you walk, step by step, into the best version of yourself. If lingering frustration with yourself or others hinders your path, now is the moment for genuine change. Choose to toss it all to the wind and get your feet planted into the real earth. Rediscover yourself and only focus on things that you can do something about. Grant yourself the blissful gift of walking a balanced path, without any burdens, fear, anger, and with no regrets.

Toes

Affirmations:

- I feel relieved to walk through life with peace of mind and love of heart.
- I clearly focus for a while and then relax for a moment and then repeat.
- I am grateful for every moment I get to be with the ones I love.
- I can't imagine thinking another negative thought again.
- I am successfully walking the path of adventure and completion.
- I enjoy the thrill of completing my tasks and accomplishing my goals.
- My stumbles don't make me crumble but give me a strong character to excel.
- I catch the fear and turn it into awareness.
- I catch the frustration and turn it into action.

Supporting Foods:

- Eat a diet of raw vegetables and juices for 3 days to help balance the acidity/alkalinity of the body
- Umeboshi (Japanese salt plum)

Tongue

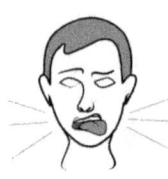

Troubled Mindset

- You are fine in the moment, but as you look back, you resent the 'forked-tongue' lying of others. In truth, you may have been in your own denial and dishonesty with yourself.
- Life is sometimes giving you a "bad taste" in your mouth because your mind and body are not aligned or in sync with how to process everything.
- You and your wants seem to be rejected by many.
- You may feel unwanted or unacceptable.
- You feel you have too much burden in your communications.
- You may be taking on too much responsibility for the reaction of others to what you say.
- When you make a mistake, it adds to the issues that show up on the tongue.
- Cankers: you blame of self or others.
- Biting your tongue: you want to stop expressing too much.
- Blotches: you judge yourself that you can't stand up for yourself.
- Tongue pimples: you believe your expression is not good enough, and you have hidden the anger towards yourself or your perceived enemy.
- Pale tongue: low energy and less motivation to deal with life.

Tongue
Troubled Mindset
(Continued)

- Geographic tongue: your emotional secrets are mounting, and you are having a difficult time assimilating everyday life.
- Red hot tongue: a hidden upset that needs to come to the surface and be handled properly.
- Fuzzy tongue: feeling powerless with a fear of the future, suppressing feelings, hiding a secret, or feeling manipulated.

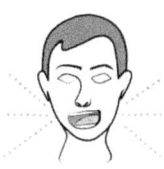

Healing Mindset

You need to exercise your tongue muscle daily by releasing your emotions gradually and respectfully. You can learn to express your thoughts and feelings in a way that honors your feelings and the feelings of others. Even if some people are closed to deeper emotional relationships, you can mature your ability to communicate with them within their emotional intelligence level.

'Be impeccable with your word.' The tongue is a muscle, as is the mind. Exercise discipline while honoring the truth that you can only take responsibility for your part. Do take responsibility for yourself, and let others take responsibility for themselves. Honor your highest and best self as you continue to share with love and compassion for yourself and others.

Tongue

Affirmations:
- I enjoy the taste of life in its vast variety and experience.
- I reach deep inside and let myself sing my emotions to anyone who wants to listen.
- I love to share the thoughts and feelings with other awesome humans.
- I think life is only bland to those who are too scared to taste another adventure.
- I thank the good Lord for the gift of taste, talk, and digestion.
- The tongue is a wonderful tool.
- I have one tongue and two ears, and I use them well in every heartfelt communication.
- I express the thoughts that come to my mind quickly before my ears can stop me from making a fool of myself.

Supporting Foods:

- Beans
- Seeds
- Yogurt
- Kefir
- Watercress
- Beets
- Sweet rice
- Cabbage
- Turnips
- Kohlrabi
- Sprouted grains
- Fresh fruits & vegetables
- Cottage cheese
- Brussel sprouts
- Green leafy vegetables
- Cauliflower
- Broccoli
- Asparagus
- Raw onions
- Rye
- Amaranth
- Quinoa
- Lemon
- Lime
- Grapefruit
- Strawberries
- Peaches
- Cherries
- Pine nuts

Tonsillitis

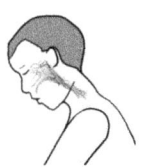

Troubled Mindset

- Your fears have built up in your throat because you can't swallow what is happening around you.
- As a child, you may not have understood the conflicts in the home, but your body could feel them.
- As an adult, you still don't understand how to deal with all the emotions and conflicts.
- You are sacrificing health, in favor of building up irritations and fears that lead to internal inflammation of feelings.
- Your subconscious thinks it must hold back because you feel vulnerable with expressing your feelings.
- You feel judged, and you don't dare express that to them.
- You wish things were different, so you become silently anxious about the conflict between your fear and anger.
- You feel stuck and lost, not knowing the power within yourself to move through your upset and fear and to finally heal.

Tonsillitis

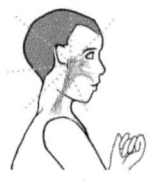

Healing Mindset

Any infection or inflammation starts somewhere, and any healing begins with you. You can change your world by expressing yourself verbally and creatively.

You can learn to take chances at being judged and start finding the courage inside to be yourself in your relationships. Even if your fears are larger than your life, you can start slowly and gradually and deal with one conflict and one fear at a time. You have plenty of energy to do this, even if you feel fatigue and pain.

The energy is not the problem; it is how you use that energy. As you respect yourself and take care of your heart, mind, and body, you will learn to work through your vulnerabilities and turn them into strengths. Ask the questions of, "Why are my fears here? What are the fears trying to protect?" Understand the vulnerability with compassion, and make a conscious choice to move through them one step at a time. Do breathing and visual meditations to release negative emotions. Simultaneously, nourish your body to help with the physical and emotional detox.

Tonsillitis

Affirmations:
- I respect my heart as it honors my core needs.
- I have the courage to speak my truth and live my life.
- I breathe into my pain and listen to its message.
- I listen to my body and intently use its wisdom.
- I trust that my words will reach the mind and heart of the authentic part of another person.
- I hope in peace while I act in truth.
- I ignore the harmful critical voice and encourage the fortifying insightful voice.
- I am good enough, strong enough, and very lovable.
- I accept the warm embrace of others.
- Sharing is caring, especially when the other is open and ready.
- I speak my peace, I talk my idea, I express my heart, and I hear my friend.

Supporting Foods:
- Eat a well balanced diet of fresh fruits and vegetables
- Whole grains
- Legumes
- Including foods high in Vit. C
- Berries
- Citrus fruits
- Leafy greens
- Asparagus
- Avocados
- Beet greens
- Broccoli
- Brussel sprouts
- Cantaloupe
- Mangos
- Onions
- Papayas
- Peas
- Sweet peppers
- Pineapple
- Rose hips
- Tomatoes

Toothache

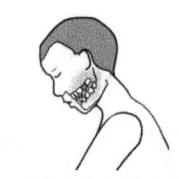

Troubled Mindset

- Your emotions are pushing your heart worries into your mouth because you tend to hold back until it is too late, and the body overreacts.
- Your suppressed emotions need a place to go, or they will fester underneath, and then they will surface when you are out of control of the situation.
- The body is not able to handle the outcome when anger turns to tears, and sadness turns to resentment.
- You want to control the outcome, but you can't because you can't see the "forest from the trees," and you can't see the end results.
- Sometimes you resist positive recognition because you feel manipulated. However, It could also indicate that you don't always feel worthy or deserving of praise.
- Fear of being vulnerable by taking chances in relationships is making you feel shame and eventually bitter because the other person is not reading your mind.
- They are not reading your mind because you are not moving your lips with positive interactive communication.
- Shame is contributing to why you are holding on to negative emotions.

Toothache

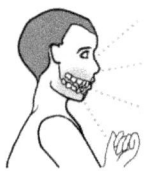

Healing Mindset

You have neglected your emotional and mental state for too long. It is time to be real and honest with yourself and face your unfulfilled expectations, undeserving self-pity, persistent blaming, and your fearful hesitations to communicate authentically.

Focus on your physical and emotional needs with compassion for where you are and what has happened. Release the negative emotions, especially shame, as you embrace who you are. Release with journaling, walking, meditating, and engaging in empowering conversations with people who can positively support you in your desire to change and transform.

Toothache

Affirmations:
- Daily, I engage in healthy conversations.
- I embrace my denial self, and cross the ocean of emotions, to find a new promised terrain of personal self-discovery.
- I give room for empowering thought and deed.
- I chew on new thoughts and refreshing insights.
- I take care to be caring for my heart and share those feelings that need to come to the surface.
- I'm enough, I'm good, and I'm happy.
- I empower myself to find the root of the problem before the problem uproots me.
- I am resourceful, creative, and productive.
- I fight for a clean, healthy, and self-healing body.

Supporting Foods:
- Raw fruits and vegetables
- Beets, steamed
- Blueberry
- Celery juice
- Chia seed, soaked
- Fig (fresh)
- Flax seed, soaked
- Grapefruit
- Lemon
- Lentils
- Lettuce
- Lime
- Orange
- Papaya
- Pineapple
- Quinoa
- Sauerkraut
- Sesame seed milk
- Watermelon
- Zucchini

Tumors

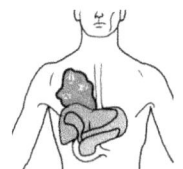

Troubled Mindset

- Old emotional and physical toxins have accumulated and clustered together.
- You have been ignoring unresolved issues for too long.
- The buildup of emotions and negative thought patterns become a major problem when major trauma hits.
- The body has less power and capacity to deal with the onslaught of problems.
- Your negative thinking and attitudes need to change.
- Your ego has taken priority over your relationships, including with your parents.
- You've felt trapped in the pains from the past as they run through your mind.
- You've felt angry and resentful, wondering if anyone really cares.
- You want to grow out of the conflict, but you didn't have tools to do it.
- You have instead 'stored' things in the 'back closet.'
- You have an unresolved trauma in your near past that is causing vibrational drama inside your body and mind.
- Taking the emotional pain and the stuck beliefs and hiding them deep inside will only feed the problem.

Tumors

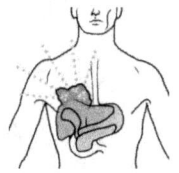

Healing Mindset

Find forgiveness and love as you travel on the pathway passing by pain, denial, old hurts, old judgments, old defenses, expectations unfulfilled, betrayals, shock, and deep grief. The pathway to healing is not easy, but it is easier if you are willing to get support from professionals, from the divine, or the universe. You can't do it alone. It is a good thing that you need others because this life is about opening up the tender side of yourself and finding a way to share your heart feelings of pain, suffering, goodness, and love.

Forgiveness to self and others comes graciously and naturally when you take a chance. Find the appropriate professionals to support you through healing in mind, heart, and body. As you improve your diet to support yourself through the release of physical toxins, also improve your mental diet to support yourself through the release of emotional toxins.

Gradually you will mend your relationships, especially with yourself, as you stay open and humble. And then fight like heavens and the earth to be strong for you, your body, and your life.

Tumors

Affirmations:
- I fight for truth, my heart, my soul, my body, and my healing.
- I stand here with open arms to the healing energy from the universe.
- I surround the enemy with a bright sun of healing energy.
- I deeply breathe into my cells, the life force that vibrates to my unique song of life.
- I resonate with the power of God's love throughout my whole body and soul.
- There is no one more grateful than me at this moment, at this time.
- I find the precious gems of wisdom in the deep caverns of my soul.
- I acknowledge and appreciate the part of myself that wants my undivided attention and love.
- My shame is free to go.
- My blame has left the building.
- My discouragement is no more.
- I am courage, I am hope, and I am strength.
- My immune system is focused, armed, ready: now go.
- I love the process of healing and transforming my life every day.

Tumors

Supporting Foods:

- Eat a diet of 50% raw fruits and vegetable
- Nuts
- Seeds
- Whole grains
- Plain yogurt
- Potato (raw)
- Garlic
- Onions
- Raw almonds
- Eat plenty of cruciferous vegetables
- Broccoli
- Bussel sprouts
- Cabbage
- Cauliflower
- Carrots
- Pumpkin
- Squash
- Kelp
- Yams
- Apples
- Berries
- Brazil nuts
- Cantaloupe
- Cherries
- Grapes
- Chickpeas
- Lentils
- Red beans
- Plums

Ulcers

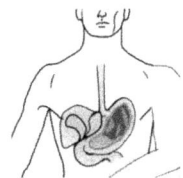

Troubled Mindset

- Slow down! Your worries run circles around you.
- You try to achieve unrealistic and perfectionistic ideals to compensate for a deeper need, including to feel 'good enough.'
- Fears of panic, anxiety, or abandonment urge you to try and 'earn' love.
- You crave 'mother love' or other types of warm and comforting emotional, mental, and physical nourishment.
- You constantly worry about everything, without the strength to face things as they are.
- Other financial and relationship stresses compound the issue.
- Gastrointestinal ulcers: Not 'letting go' of the gunk. You may struggle to decipher what is important and what is not.
- Stomach ulcers: You are not nourishing yourself emotionally and physically. Your negative perspective makes everything look bleak.
- Peptic ulcers: You're racing around. Your body is saying, "SLOW DOWN!" Your mind and your heart need to slow down with the rest of you.

Ulcers

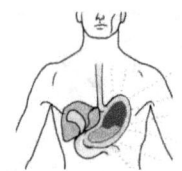

Healing Mindset

Have respect for yourself. You deserve better than this self-destructive form of coping. You are stuck on a lower level of awareness. Your body is trying to help you deal with that which is unsolvable by the gut, intestines, or any other body part.

Your 'out of control' fear is being mixed with worry and anger. You suppress the anger and show the cycle of fear, worry. You try, but you need to realize that your wishes and resentment of what is happening is lurking right below the surface. Burning away your insides will only exacerbate the problem. You crave warmth and love, safety, and security, but you stand there, pushing it away because you don't know if it is truly safe. Pause for the moment. The present is the only thing that you can experience without any negative consequence.

Ulcers

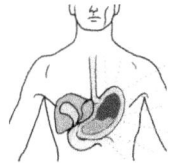

Healing Mindset
(Continued)

Stop trying to hold onto the spinning wheel of worry. It is cutting your insides up because your worry has tiny chards of fears, regrets, anger, and criticisms (to self and others).
It is time to take your best self and calm that part down to the reality of what is possible so you can enjoy what is happening.

There is no sense in pushing the river that can't move in your fantasized direction. Get with the flow and move with it as you change directions with the state of positive motivation, fun encouragement, mature understanding, and enlightening progression. Every event is a possible growth when you are not digging away at yourself. It is time for self-love and self-care.

Ulcers

Affirmations:
- I run and walk in synchronization with life.
- I am safe to be.
- Money is my friend.
- I can slow down and work through this.
- God wants the best for me.
- I give myself permission to feel what is best.
- I trust my intuition.
- I notice when my thoughts are running away from me.
- I thank them for trying to fix something.
- I invite them back and restart the moment with a breath, with simple movements, and with a calm thought of I am doing my best, and enjoy the rest.
- I am prepared for the day because I live in the present, make simple goals for the future, and relish the enriching past for its growth and wisdom.
- I honor and respect my body with positive thoughts, caring feelings, and positive challenges that build and enhance my physical body.
- I am real with taking time to be true to my intuition and learn to become synchronized with body, mind, heart, and spirit.

Ulcers

Supporting Foods:

- Dark green leafy vegetables
- Seaweed
- Fresh cabbage juice
- Barley juice
- Wheat juice
- Alfalfa juice
- Drink plenty of water to dilute stomach acids
- Eat frequent small meals
- Millet
- Rice or rice congee
- Raw goat's milk or almond milk
- Soured products such as plain yogurt, cottage cheese and kefir.

Ulcerative Colitis or Colitis

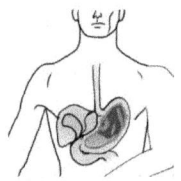

Troubled Mindset

- You live in worry and grief that is suppressing other emotions including the frustration about your relationships; wondering why others are so non-responsive and lack respect to helpful and caring communication.
- Internally, you feel sad, guilty, angry, and afraid to speak up and speak out, so your gut claws and inflames.
- Unsuspecting irritations from others surprise you all too often.
- You wish the other person would just get a clue about what they are doing to you, but they don't and probably won't. Meanwhile, you still labor through each day, holding on to a thread of hope and a rope of inner trouble.
- You can't understand why people act that way.
- People that you worry about or have resentments towards are stuck in their own self-centered problems. Recycling their own childish pain by adding problems for others.

Ulcerative Colitis or Colitis

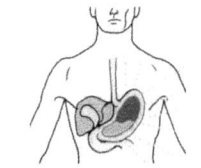

Healing Mindset

You just want to be loved, but you have a hard time truly loving yourself. You think that if you were a better person—more capable, more understanding, smarter, more beautiful, or just different—then things would be better. That is where you start—accept who you really are, acknowledge your true gifts, and identify what is most important to you. Instead of placing value on what you can't control, find your true value and invest trust and effort there.

You have to be careful of your diet and what you consume. Likewise, you have to be careful with your mental and emotional diet of what passes through your mind and heart. The very thought of pushing your frustration onto them leaves your gut with more agitation and despair.

This life is not meant to have inner storms all the time. Finding a place of peace inside could be as important as a piece of food that is calming to your body. Turning your worry into a few moments a day of quiet trust in something that is simple and understandable.

Ulcerative Colitis or Colitis

Affirmations:

- I am free to be me.
- I accept what is and live with authentic hope.
- I turn my pain upside down and transform it into a positive challenge.
- I stop the churning and burning and find a reason to be me.
- I am losing my guilt and fear and finding reason for each season of life's experiences.
- I hope, I pray, I act, and I experience.
- I am grateful for the small stuff.
- I forgot it isn't all my fault and I am not going to remember that any more.
- Look, I see some bright sunshine waiting to enter my heart.

Supporting Foods:

- Applesauce
- Apples, peeled and steamed
- Avocado
- Banana
- Brown rice
- Chicken slowly cooked
- Cucumbers, steamed
- Millet
- Oats (gluten free)
- Pears, peeled
- Soft foods
- Vegetables, peeled and steamed
- Yam
- Zucchini
- Chew food slowly
- Eat in small amounts
- Never eat late

Underweight

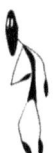

Troubled Mindset

- You are weak in the physical but strong in the emotional.
- You are sensitive to life but resistant to grow with it.
- You are both weak and strong of heart and mind.
- You have so much going on inside your head that your body can't keep up with you.
- You battle the demons inside of past conflicts and won't let those recycling mental stories go in order to give your soul some peace of mind.
- Your anxiety is running your adrenals to the ground and burning everything up.
- You run from one drama/trauma to the next.
- You are reactive to the drama of others, which makes you too immersed in your own issues.
- You have a difficult time distinguishing which energy, belief, story, or emotions are yours and which ones are theirs.
- You feel picked on when others start to blame you.
- You are effective at dodging blame.
- You have a difficult time being authentic when dealing with interpersonal issues.

Underweight

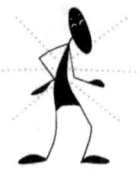

Healing Mindset

You seek answers, but you question the solutions that come your way. So, take off that shirt of denial and try to eat some yummy humble pie. It might be hard to swallow at first, but accept that you can take some of the responsibility of a conflict within your relationships.

Sometimes you take a little responsibility, and other times you take too much of the burden. You are either the villain or the hero, and you don't recognize your victim. Become aware of how you live your drama in life.

If you want to find the joy of living, then rise above the drama. To transform the traumas and drama, find the value of your life experiences, and look at the opportunities of life. Allow yourself to heal from what has happened in your own life.

Underweight

Affirmations:
- Whatever I think or feel, I know there is love in the universe waiting for my heart to receive.
- I appreciate each and every moment that life gives me.
- I am free to see and sense the beauty of life all around me.
- Everyone is my teacher, including my inner core self.
- I let go of judgments and make room for unconditional love.
- I open my mind to new possibilities, including feeling the warmth of love.
- I end the behavior of resistance and open my heart and mind to others in my life.

Supporting Foods:
- Eat at 2,500 - 3000 calories a day including complex carbs
- Whole grain breads
- Fruit and vegetable juices
- Drink herbal teas
- Soy based cream soups
- Soymilk
- Pasta
- Cereals
- Turkey
- Chicken
- Fish
- Eggs
- Olive oil
- Avocados
- Raw cheeses
- Bananas
- Yogurt
- Nuts
- Nut butters
- Seeds

Urinary Tract Infections (UTI)

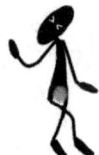

Troubled Mindset

- You are feeling irritated, upset, and embarrassed, which makes it difficult for your body to process.
- You don't usually express your suppressed feelings, so they build up and become toxic to you. This toxic state is very irritating to your body.
- It causes further pressure to either push the emotions down deeper or to eventually get angry and burst them out.
- You want to get rid of your problems, but the need for secrecy gives you the illusion that you can hide your embarrassments.
- The urgency is trying to get you to release the pressure you have placed on yourself.
- Your irritations signify that it is someone else's fault, and you expect others to change. However, you are filled with guilt and feel a bit of shame that you might be part of the problem. Yet, you don't want to see or admit to your part.
- It's terrifying because deep down, you think there might be something fundamentally wrong with you.
- You fear being left alone or abandoned.

Urinary Tract Infections (UTI)

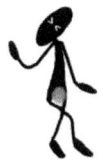

Troubled Mindset
(Continued)

- You are constantly running, and your reserves are depleted. "I just can't do this anymore."
- Your fear kept you from learning how to stand up for yourself in a calm, yet firm way.
- You end up easily manipulated or controlled.
- You have avoided loving the most tender and vulnerable parts of yourself.

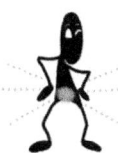

Healing Mindset

Start by nourishing yourself with kindness at the darkest and most distressing times. That is where you have the most power to have an impact that will make a transformative difference.

Nourish yourself physically as you strengthen your resolve to turn away from the angry thoughts and return to love again, and again. Be more open with other people. Hiding doesn't heal. Usually, dread and lack of support precede this problem. Find the path of courage, action, and positive self-expression to help you.

Urinary Tract Infections (UTI)

Affirmations:
- I flow with life through the dark and the light.
- I take the time for me, myself, and my heart.
- I listen to the whisperings and sensations of my body.
- I honor and respect my precious and beautiful body.
- I find any negative feeling or thought and flush it out and away to be repolarized into joy, peace, and action.
- I trim off the hatred and bring in understanding.
- I cut out dread and bring in curiosity.
- I let go of fear and enliven my heart.
- I push out the anger and courageously be myself in action and deed.
- I consciously flow through the negative moments into the progressive changes of my life.

Supporting Foods:

- Water/Get hydrated
- Garlic
- Turmeric
- Pure unsweetened cranberry juice
- Fresh celery juice
- Celery
- Parsly juice
- Parsley
- Watermelon

Varicose Veins

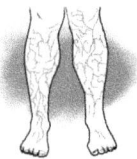

Troubled Mindset

- You are frustrated with life and its challenges.
- You think that you have tried everything, and it's still not working.
- You feel cornered with no way out of your situation.
- You are unsure which direction to go or where to get resources that will support you because you don't trust them.
- You resist love in the form of verbal, emotional, physical, or intimate affection because of this lack of trust.
- You regret the past and feel the future is a burden.
- You carry the burdens of others, wishing they would change, but wondering if they ever will.

Varicose Veins

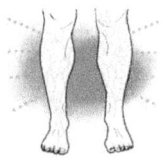

Healing Mindset

You spend too much time wishing you were on another life path, or that others would be different on their path. You have not been given exactly what you wanted, and the hidden suffering is causing your body to work too hard.

Seek to challenge yourself to be present while on the path you are living. It is debilitating to carry regret and to be constantly wishing for the other side of the fence. It is empowering to embrace the stress as an opportunity for growth. Reach into your past to discover the misunderstandings that lead you to resist love. Review those reasons from your adult perspective to help you find a resolution that will calm your fears. Be flexible with your mindset and opinions to allow you to gain a new perspective on which direction will be the best option for you in your life.

Varicose Veins

Affirmations:

- I am able to understand the value of surrendering what is not mine.
- I get to choose for myself what I carry in my life.
- I choose to care deeply instead of carrying heavy.
- I ask myself, "Why choose to resist the release of burden when I can be free?"
- I replace my vanity with purity of self-love and gratitude.

Supporting Foods:

- Water/Stay hydrated
- Eat a diet low in fat and refined carbohydrates
- Eat plenty of fresh fruits, and vegetables
- Fish
- Whole grain
- Legumes
- Asparagus
- Broccoli
- Cantaloupe
- Kale
- Spinach
- Papayas
- Sweet peppers
- Citrus fruits
- Berries
- Tomatoes
- Eggs
- Brown rice
- Oatmeal
- Soybeans
- Sweet potatoes
- Wheat germ

Venereal Disease (STD's)

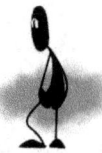

Troubled Mindset

- You haven't had it easy, so having this happen stops you in your tracks.
- You were not thinking of all the consequences in life.
- The emotions are rampant and deep.
- At one time, you may have been self-centered, careless, wanting to rebel, upset at authority, and/or felt a need for secrecy.
- Now you have fear, embarrassment, anger, a great deal of guilt and shame, self-judgment, and resentment to others and God.
- You feel it is not fair, and you may be correct; however, regret and blame make matters worse.
- You feel embarrassed and responsible for the shame and pain of others.
- You feel deep rejection from your partner, others, and yourself.
- Embarrassed and angry, you feel you've made a huge mistake.
- You are punishing yourself.

Venereal Disease (STD's)

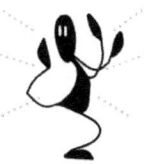

Healing Mindset

It is time to stop holding your guilt as a punishment to your body. It is not the fault of your body. Give your body a chance to be healed. The worse you can do is wallow in your self-pity and hatred. Allow the punishing reflection of your self-judgment to be transformed into taking responsibility for what is, and what can be done. Change regret and resentment into making a difference in the lives of others, and you will find healing to your soul.

Every part of your body is divine. Cherish the many gifts your body offers. Be grateful for everything your body does for you. Your eyes see. Your ears hear. Your organs allow you to be nourished and strengthened. Your lungs bring in life-giving breath each moment of every day.

Embrace the sexual components of yourself in the same way. They bring the opportunity for bliss into your mind and life. Be wise. Understand your vulnerabilities, and don't compromise yourself to please someone else. Take full responsibility for your choices so you can be empowered and sustained. Allow yourself to be loved in deeply nourishing ways so you can become your highest and best self in mind, body, and spirit.

Venereal Disease (STD'S)

Affirmations:

- I have the hope that by making a difference in another's life, I will find peace in mine.
- I realize that wishing is just fishing for an illusion.
- I hope from my core soul to reap the benefits from deep healing.
- I empathize with the pain of others, and I send them love.
- My body has deep healing powers.
- My courageous will is supported by the wisdom of the universe.
- I release the temptation to blame or regret.
- I embrace the opportunity to change my inner self for the better.
- I am super energized to make a difference every day of my life.
- I choose life, health, caring, and oneness.

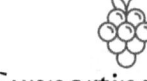

Supporting Foods:

- Herbal teas
- Whole grains
- Legumes
- Raw seeds
- Raw nuts
- Garlic
- Kelp
- Seaweed
- Asparagus
- Broccoli
- Cantaloupe
- Kale
- Spinach
- Papayas
- Sweet peppers
- Citrus fruits
- Berries
- Tomatoes
- Soybean
- Eggs
- Fish
- Eat a well balanced diet of fresh fruits and vegetables

Viruses

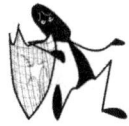

Troubled Mindset

- First, you are overwhelmed, and then you felt attacked.
- You are on the lookout too much, and your body's defenses are in too many places at the same time.
- You wish you could get a break in life, but life is breaking you.
- You feel victimized by the gloom and doom of life.
- Life struggles are the overshadows of life's joys.
- You tend to expect to get the short end of the stick.
- You have someone in your life you don't want to stand up to, so you are hiding your real emotions.
- Your immune system is challenged with emotional conflict, secrets, dark feelings, overwhelm, worry, anger, resentment, and/or blame.
- When the emotions cause immune challenges, viruses have a door into your world.

Viruses

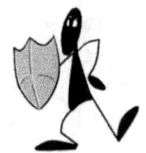

Healing Mindset

Challenge your beliefs that cause you to feel like a victim in your circumstances. For you to feel weak and sick, there is some belief that causes you to blame without seeing a solution to the problem. Decide today to be proactive in moving through your frustration. Allow your emotional pain some movement with meditation, writing, or expressing it to someone who has the capacity to listen intently.

Be attentive to your own mental and emotional needs, and don't wait for others to change in order for you to happy and content. You can create your own positive experience. Don't rely on the expectations of others. Let go of the beliefs that don't serve you. Strengthen your mind and body to become your highest, best, and awesome self. Choose now to distinguish yourself from those around you. Be you and be happy, beginning and end of the story.

Viruses

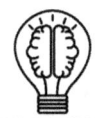

Affirmations:

- I am watchful of my actions so that I can choose my thoughts in the moment.
- I am aware of my emotions so that I can stay focused on the task in the moment.
- I am grateful for my experiences so that I can be free in the moment.
- I am hopeful in my healthy quest so that I can stay strong in my immune system.
- I catch the random negative thoughts and toss them out to the wind of emotions.
- I am discovering the empowering courage within my soul to be true to my core values.
- I am infusing insight into the nucleus of my cells to powerfully distinguish between "the self" and the "non-self."
- I choose to be me and heal now.

 ## Supporting Foods:

- Micro-greens
- Fermented foods
- Steamed broccoli
- Steamed cauliflower
- Warm broth soups
- Steamed red beets
- Turkey soup with healing spices
- Cinnamon spice
- Clove spice
- Ginger spice
- Thyme spice
- Celery juice
- Carrot juice
- Celery juice
- Congee (Extra slow cooked rice)
- Squash
- Watermelon
- Asparagus
- Chicken soup
- Garlic
- Green onions
- Parsley
- Jicama

Virus, Corona

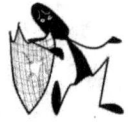

Troubled Mindset

- Your normal shields are down.
- The world is pushing you until you can't take the pressure anymore.
- There is a gap in the heart and the lungs.
- You have been slapped with disapproval or betrayal.
- Your capacity for the love you normally can give has greatly diminished because of your fears and pain.
- Surviving another day with enough light, air, and water includes being real with what can happen, and what really did.
- You forgot that life is sensitive, fragile, and precious.
- You needed a reminder to come back home to your real self and let go of the negative effects of blame, fear, frustration, and resentment.
- You have some residual polluted feelings that have gradually come to the surface and made you vulnerable.
- Or you have been a hero to others who carry polluted feelings.
- You have grief that has turned into regret.
- The trapping feeling of worry, fear or anger won't let go until you responsibly face them.

Virus, Corona

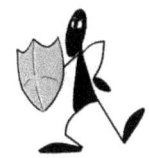

Healing Mindset

You can do something with your unproductive thoughts about your condition. In the past you lacked awareness and then you pushed to discover truth. Now you have awareness, but you still lack inner truth. Look inside to find the core values that are based on an inner light that has no negative connections.

The messages around you have been polluted with negativity, fear, and resentment. Clean your inner house and bring your true heart home. Breath is easy and precious. However, breathing is labored when you are worried, concerned, and overwhelmed. Often the body will take your breath to get your attention. So, do it. Give your body attention and calmly take each moment with a breath that is full of newness, light, boldness, and strength.

Be excited about the challenge and clear your focus. Strengthen the mind, ground with courage, truth, and hope.

Virus, Corona

Affirmations:

- I give myself permission to face the challenges of this day with courage and hope.
- When I feel trapped, I find peace in calming my breath and relaxing my thoughts.
- I focus on what is real and release all else.
- I strengthen my mind, ground my body, encourage my heart, and enliven my soul.
- The hope of breath is simple because I envision my cells receiving strength and support.
- I give my amazing immune system my faith, vision, support and love.
- I am so grateful for every part of my immune system.
- My kidneys move the shadows to the earth and receive the light of the heavens.
- I embrace the challenge to heal all my griefs, my losses, and sufferings.
- Old regrets are transforming into new learnings and wisdom.

Virus, Corona

Supporting Foods:

- Cinnamon spice
- Clove spice
- Ginger spice
- Thyme spice
- Micro-greens
- Fermented foods
- Squash
- Jicama
- Celery juice
- Carrot juice
- Celery juice
- Warm broth soups
- Watermelon
- Asparagus
- Steamed broccoli
- Steamed cauliflower
- Chicken soup
- Garlic
- Steamed red beets
- Green onions
- Parsley
- Turkey soup with healing spices
- Congee (Extra Slow cooked Rice)

Vitiligo

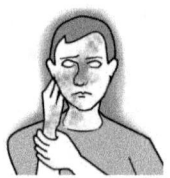

Troubled Mindset

- You don't get to do what you want to do so you let it pester and agitate your mind and heart until the body can't stand it anymore and takes it out on your skin.
- Being angry about things that you can't control is taking the color out of your life and your skin.
- You crave love, but you want respect more.
- "If only they would listen and consider my view," runs through your mind.
- You don't trust anyway, so even if respect comes, you are hesitant to open your heart fully because they might betray you someday anyway.
- You are mixing fear and sadness with a lot of anger, all churning inside until you explode under major stress and overwhelm.
- Your inner critic needs a rest, it is working way too hard.

Vitiligo

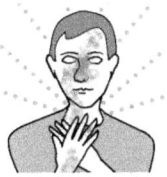

Healing Mindset

Bring back the true colors of life with one moment at a time. Step slowing and methodically. Take your apprehension and turn it upside down to positive expectation.

Of course others will make mistakes and forget to give you what you want and cherish. But if your 'precious' is for them to change, then you will be internally in pain and discomfort for a *long time* and your volcano will spew out the wrong colors leaching your skin and body of life.

What if your experience is for your good and growth? What if the other person doesn't change, can you still find joy, peace, fun, clarity, communication, connection, and sharing? Their obstacle can be your positive challenge and opportunity to channel your mental judgments and emotional fatigue into new and rewarding character strength.

Your body needs some rest. It is very tired from the constant thoughts and negative feelings. Provide it with a break three times a day, lasting 5 to 10 minutes each. Share your heart with those that are safe in order to rebuild and nourish your heart.

Vitiligo

Affirmations:
- I nourish my heart and soul first before I share what's on my mind.
- I release the suffering and pain of the past and make room for healing.
- I am focused on the simple and the predictable.
- I allow nature to feed my soul and heart.
- I honor my true value and respect the value in others.
- I turn difficult conflict over and use it as a stepping stone.
- I color my life with fresh ideas, joyful moments, and positive expectation.

Supporting Foods:
- Beetroot
- Black dates
- Carrot
- Chickpeas
- Garlic
- Lemon
- Orange
- Fermented foods
- Romaine lettuce
- Green leafy vegetables
- Red radish
- Spinach
- Seeds
- Ginger
- Broccoli
- Avocado
- Squash
- Papaya

Vomiting

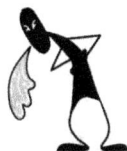

Troubled Mindset

- You may be feeling embarrassed, sick and tired, stuck, or afraid to go forward.
- You may be feeling some disgust with your situation.
- You feel something is revolting and/or very disgusting.
- You are intensely rejecting your emotions about what has happened in your life, or you believe that something harmful could happen.
- Your body received harmful feelings from others or yourself long ago, and that memory is triggering the current reaction because the body is trying to protect you from future harm or embarrassment.
- You feel the harm could be offensive, and more than your body can handle.
- You feel like you have to figure this out and make up for what has happened all on your own.
- Your mind and body are not connected because you are rejecting being a part of that horrible feeling.

Vomiting

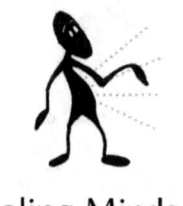

Healing Mindset

Clearing your energy and finding a way to ground to mother earth is essential. Give your belly a rest, and don't challenge it with food.

Likewise, give your heart moments to come back to your real self. You need to identify your dread and fears before starting up again. You need to not accept the blame from others, including self-blame. Notice how easy self-blame happens, then choose to learn quickly, and then go on.

Work through struggles with those around you. Support yourself with calming breath as you face things as they are.

Vomiting

Affirmations:
- I find the bliss between the moments of life.
- I act, instead of react to my situations.
- All my experiences are for my good as I calmly relax my body and mind.
- This too shall pass, as I let go of the fear of the unknown, and act with courage.
- I find comfort in breathing deeply to my toes, and to the earth.
- I find strength in bringing myself back into my body.
- I pass the blame of others to the wind and fill my mind and soul with comfort, hope, and courage.

Supporting Foods:
- Apple cider vinegar
- Freshly cut ginger
- Bone broth
- Applesauce
- Bananas
- Squash
- Zucchini
- Dry crackers
- Ginger tea
- Raspberry leaf tea
- A little salt water

Warts

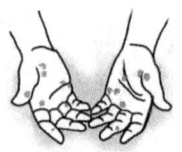

Troubled Mindset

- You feel something strange about yourself.
- Sometimes you feel disgusted with yourself; then you reject yourself.
- You feel ugly or loathsome.
- You don't believe that you are lovable.
- Your excessive self-criticism has lead you to a pessimistic view towards life.
- The problem of your negative thoughts is that they sometimes take on a life of their own, and they repeat themselves all too often.

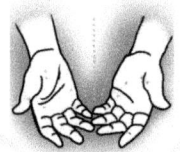

Healing Mindset

The seeds of your issues don't come from the outside, but digging at them only causes you to become more bitter. Let's go for the positive parts of yourself. Focus in and bring out the things you love about yourself. Heal the deep hurts with nourishing kindness towards yourself. The most important and impactful time is when it's the hardest to do. Be there for yourself when things are the darkest and most difficult.

Warts

Affirmations:

- I enjoy the expression on their face when I smile with a twinkle in my eye.
- I love my uniqueness.
- It is awesome to be me.
- I am not different; I am an original.
- I have what it takes, so look quickly, because I'm expressing the real me now.
- I am gorgeous and beautiful, just wait until you meet the other side of myself.

Supporting Foods:

- Pumpkin
- Carrots
- Papaya
- Mangos
- Apricots
- Kale and other green leafy vegetables
- Broccoli
- Bell peppers
- Pineapple
- Berries
- Figs
- Rose hips
- Garlic to boost your immune system
- Eat more foods with sulfur-containing amino acids such as asparagus, citrus fruits, eggs, and onions.

Wrist Problems

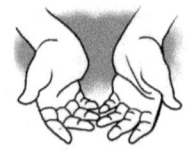

Troubled Mindset

- It's hard to follow through with your intentions gracefully.
- You are conflicted because you are not doing what you think you ought to be doing.
- You have a tug-a-war between following through with what you prefer to do and believing that it's the wrong thing to do.
- You can't sort out the appropriate balance with serving others and being committed to yourself.
- You may believe it is selfish to care for your own needs and personal desires.
- You go about fulfilling your responsibilities, but resentfully, wishing your work was more appreciated.
- The left wrist has to do with you limiting yourself and your needs or desires.
  - You struggle to decipher how to prioritize your values for yourself and your group responsibilities.
- Your right wrist has to do with a lack of certainty about how to make what needs to happen, happen.
  - You don't have confidence in your abilities, and you are concerned that others may notice.

Wrist Problems

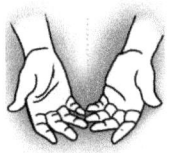

Healing Mindset

You have a double heart for yourself and others. Take that heart, and thank it for trying to make everyone happy, but help your big inner 'hero-self' to understand that your hands can't serve two masters.

Conflicts make matters worse for the wrist. Decide today to be confident and firm about your needs and serve others within your capacity and within your desires. There is always a negative consequence if you try to match their expectations while over-sacrificing yourself.

It is time to take a hold of yourself and rethink what you are doing. Blame will come from them, or from you to them, then pain and frustration follow. Find a way to take care of your needs first, and watch out for expectations that are not possible. Honor and respect your body and heart, and then you can help others.

Be sure to notice if you are feeling resentful when you share your time and efforts with others. Pause and let the judgments go, or stop helping so that you can let the negative thoughts "get off the bus."

Wrist Problems

Affirmations:

- I am confident, courteous, and generous.
- I am flexible with a firm grip on the outcome.
- I am clear with my goals, so that I can direct my actions.
- No longer do I please to appease.
- I am a positive, creative, and helpful person.
- I appreciate the gift of my hands give me everyday.
- I can greet life, people and my projects with creative possibilities.
- I am flexible and strong.
- I have confident personal power.
- I create amazing experiences.
- I share my heart with positive boundaries and clear mind.
- I value the force for good and the will for change.
- I encourage myself to turn any overwhelm into an intriguing adventure.
- I grasp the problem with clear awareness and take action within my capacity.

Wrist Problems

Supporting foods:

- Brewers yeast
- Nuts
- Oatmeal
- Plums
- Spirulina
- Watercress
- Peas
- Pork

- Poultry
- Brown rice
- Legumes
- Liver
- Carrots
- Sunflower seeds
- Wheat germ
- Whole wheat

- Avocado
- Bananas
- Soybeans
- Dairy products
- Kelp
- Leafy greens

- Eat fresh pineapple daily to reduce pain and swelling
- Drink plenty of water/stay hydrated
- Eat a well-balanced diet
- Foods high in B vitamins

About the Author

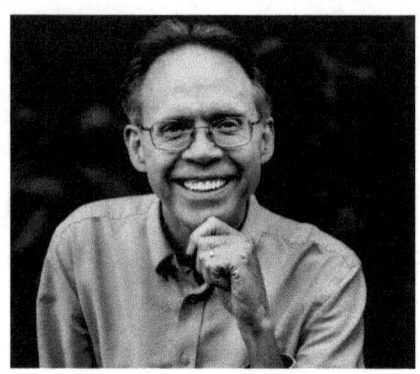

Ronald B. Wayman has devoted the past three decades to passionately coaching individuals to empower their inner storyline to become their best selves. As an Empowerlife Brain Integration Specialist, a licensed massage therapist, Empowerlife Kinesiologist and Emotional Coach, Neuro-Energetic Kinesiologist, and Food Enzyme Consultant, Ron underscores the significance of empowerment and congruency within the heart, mind, body, and soul. He wrote a brain integration and mindfulness self-help book called Life Centering. He enjoys teaching Life Centering techniques to family, friends, and clients. He is founder of the Sensory Dynamics Center, and co-founder of Empowerlife Kinesiology; a body and mind energy school. He helped create a spice blend, herbal blends, and essential oil blends for health and brain/body integration.

Ronald Wayman and Denise Wayman Scholes are co-founders of Mindbody Dictionary, which helps bridge the gap of understanding the powerful connection between the mind and the body.

Ron's extensive work integrates applying breakthroughs in body energy systems, integrated body movements, brain neuroscience, nutrition, sensory integration, focused emotional processing, and motivational heart-mind empowerment. Constantly exploring new techniques rooted in traditional eastern healing methodologies, he empowers practitioners to experience and facilitate remarkable physical, emotional, and energetic alchemy. He wants people to find the truth within their body, heart, and mind, which brings one back to their authentic soul.

Ron and his wife, Janette, are proud parents of six children and grandparents of 18.

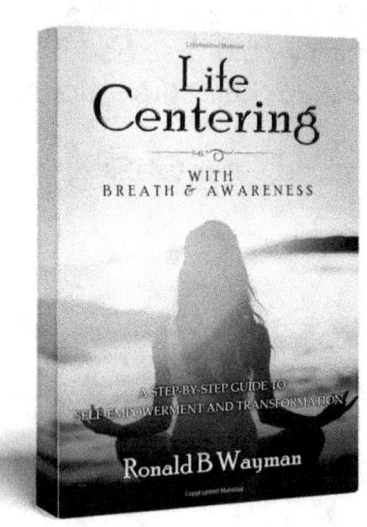

Find
"Life Centering"
By Ronald B. Wayman
on Amazon

Go to
Empowerlife.com
to find products, courses and more.

About the Contributing Author

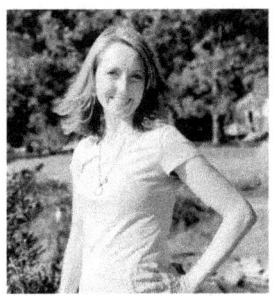

Denise Wayman Scholes, a lifelong student and mentee of Ron, embodies the profound impact of Neuroenergetic Kinesiology. As the owner of Core Light Connection, LLC, she applies her Empowerlife studies to guide clients nationwide towards greater connection, healing, and alignment.

Denise's journey into Energy Healing began when she recognized the deep connection between her body and mind. This realization led her to delve into the mind-body connection, uncovering the incredible intelligence and wisdom embedded in the body's messages. Her awakening fueled a passion for understanding, listening, and aligning with the insights provided by our bodies.

Denise, who enjoys writing poetry that captures the essence of healing, shares her reflections in *Insights from Healing Journey: Short Stories and Poems*. Additionally, she has crafted a children's book titled *Reaching: A Seedling's Journey of Growth*. More books are in the works.

Alongside her husband Aaron, Denise is a homeschooling parent to four vibrant children. They are deeply grateful for the opportunity to raise their children with this additional knowledge, guiding and supporting their well-being.

Additional Resources

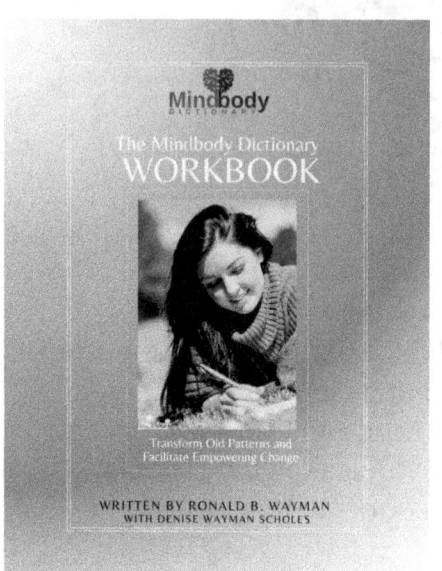

Facilitate a process and routine that will create a pattern of
- Deepening your awareness
- Taking responsibility
- Empowering change
- Transforming old patterns into aligned consciousness.

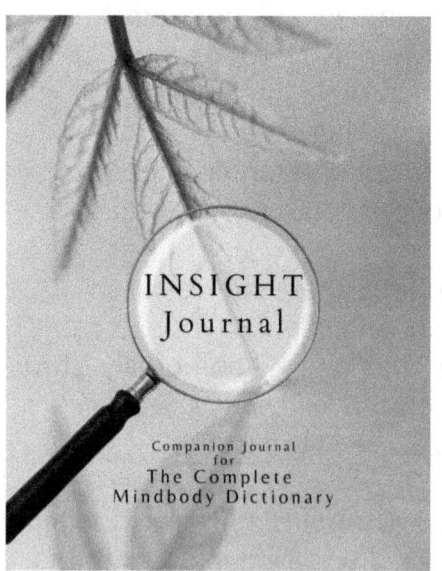

Your companion for journaling personal insights from "The Complete Mindbody Dictionary," designed to empower you to reflect, gain insights, and deepen your understanding on your healing journey.

Additional Resources

Free Download on Apple and Android

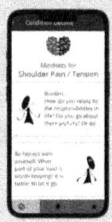

- Troubled Mindset
- Healing Mindset
- Foods
- Products
- Resources

For more information about classes, resources and products.

mindbodydictionary.com

The Complete Mindbody Dictionary, with its accompanying Workbook and Journal, will provide a format for deeply transformational soul healing like nothing else.

Mindbody Movements

**Move your body.
Reconnect your mind.
Transform your health.**

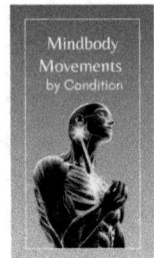

Mindbody Movements are thoughtfully designed, mindful exercises that support brain-body integration and address the emotional and physical roots of imbalance as outlined in *The Complete Mindbody Dictionary.*

These movements go beyond traditional exercise—they work with your body's energy systems, including the acupuncture meridians, to help your mind and body stop fighting and start working together.

Whether you're dealing with fatigue, anxiety, brain fog, low energy, emotional stress, or chronic tension, these simple yet powerful movements are a supportive tool for clarity, vitality, and inner harmony.

Start by identifying your condition in *The Complete Mindbody Dictionary*, then use the corresponding Mindbody Movements and affirmations to create a personalized path toward healing.

Perfect for all ages and fitness levels, these movements require no equipment—just your presence and willingness to reconnect.

If you're feeling tired, stuck, overwhelmed, or emotionally weighed down, **Mindbody Movements** may be the missing piece to help you feel more like you.

www.ingramcontent.com/pod-product-compliance
Lightning Source LLC
Chambersburg PA
CBHW051105230426
43667CB00014B/2451